Essentials *of* *Medical* *Transcription*

A MODULAR APPROACH

Essentials *of* Medical Transcription

A MODULAR APPROACH

CINDY DESTAFANO, BSBa, RT(R)
Consolidated School of Business
York, Pennsylvania

FRAN M. FEDERMAN, MSEd
Central York High School
York, Pennsylvania

W.B. SAUNDERS COMPANY
A Harcourt Health Sciences Company
Philadelphia London Toronto Montreal Sydney Tokyo

W.B. SAUNDERS COMPANY
A Harcourt Health Sciences Company

The Curtis Center
Independence Square West
Philadelphia, Pennsylvania 19106-3399

Acquisitions Editor: Maureen Pfeifer
Developmental Editors: Tamara Myers and Scott Weaver
Project Manager: Linda McKinley
Production Editor: Ellen Forest
Book Design Manager: Gail Morey Hudson
Designer: Stephanie Foley
Cover Design: Jennifer Chapman

Library of Congress Cataloging-in-Publication Data

Destafano, Cindy.

Essentials of medical transcription: a modular approach/Cindy
Destafano, Fran M. Federman.

p.; cm.

Includes bibliographical references and index.

ISBN 0-7216-8694-X

1. Medical transcription.   I. Federman, Fran M.   II. Title.

[DNLM: 1. Medical Records.   2. Medical Secretaries. W 80
D476e2001]

R728.8.D45 2001

653'.18—dc21

00-057377

Essentials of Medical Transcription

ISBN 0-7216-8694-X

Printed in the United States of America

Last digit is print number: 9   8   7   6   5   4   3   2   1

Reviewers

Jerri Adler
Lane Community College
Eugene, Oregon

Barbara Cowan
Southern Utah University
Cedar City, Utah

Laura Southard Durham
Forsyth Technical Community College
Winston-Salem, North Carolina

Rhonda Faul
Community College of Southern Nevada
Las Vegas, Nevada

Savanna Garrity
Madisonville Technical College
Madisonville, Kentucky

Bonita Makin
Cambria-Rowe Business College
Indiana, Pennsylvania

Geralyn A. Matejcek
North Dakota State College of Science
Wahpeton, North Dakota

Glen McCreary
DPT Business School
Philadelphia, Pennsylvania

Lori Ann Raith-Andreucci
Gateway Technical College
Racine, Wisconsin

Dedication

I give special thanks to the most important person in my life—my husband, **Izzy**—without his unending devotion, support, and encouragement, this textbook would not be realized. I also want to thank my children, **Gwenn, Ben,** and **Allan,** who sacrificed home-cooked meals; my mother-in-law, **Anna,** for allowing me to disturb her sleep during the many hours I spent in front of the computer; my **students** and **staff** at Central York High School for their ongoing enthusiasm over this project; and my many **friends** and **family members** who have lent their support as well. Of course, one of the most wonderful experiences that resulted from this project is the warm friendship and comradeship that developed between me and my co-author **Cindy.** Thank you all.

Finally, this textbook is also dedicated to the memories of special people who had a profound influence on me: my mother and father, **Albert** and **Cynthia Dobbins,** and my father-in-law, **Morris Federman.**

Fran M. Federman

In the ocean of life we constantly battle the storms, occasionally ride the waves, but mostly we tread water. Deep appreciation and much love go to my family and friends who keep my boat afloat: **Dave,** my husband, my co-captain, and my anchor; **Matthew** and **Kate,** my children, who always rock the boat but are the wind beneath my sails; **Jenny,** my great stepdaughter, who's about to set sail on her own adventure; my **parents,** my lighthouse in a storm; my **friends,** the rudders in my life, who help keep my oars (or try to) in the water; **Fran,** my friend and shipmate in this uncharted adventure; and you, the **student,** the reason for the journey.

A medal of valor goes to my good friend, **Bunny Best,** who withstood my endless torrents of frustration, elation, tedium, and hope.

This textbook is dedicated to **Richard F. Geiger,** *my mentor, my guide, my father (December 6, 1928, to July 19, 1999).*

Cindy Destafano

Preface

Notes to the Student

In *Essentials of Medical Transcription,* you will work with the textbook, accompanying CD-ROM, and audiocassettes (available separately). The textbook is divided into two units. Unit I emphasizes medical terminology, keyboarding, and proofreading skills. A variety of reference materials will be discussed and you will learn to use them. Audiocassettes provide a list of medical terms that are pronounced, spelled, and defined, followed by keyboarding exercises for seven different medical specialties. It is important that you listen to the pronunciation of the terms before starting to transcribe the report. You may also wish to practice spelling the terms as you listen to each term pronounced. Listening to a medical term and then correctly spelling that word are critical skills.

In Unit II, each chapter will discuss a different medical specialty that includes a glossary of medical terms with their respective phonetic pronunciation and definition. You will assume the role of a medical transcriptionist employed at the fictitious FedDes Wellness Center. You will be directed to complete several outpatient reports pertinent to the medical specialty presented in the chapter. A list of the patient's name and the type of report is included. All chapters contain review worksheets and timed transcription exercises to assess your understanding of presented medical terms and concepts.

EVALUATION

Your mastery of transcription skills in Unit I is assessed through worksheets, "Check Your Progress," keyboarding exercises, and the error analysis chart. In Unit II, your mastery is assessed through worksheets, timed transcription exercises, the error analysis chart, and the Production for Pay summary. All medical transcriptionists employed at the FedDes Wellness Center are required to proofread, correct, and analyze their own transcribed documents. After transcribing a report, you will proof-read your work and correct any errors. Then you will compare your proofread work against a master transcript (found in the back of the text and the end of the CD-ROM), categorize all errors, and tabulate the errors on the error analysis chart. The Production for Pay summary correlates your production to the FedDes Wellness Center pay scale, which is based on industry compensation standards. The scale is also linked to your grade. Some exercises are also on the CD-ROM in a format that records your transcription time, corrects your errors, and displays both the error analysis chart and the Production for Pay summary. This system allows you to assess your mastery of transcription skills in a real-world scenario.

Medical transcription is a difficult skill to master. Be patient with yourself and work diligently.

Notes to the Instructor

Essentials of Medical Transcription: a Modular Approach is a skill development textbook that was conceived as a result of actual classroom experiences witnessing students' frustrations with current textbooks. This modular-based textbook focuses on the development of transcription skills through a building block format. The student will work with the textbook, CD-ROM, and accompanying audiocassettes. The textbook follows a student-driven approach to learning in which the instructor assumes the role of a coach and facilitates the learning process. The CD-ROM provides self-correcting and assessment features. The audiocassettes contain dictation from outpatient specialty practices. As a programmed learning textbook, all answer keys for respective exercises are found in the textbook and CD-ROM, providing immediate feedback. Textbook worksheets, exercises, and transcription tips guide the student in the development of critical thinking skills. Check points are built into the text to allow the student to assess mastery of each presented skill. Thus students obtain immediate feedback of their skill development. Students are cautioned not to proceed to the next skill development level until competency is achieved. Because this is a beginning transcription course, the audio transcriptions are presented in a controlled environment with no variation of accents or background noises, as might appear in real-world dictation. Variation in accents only befuddle the beginning student, who is still trying to grapple with the synthesis of multiple, newly learned skills.

The textbook is divided into two units. Unit I (Chapters 1-4) presents the fundamental skills and knowledge necessary for medical transcription practice. Unit I includes a discussion of the profile of the medical transcriptionist, different types of reports and their formats, and selected transcription guidelines.

Unit II (Chapters 5-11) presents a chapter for each of the seven specialties: family practice, orthopaedics, urology, pulmonary medicine, gastroenterology, cardiology, and diagnostic imaging. Unit II uses an innovative approach to the integration of visual and auditory learning with the development of transcription skills. These skills are developed through keyboarding exercises rather than the traditional approach of simply reading through the chapter. The learning activities move the students from visual keyboarding exercises to auditory transcription exercises. Each chapter is subdivided into three parts. In "Part I: Getting Close to the Real Thing," the student masters the fundamentals by keyboarding medical terms and their definitions, spelling medical terms, and transcribing medical sentences. In "Part II: Proofreading and Error Analysis," the student proceeds to transcribe reports and develop proofreading skills. "Part III: You Are There" combines theory, medical terminology, and keyboarding and proofreading skills by having the student transcribe complete medical reports. Concepts and skills are presented one at a time, which allows the student to progress sequentially from one skill to the next, instead of immediately being thrust into a situation that requires the use of multiple skills and concepts to produce a medical report. In Unit II, the student assumes the role as a medical transcriptionist employed at the fictitious FedDes Wellness Center. Students are directed to follow the transcription guidelines of the FedDes Wellness Center as described in Chapter 4.

The case studies are developed from actual medical records.

Students transcribe medical documents using the error analysis chart. The error analysis chart was developed to categorize and track undetected errors. A transcription error analysis chart for each document helps the student and instructor prescribe a remedy for each error. Observation of the occurrence of repeated mistakes through charting will improve the student's transcription skills. The chart is divided into two major categories: Medical Language and English Language. The medical language errors are weighted heavier because medication and allergy errors and incorrect patient identification adversely affect patient care. The traditional evaluation process is replaced with a motivational Production for Pay summary sheet linked to a grading grid. Net words of production are calculated to a monetary value. Students experience the real-world accountability of earning a paycheck.

Chapters with a "Pretest" allow students to assess their mastery level for each of the three parts of a chapter. A score below 90% on the pretest for each part indicates the student has not mastered the material and should complete all activities included in the chapter. A score above 90% indicates a level of mastery of the chapter's contents. The instructor may choose to follow or modify the directions given for the pretest. Each part also includes a "Check Your Progress" activity. The purpose of this activity is to provide immediate competency assessment of the objectives for each part of the chapter.

PREREQUISITES

Students should be proficient in keyboarding and have a strong background in medical terminology, basic anatomy and physiology, pharmacology, laboratory and diagnostic tests, and procedures before beginning this course. Students must also understand and be able to use computer word processing software.

OBJECTIVES

Upon successful completion of this course, students should be able to do the following:

1. Understand the content and purpose of chart notes, history and physical examination reports, letters, x-ray reports, and consultations.
2. Use reference resources.

3. Transcribe medical reports using correct report format.
4. Transcribe medical reports using correct capitalization, numbers, punctuation, abbreviations, symbols, and metric measurement rules.
5. Correctly spell both the English and the medical terms and abbreviations presented in the dictation tapes and textbook.

6. Produce correct and accurate medical transcription reports within given time constraints.
7. Proofread and edit medical documents.
8. Demonstrate critical thinking and decision-making skills.

Acknowledgments

This textbook is a result of the combined talents of many outstanding individuals. We are deeply grateful to Maureen Pfeifer, Senior Acquisitions Editor; Tamara Myers, Associate Developmental Editor; and Scott Weaver, Senior Developmental Editor, for their vision, encouragement, and patience in working with us to create this textbook. We also wish to acknowledge Bunny Best, Senior Career School Sales Representative, the catalyst for this project, and the helpful and talented Harcourt Health Sciences production team: Stephanie Foley, Book Designer, and Gail Morey Hudson, Book Design Manager, for the interior and cover designs; Sharon Iwanczuk, Senior Illustrator, for the creation of the medical illustrations; and Ellen Forest, Production Editor, for copy editing and overseeing the production process along with Linda McKinley, Project Manager. It has been an exciting adventure for us.

We extend tremendous appreciation for the support and contributions of Charlotte DiCola, Karen Branner, Sandy Deitz, Dr. Bruce Frantz, and Rachel Damoth.

Contents

UNIT I

Fundamentals of Medical Transcription

What Is Medical Transcription?

OBJECTIVES

At the completion of Chapter 1, you will be able to do the following:

1. Identify the skills and knowledge necessary to be a successful medical transcriptionist.

2. Identify the personal attributes of a medical transcriptionist.

3. Understand the career outlook and overall job environment for a medical transcriptionist.

4. Understand the job description of the medical transcriptionist.

5. Evaluate your own skills, knowledge, and personal attributes for a career in medical transcription.

What's Ahead

Career Outlook

Profile of the Medical Transcriptionist

Personal Attributes, Skills, and Knowledge

Becoming a Medical Transcriptionist Using the *Essentials of Medical Transcription* Method

Chapter 1 ▪ Activity 1: So You Want to Be a Medical Transcriptionist

3

Career Outlook

According to *Occupational Outlook Handbook,* the demand for medical transcriptionists is expected to increase with the growth of healthcare services and the industries that provide it. Growing numbers of medical transcriptionists will be needed to amend patients' records, edit for grammar, and discover discrepancies in medical records.[1]

Transcriptionists work in hospitals, doctors' offices, insurance companies, clinics, government medical facilities, and medical transcription services. An increasing number of medical transcriptionists work from home-based offices as subcontractors for hospitals and transcriptionist services. Many medical transcriptionists work a standard 40-hour week, although one in four transcriptionists works part time. A substantial number of medical transcriptionists, however, are self-employed, which may result in irregular working hours. Earnings depend on education, experience, and geographic location.[2]

The career outlook for experienced medical transcriptionists includes a wide choice of opportunities, including supervisor or manager, quality assurance expert, instructor, author, editor, consultant, as well as business entrepreneur. You are now ready to step through the door into the exciting world of medical transcription.

Profile of the Medical Transcriptionist

The healthcare team includes many of the obvious professionals: physician, nurse, technicians, and therapists, as well as the not-so-obvious accountant, social worker, and medical transcriptionist.

Medical transcriptionists transcribe dictated medical information that describes the condition, care, and treatment of a patient. Such documents may include office chart notes, history and physical examinations, consultations, letters, memos, admission notes, operative reports, discharge summaries, and many laboratory and diagnostic tests. All of these documents comprise the patient's medical record, which becomes the communication medium for patient treatment and care, insurance and reimbursement, legal documentation, and research support. Figure 1.1 shows several model reports typically used in an outpatient facility.

A model job description developed by the American Association of Medical Transcription (AAMT) is

SAMPLE CHART NOTE USING SOAP NOTE STYLE

CHART NOTE

Patient Name: Felter, Michael

Date of Birth: July 3, 1954

Examination Date: *current date*

SUBJECTIVE: Patient complains of right elbow pain for past three months. He has been playing tennis once a week over the summer with gradually worsening pain.

OBJECTIVE: Tenderness over right medial epicondyle. Pain radiates to the forearm and back of the hand with flexion and supination.

ASSESSMENT: Epicondylitis.

PLAN: Advised patient to stop playing tennis for three weeks and rest elbow until inflammation subsides. Prescribed Motrin 200 mg p.o. q.i.d. Urged the patient to wear an elastic strap for support, when playing tennis in the future.

Harry A. Medulla MD
Harry A. Medulla, MD/xx

A

SAMPLE X-RAY REPORT

X-RAY REPORT

Patient Name: Farley, Cassandra

File Number: 5690341

Date of Birth: February 1, 19xx

Examination Date: *current date*

Ordering Physician: Izzy Sertoli, MD

Examination: PA AND LATERAL CHEST X-RAY

HISTORY: This is a 57-year-old female with a history of lung cancer and increased shortness of breath for one week.

FINDINGS

CHEST: There is mild fibrotic change at both lung bases, over the left lung apex, and along the left chest wall laterally. There is some deformity to the left rib cage, apparently reflecting several old, healed rib fractures. There are some increased markings at the left lung base.

IMPRESSION: Early pneumonia, superimposed upon the underlying fibrotic changes. The heart size is normal.

Adam Valence MD
Adam Valence, MD/xx

B

FIGURE 1.1 Medical reports typically used in outpatient facilities. **A,** Sample chart note using SOAP style. **B,** Sample X-ray report.

SAMPLE CHART NOTE USING HISTORY AND
PHYSICAL STYLE

CHART NOTE

Patient Name: Schaeffer, Carolyn

Date of Birth: April 18, 19xx

Examination Date: *current date*

CHIEF COMPLAINT: Chest pain

HISTORY OF PRESENT ILLNESS: Carolyn is a 52-year-old white female who experienced chest pressure, palpitations, heart racing, numbness and weakness in her right arm while at church services this morning. This episode lasted approximately four minutes. She also felt somewhat nauseated and clammy. Patient cardiac risk factors include tobacco abuse, hyperlipidemia, and obesity.

PAST MEDICAL HISTORY: Vaginal hysterectomy in 1975 for excessive bleeding. Hyperlipidemia with triglycerides in the 350 range and cholesterol over 300. While taking Lopid, cholesterol fell to approximately 252 and triglycerides were 183.

PHYSICAL EXAMINATION

GENERAL: She is a very pleasant and cooperative patient in no acute distress.

HEENT: She is wearing corrective lenses. Sclerae anicteric, tympanic membranes clear. Nose clear. Throat normal. She has a normal gag reflex. She has multiple filled caries.

NECK: Supple without thyromegaly or lymphadenopathy. Carotids 2+ bilaterally without bruits.

CHEST: Clear to auscultation anteriorly and posteriorly.

HEART: Regular rate and rhythm with a grade I/VI systolic murmur heard best at the aortic region.

ABDOMEN: Mildly obese. Normoactive bowel sounds. Nontender, no organomegaly.

BREASTS/PELVIC/RECTAL: Deferred as these were done at the office one month ago and were normal.

EXTREMITIES: Without clubbing, cyanosis, or edema. Pulses 2+ in the upper and lower extremities.

NEUROLOGICAL: No focal neurologic deficits.

ASSESSMENT:
1. Chest pain.
2. Hypothyroidism.

PLAN:
1. Obtain serial EKGs and cardiac enzymes to rule out myocardial infarction.
2. Obtain echocardiogram and stress thallium test.

Adam Valence MD
Adam Valence, MD/xx

C

SAMPLE HISTORY AND PHYSICAL EXAMINATION

HISTORY AND PHYSICAL EXAMINATION

Patient Name: Rouf, Andrea

File Number: 2348901

Date of Birth: April 10, 19xx

Examination Date: *current date*

Physician: Gwenn Maltese, MD

HISTORY

CHIEF COMPLAINT: Abdominal pain, RLQ for three days.

HISTORY OF PRESENT ILLNESS: The patient is a 27-year-old legal secretary, who first noted the onset of colicky lower abdominal pain situated slightly to the right of midline, below the umbilicus and above the pubic bone three days ago.

PAST HISTORY: The patient had varicella at age 2 and the mumps at age 4. She had a tonsillectomy and adenoidectomy at age 11. There is no family history of diabetes.

REVIEW OF SYSTEMS:

HEENT: Mild upper respiratory infection two weeks prior to present illness manifested by rhinitis and sore throat.

GENITOURINARY: Gravida II, para II, ab 0. No frequency, hematuria, or nocturia.

PHYSICAL EXAMINATION

GENERAL: The patient is alert, oriented and in moderate distress. BP 120/80, pulse 106 and regular, temperature 37.2 C, respirations 14/min.

LUNGS: Clear to P&A.

HEART: Normal sinus rhythm, no cardiomegaly, no murmurs, gallops, or thrills.

ABDOMEN: Flat. Tenderness with muscle guarding in right lower quadrant. Rebound tenderness was present. Bowel sounds are normal. No organomegaly.

PELVIC: Bartholins, urethral, and Skene's gland normal. Adnexa normal. Uterus not enlarged.

EXTREMITIES: Within normal limits. No edema. Good range of motion.

NEUROLOGICAL: Grossly intact.

IMPRESSION: Acute appendicitis.

PLAN: Refer to John Smithson, MD for surgical consult.

Gwenn Maltese MD
Gwenn Maltese, MD/xx

D

FIGURE 1.1—CONT'D **C,** Sample chart note using history and physical style. **D,** Sample
history and physical examination.   *Continued*

FedDes Wellness Center
Diagnostic Imaging Division, Suite 157
101 Wellness Way Drive
New York, NY 10036

SAMPLE CONSULTATION REPORT (INFORMAL STYLE WITH HEADINGS)

CONSULTATION REPORT

Patient Name: McWilliams, Betty

File Number: 5678123

Date of Birth: February 2, 1949

Examination Date: *current date*

Requesting Physician: Charles P. Davis, MD

E

HISTORY OF PRESENT ILLNESS: Ms. McWilliams appears to be more stable with the supportive measures already instituted. The respiratory rate is still rapid, but her color is better. There are no signs of congestive heart failure.

IMPRESSION/RECOMMENDATIONS: Review of the clinical picture, chest x-ray, and lung scan point definitely toward a pulmonary embolus. I would recommend checking the blood gases, maintaining the oxygen and supportive measures, and starting her on anticoagulation with heparin. She should be maintained on the EKG monitor.

I feel she also has evidence of thrombophlebitis of the left leg and should be treated with elevation and soaks to this extremity. Thank you. I will follow.

Adam Valence MD
Adam Valence, MD/xx

c June Davis, MD

Current date

Charles P. Davis, MD
FedDes Wellness Center
Family Practice Division, Suite 300
101 Wellness Way Drive
New York, NY 10036

Re: Betty McWilliams
    Date of Birth: February 2, 1949
    Examination: RIGHT BREAST SONOGRAM

Dear Dr. Davis

F

Comparison is made to the prior mammogram dated January 25, 20xx. An 18 x 8 x 20 mm well-demarcated simple cyst is demonstrated within the central 12 o'clock position of the right breast corresponding to the well-demarcated density noted on mammography in this region.

IMPRESSION: The two densities noted in the right breast on the recent mammogram correspond to simple cysts as described.

Thank you for this referral.

Sincerely yours

Potter T. Bucky MD
Potter T. Bucky, MD

xx

FIGURE 1.1—CONT'D   E, Sample consultation report (informal style with headings). **F,** Sample diagnostic imaging letter.

SAMPLE CONSULTATION LETTER
(FORMAL STYLE WITHOUT HEADINGS)

FedDes Wellness Center
Diagnostic Imaging Division, Suite 157
101 Wellness Way Drive
New York, NY 10036

Current date

Charles P. Davis, MD
FedDes Wellness Center
Family Practice Division, Suite 300
101 Wellness Way Drive
New York, NY 10036

Re: Betty McWilliams
    Date of Birth: February 2, 1949

Dear Dr. Davis

G   Ms. McWilliams appears to be more stable with the supportive measures already instituted. The respiratory rate is still rapid, but her color is better. There are no signs of congestive heart failure.

Review of the clinical picture, chest x-ray, and lung scan point definitely toward a pulmonary embolus. I would recommend checking the blood gases, maintaining the oxygen and supportive measures, and starting her on anticoagulation with heparin. She should be maintained on the EKG monitor.

I feel she also has evidence of thrombophlebitis of the left leg and should be treated with elevation and soaks to this extremity. Thank you. I will follow.

Sincerely yours

Adam Valence MD
Adam Valence, MD

xx

c June Davis, MD

FIGURE 1.1—CONT'D   G, Sample consultation letter (formal style without headings).

shown in Figure 1.2. AAMT is a membership organization for the medical transcription profession. Although it does not offer program accreditation or evaluation, it does publish recommendations for model curricula and code of ethics, journals, reference materials, such as *The AAMT Book of Style for Medical Transcription,* and other items of interest to the medical transcriptionist.

AAMT awards the voluntary designation of certified medical transcriptionist (CMT) to those who earn passing scores on written and practical examinations. As in many other fields, certification is recognized as a sign of competence in medical transcription. To retain this credential, certified medical transcriptionists must obtain at least 30 continuing education credits every 3 years.[3] Further information about AAMT and its certification process can be obtained by contacting AAMT directly.

American Association for Medical Transcription
PO Box 576187
Modesto, CA 95357-6187
Tel: (209) 551-0883
Fax: (209) 551-9317
E-mail: aamt@sna.com

Although medical transcriptionists do not have the glamour of emergency room physicians or hold the spotlight in popular TV shows, they provide a vital service to the patient and medical community.

Personal Attributes, Skills, and Knowledge

Successful medical transcriptionists are organized, work independently with little or no supervision, are interested in medical language, are disciplined to work within time constraints, are inquisitive and enjoy learning new concepts, can concentrate for long periods of time, possess common sense and sound judgment, enjoy detail and precision, and are discreet in handling confidential information.

Medical transcription is both a skill-based and knowledge-based profession. Skills needed include keyboarding, computer literacy, and English language mastery. Specifically, you need the following:

- Computer and word processing skills
- Fast and accurate keyboarding skills
- Proofreading skills
- Critical thinking skills
- Hearing acuity

AMERICAN ASSOCIATION
FOR MEDICAL TRANSCRIPTION

AAMT Model Job Description:
MEDICAL TRANSCRIPTIONIST

The *AAMT Model Job Description* is a practical, useful compilation of the basic job responsibilities of a medical transcriptionist. It is designed to assist human resource managers, department managers, supervisors, and others in recruiting, supervising, and evaluating individuals in medical transcription positions.

The *AAMT Model Job Description* is not intended as a complete list of specific duties and responsibilities. Nor is it intended to limit or modify the right of any supervisor to assign, direct, and control the work of employees under supervision. The use of a particular expression or illustration describing duties shall not be held to exclude other duties not mentioned that are of a similar kind or level of difficulty.

Position Summary: Medical language specialist who interprets and transcribes dictation by physicians and other healthcare professionals regarding patient assessment, workup, therapeutic procedures, clinical course, diagnosis, prognosis, etc., in order to document patient care and facilitate delivery of healthcare services.

Knowledge, skills, and abilities:
1. Minimum education level of associate degree or equivalent in work experience and continuing education.
2. Knowledge of medical terminology, anatomy and physiology, clinical medicine, surgery, diagnostic tests, radiology, pathology, pharmacology, and the various medical specialties as required in areas of responsibility.
3. Knowledge of medical transcription guidelines and practices.
4. Excellent written and oral communication skills, including English usage, grammar, punctuation, and style.
5. Ability to understand diverse accents and dialects and varying dictation styles.
6. Ability to use designated reference materials.
7. Ability to operate designated word processing, dictation, and transcription equipment, and other equipment as specified.
8. Ability to work independently with minimal supervision.
9. Ability to work under pressure with time constraints.
10. Ability to concentrate.
11. Excellent listening skills.
12. Excellent eye, hand, and auditory coordination.
13. Certified medical transcriptionist (CMT) status preferred.

Working conditions:
General office environment. Quiet surroundings. Adequate lighting.

Physical demands:
Primarily sedentary work, with continuous use of earphones, keyboard, foot control, and where applicable, video display terminal.

AAMT gratefully acknowledges Lanier Voice Products, Atlanta, Georgia, for funding the development of the *AAMT Model Job Description: Medical Transcriptionist*.

For additional information, contact AAMT, PO Box 576187, Modesto, CA 95357-6187. Telephone 209-551-0883. Fax 209-551-9317. Web site: http://www.aamt.org/aamt. E-mail: aamt@sna.com.

FIGURE 1.2 AAMT model job description. (Courtesy American Association for Medical Transcription, Modesto, Calif., 1990, The Association.)

AAMT Model Job Description: Medical Transcriptionist

Job responsibilities:

1. Transcribes medical dictation to provide a permanent record of patient care.

2. Demonstrates an understanding of the medicolegal implications and responsibilities related to the transcription of patient records to protect the patient and the business/institution.

3. Operates designated word processing, dictation, and transcription equipment as directed to complete assignments.

4. Follows policies and procedures to contribute to the efficiency of the medical transcription department.

5. Expands job-related knowledge and skills to improve performance and adjust to change.

6. Uses interpersonal skills effectively to build and maintain cooperative working relationships

Performance standards:

1.1 Applies knowledge of medical terminology, anatomy and physiology, and English language rules to the transcription and proofreading of medical dictation from originators with various accents, dialects, and dictation styles.
1.2 Recognizes, interprets, and evaluates inconsistencies, discrepancies, and inaccuracies in medical dictation, and appropriately edits, revises, and clarifies them without altering the meaning of the dictation or changing the dictator's style.
1.3 Clarifies dictation which is unclear or incomplete, seeking assistance as necessary.
1.4 Flags reports requiring the attention of the supervisor or dictator.
1.5 Uses reference materials appropriately and efficiently to facilitate the accuracy, clarity, and completeness of reports.
1.6 Meets quality and productivity standards and deadlines established by employer.
1.7 Verifies patient information for accuracy and completeness.
1.8 Formats reports according to established guidelines.

2.1 Understands and complies with policies and procedures related to medicolegal matters, including confidentiality, amendment of medical records, release of information, patients' rights, medical records as legal evidence, informed consent, etc.
2.2 Meets standards of professional and ethical conduct.
2.3 Recognizes and reports unusual circumstances and/or information with possible risk factors to appropriate risk management personnel.
2.4 Recognizes and reports problems, errors, and discrepancies in dictation and patient records to appropriate manager.
2.5 Consults appropriate personnel regarding dictation which may be regarded as unprofessional, frivolous, insulting, inflammatory, or inappropriate.

3.1 Uses designated equipment effectively, skillfully, and efficiently.
3.2 Maintains equipment and work area as directed.
3.3 Assesses condition of equipment and furnishings, and reports need for replacement or repair.

4.1 Demonstrates an understanding of policies, procedures, and priorities, seeking clarification as needed.
4.2 Reports to work on time, as scheduled, and is dependable and cooperative.
4.3 Organizes and prioritizes assigned work, and schedules time to accommodate work demands, turnaround-time requirements, and commitments.
4.4 Maintains required records, providing reports as scheduled and upon request.
4.5 Participates in quality assurance programs.
4.6 Participates in evaluation and selection of equipment and furnishings.
4.7 Provides administrative/clerical/technical support as needed and as assigned.

5.1 Participates in inservice and continuing education activities.
5.2 Provides documentation of inservice and continuing education activities.
5.3 Reviews trends and developments in medicine, English usage, technology, and transcription practices, and shares knowledge with colleagues.
5.4 Documents new and revised terminology, definitions, styles, and practices for reference and application.
5.5 Participates in the evaluation and selection of books, publications, and other reference materials.

6.1 Works and communicates in a positive and cooperative manner with management and supervisory staff, medical staff, co-workers, and other healthcare personnel, and patients and their families when providing information and services, seeking assistance and clarification, and resolving problems.
6.2 Contributes to team efforts.
6.3 Carries out assignments responsibly.
6.4 Participates in a positive and cooperative manner during staff meetings.
6.5 Handles difficult and sensitive situations tactfully.
6.6 Responds well to supervision.
6.7 Shares information with co-workers.
6.8 Assists with training of new employees as needed.

FIGURE 1.2—CONT'D For legend, see opposite page.

The act of listening to an oral dialogue of a person's medical condition and then transcribing it requires the transcriptionist to have an extensive understanding of the following medical subjects:

- Medical terminology
- Anatomy and physiology
- Pharmacology
- Human diseases and conditions
- Surgical procedures
- Diagnostic studies
- Therapeutic treatments
- Laboratory tests

Many of us are visual learners, so the act of listening and then transcribing what we hear is a new and very different course of study. Most students have never encountered a class where they were required to coordinate multiple mental and physical skills to produce a document. It requires the coordination of your eyes, ears, fingers, and foot as you transcribe medical terms that are presented in terse phrases and seemingly incoherent style of prose. It often frustrates even the most enthusiastic and earnest student. The presentation of this textbook allows you to sequentially build your medical transcription skills. This method will still require your commitment and effort, but it should make learning a positive experience. You have chosen a noble profession that plays a vital role in providing quality patient care.

Becoming a Medical Transcriptionist Using the *Essentials of Medical Transcription* Method

This textbook is designed to introduce you to medical transcription skills that are basic to the profession. In Unit I, you will be exposed to medical reports that are fundamental to ambulatory care, related medical terminology, a discussion of appropriate formatting styles, selected specialized rules of grammar and punctuation peculiar to dictated medical reports, and proofreading and transcription process and techniques. A variety of reference materials will be discussed, and you will learn how to use them.

In Unit II, you will apply these principles discussed in Unit I as you transcribe medical reports from seven different specialties relating to a fictitious outpatient healthcare facility, FedDes Wellness Center. Accompanying audiocassettes and the CD-ROM provide a list of medical terms that are pronounced, spelled, and defined, followed by keyboarding exercises. It is important for you to listen to the pronunciation of the terms before starting to transcribe the report. You also may wish to practice spelling the terms as you listen to each term pronounced. Listening to a medical term and then correctly spelling it are critically necessary skills. A list of the patient's name and the type of report, transcription tips, and error analysis and production pay charting are included for each specialty. You will be able to assess your mastery of transcription skills in a real-world scenario.

Checkpoints are included in each chapter to allow you to assess your mastery of each presented skill. As a programmed learning textbook, answers to all exercises are found at the end of this textbook, providing immediate feedback.

So you are interested in becoming a medical transcriptionist—let's begin our journey using the *Essentials of Medical Transcription* as your guide!

REFERENCES

1. *1998-99 Occupational outlook handbook,* p. 4. Available online at www.stats.bix.gov/oco/ocos/152.htm.
2. *1998-99 Occupational outlook handbook,* p. 5. Available online at www.stats.bix.gov/oco/ocos/152.htm.
3. *1998-99 Occupational outlook handbook,* p. 3. Available online at www.stats.bix.gov/oco/ocos/152.htm.

ACTIVITY 1 / SO YOU WANT TO BE A MEDICAL TRANSCRIPTIONIST

Directions: Let's assess your knowledge, aptitude, and ability to become a successful medical transcriptionist. Answer "yes" or "no" to the following questions. If most of your answers are "yes," you are well on your way to becoming a medical transcriptionist.

1. Y or N   Do you have proficient keyboarding skills? Can you type at least 50 words per minute (wpm)?

2. Y or N   Do you have excellent English usage, punctuation, grammar, and spelling skills?

3. Y or N   Are you able to use dictionaries and reference books? Could you find the correct spelling and classification of a prescription drug?

4. Y or N   Do you have a mastery of anatomy and medical terminology? Do you know that the prostrate is not an organ of the male anatomy or that the word *mole* could be a pigmented nevus or a uterine neoplasm?

5. Y or N   Are you competent in a word processing software?

6. Y or N   Do you have excellent proofreading skills?

7. Y or N   Can you sit in one place for extended periods of time?

8. Y or N   Do you like medical topics?

9. Y or N   Do you have hearing acuity and medical language discrimination skills? Can you distinguish words that sound alike and then select the one with the correct meaning, or catch and correct inconsistencies within a report?

10. Y or N   Are you detail-oriented?

11. Y or N   Are you able to work with little supervision?

12. Y or N   Are you able to work under time constraints and production demands (quantity and quality)?

13. Y or N   Are you logical and organized?

14. Y or N   Do you have critical thinking and decision-making skills?

15. Y or N   Are you able to concentrate for long periods of time?

16. Y or N   Do you have excellent eye, hand, and auditory coordination?

17. Y or N   Do you want to be a member of a professional healthcare team?

18. Y or N   Can you be discreet in handling confidential information?

19. Y or N   Do you perform tasks completely and comprehensively?

20. Y or N   Do you take pride in your work?

Chapter 2

Understanding Medical Documents

OBJECTIVES

At the completion of Chapter 2, you should be able to do the following:

1. List the basic information found in chart notes, history and physical examinations, diagnostic reports, and procedure reports.

2. Identify the types of information that appear in chart notes, history and physical examinations, consultation letters, diagnostic reports, and procedure reports.

3. Explain the difference between the two styles of chart notes.

4. Apply a statement to the correct medical report or portion of a chart note.

5. Make a template for the major medical reports.

6. Format and type model medical chart notes, history and physical examinations, consultation letters, diagnostic imaging reports, and procedure reports.

12

Pretest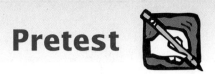

Let's find out if you understand medical documents by scoring 90% or better.

Textbook Users

Select the best answer for each question or statement concerning medical reports.

Refer to the answer key for immediate feedback.

If you score below 90%, continue on to *Activities 1–2: Understanding Medical Document Worksheets.*

If you score 90% or above, congratulations! You have mastered the material covered in Activities 1 and 2. If you wish, you can immediately move on to *Activities 3–5: Keyboarding Medical Documents.*

Software Users

Click on *Chapter 2, Pretest.*

Key the appropriate answer to each question or statement concerning medical reports.

When you are finished, click on *End Test.*

A pop-up screen will reveal your score.

If you score below 90%, continue onto *Activities 1–2: Understanding Medical Document Worksheets.*

If you score 90% or above, congratulations! You have mastered the material covered in Activities 1 and 2. If you wish, you can immediately move on to *Activities 3–5: Keyboarding Medical Documents.*

PRETEST

Directions: Select the best answer for each question or statement concerning medical reports.

1. T or F There are three parts in a SOAP note.

2. T or F The history and physical examination format is found in a chart note.

3. T or F Findings from a consultation can be dictated in letter format.

4. T or F Allergies in a medical report are formatted in such a way as to draw attention to their importance.

5. T or F The medical record is a legal record.

6. T or F Templates are never used in medical transcription.

7. T or F All medical reports include the patient's name.

8. T or F Ultrasound uses low-frequency sound waves to image the body.

9. T or F The average chart note is four pages in length.

10. T or F Abbreviations and phrases are used often in a chart note to save space.

11. T or F Many healthcare facilities have their own manual of style.

12. T or F CAT is also referred to as *computerized axial tomography.*

13. T or F Chart notes do not include a signature line.

14. T or F Usually 1-inch margins are used to format a consultation letter.

15. T or F Dictation for medical reports usually is cryptic.

16. T or F Complete sentences are normally found in history and physical examination reports.

17. T or F The history and physical examination reports are divided into three sections.

18. T or F The abbreviation *HEENT* means *head, ears, eyes, nose, and throat.*

19. T or F In a history and physical examination report, lifestyle habits would be dictated under the "Family History" section or topic.

20. T or F *Noncontributory* means nothing significant was discovered when review of systems (ROS) was performed by the physician.

21. T or F The abbreviation *HPI* means *health program information.*

22. T or F The first page of statistical data in a diagnostic imaging report is the same as in other reports.

23. T or F The military-style dateline is never used in consultation letters.

PRETEST *continued*

24. T or F   Minimally, three perpendicular projections are taken during a medical imaging procedure.

25. T or F   Templates are identified with the *.dot* file extension.

26. Medical reports are vital in which of the following?
    (a) Research
    (b) Compiling statistics
    (c) Evaluating our healthcare delivery system
    (d) All of the above

27. Which of the following are the basic four medical reports in medical offices?
    (a) Consultation letter, chart note, history and physical, and pathology
    (b) Chart note, history and physical, diagnostic, and consultation
    (c) Chart note, history and physical, SOAP, and consultation
    (d) Consultation letter, SOAP, history and physical, and pathology

28. The acronym *SOAP* includes which four topics?
    (a) Symptom, objective, assessment, progress
    (b) Symptom, objective, assessment, plan
    (c) Subjective, objective, assessment, plan
    (d) Subjective, objective, assessment, progress

29. The dictated sentence, "Discontinue use of perfumed body lotion," would be found in a chart note under which topic?
    (a) Subjective
    (b) Chief complaint
    (c) Plan
    (d) Assessment

30. The dictated sentence, "Smooth, erythematous rash over neck extending over trunk and back," would be found in a chart note under which topic?
    (a) Subjective
    (b) Objective
    (c) Assessment
    (d) None of the above

31. The dictated sentence, "My head and throat hurts," would be found in a chart note under which topic?
    (a) Subjective
    (b) Objective
    (c) Assessment
    (d) Symptom

32. The dictated sentence, "BP 120/82" would be found in a chart note under which topic?
    (a) Subjective
    (b) Objective
    (c) Assessment
    (d) Progress

33. The dictated sentence, "Acute otitis," would be found in a chart note under which topic?
    (a) Subjective
    (b) Objective
    (c) Assessment
    (d) Plan

34. The dictated sentence, "Bactrim b.i.d. $\times$ 10 days," would be found in a chart note under which topic?
    (a) Subjective
    (b) Objective
    (c) Progress
    (d) Plan

PRETEST *continued*

35. Which of the following is the usual spacing between each heading in a history and physical examination report?
    (a) Single spacing
    (b) Double spacing
    (c) Triple spacing
    (d) Quadruple spacing

36. The dictation style of a history and physical examination report include which of the following?
    (a) Recurrent phrases and terms
    (b) More negative than positive statements
    (c) Clipped sentences
    (d) All of the above

37. The history section of the history and physical examination reports include which of the following?
    (a) Chief complaint
    (b) Medications
    (c) Review of systems
    (d) All of the above

38. In a history and physical examination report, the physician's comments concerning a guaiac test would be found under which topic?
    (a) Neck
    (b) Heart
    (c) Rectal
    (d) Pelvic

39. Most transcriptionists create a template to include which of the following?
    (a) Margins
    (b) Commonly used topics
    (c) Tab stops
    (d) All of the above

40. In a history and physical examination, the dictated sentence, "The patient is a 2-year-old female," would be found under which topic?
    (a) Past history
    (b) Treatment/plan
    (c) History of present illness
    (d) None of the above

41. In a history and physical examination, the dictated sentence, "She had lower back/spine surgery in 1979," would be found under which topic?
    (a) Past history
    (b) History of present illness
    (c) Chief complaint
    (d) None of the above

42. In a history and physical examination, the dictated sentence, "Her father died at age 75 of what sounded like a heart aneurysm," would be found under which topic?
    (a) Heart
    (b) Family history
    (c) Social history
    (d) Past history

43. In a history and physical examination, the dictated sentence, "Nasal and oral mucosa was normal with oral mucosa pink and moist," would be found under which topic?
    (a) HEENT
    (b) Abdomen
    (c) Would not be included in this report
    (d) Would be included in an x-ray report

PRETEST *continued*

44. In a history and physical examination, the dictated sentence, "Both tympanic membranes are clear," would be found under which topic?
    (a) HEENT
    (b) Heart
    (c) Neck
    (d) None of the above

45. In a history and physical examination, the dictated sentence, "Micronase 2.5 mg b.i.d., Voltaren 75 mg daily, and Lescol 20 mg daily," would be found under which of the following?
    (a) HPI topic
    (b) HEENT topic
    (c) Would not be included in a history and physical examination report
    (d) None of the above

46. In a history and physical examination, the dictated sentence, "DJD of the left hip," would be found under which topic?
    (a) HPI
    (b) HEENT
    (c) Impression
    (d) Plan

47. In a chart note, the dictated sentence, "With his left hand occupied, he slipped and fell backward striking the dorsum of his left hand with the wrist flexed," would be found under which topic?
    (a) Subjective
    (b) Objective
    (c) Assessment
    (d) Plan

48. In a history and physical examination, the dictated sentence, "Early osteoarthritis affecting mainly the right hip but also the left hip and lumbar spine," would be found under which topic?
    (a) Impression
    (b) Plan
    (c) Objective
    (d) Treatment

49. In a chart note, the dictated sentence, "This patient presents with pain, redness, and tenderness in the right great toe," would be found under which topic?
    (a) Chief complaint
    (b) Lab
    (c) Assessment
    (d) Plan

50. In a history and physical examination, the dictated sentence, "There is a slight tenderness to palpation over the left trapezius," would be found under which topic?
    (a) Heart
    (b) Neck
    (c) Lungs
    (d) Extremities

Medical Reports

To become proficient in transcribing medical reports, it is important that you understand the format of the transcribed reports. You also should be able to identify the various sections of a report and understand the link between the sections or topic headings and their contents. Some physicians do not dictate a report into its correct sections, or they fail to identify the headings. As you read through this chapter, take particular notice to the design, headings, topics, and formats of the different medical documents.

The transcribed medical report is a legal medical document that communicates the patient's health status to others. It must be transcribed accurately and completely. Any error, no matter how small, may jeopardize the patient's health. The attending physician, as well as any involved specialist, therapist, or technician, will base their assessment and recommendations for care and treatment of the patient on the medical transcripts they receive and review.

Medical records also provide documented evidence of a patient's medical treatment to insurance companies, along with information necessary for federal and state regulatory requirements. They play a vital role in research, compiling statistics, and evaluating our healthcare delivery system. Quality-assurance issues and consumer concerns about access to care rely heavily on statistics and data acquired from medical records to address these problems.

Medical records are vital records for your employer's accounting department. Procedure codes (CPT) and diagnostic codes (ICD-9-CM) reported on the patient's health insurance claim form are based on the documentation in the medical record and are used in billing.

Medical reports are dictated by physicians in all medical specialties, even some that do not readily come to mind, such as ophthalmology, dentistry, chiropractic, pathology, psychiatry, and veterinary medicine.

Medical reports dictated in office practice, hospital, and inpatient facilities have similarities and differences. The four reports that form the basis of a patient's medical record in the inpatient setting (such as a hospital or rehabilitation center) include the history and physical examination, operative report, consultation, and discharge summary. These records are frequently referred to as the "big four."

Consultations letters, chart notes, history and physical examination reports, diagnostic imaging reports, and procedure reports form the fundamental group that make up a patient's medical record in the outpatient setting, such as a private or group practice.

Each report always must include information for identification, such as the patient's legal name, date of birth, and a file number that may be a social security number (SSN) or another institutionally assigned number. Healthcare facilities that adhere to Joint Commission on Accreditation of Health Organization (JCAHO) standards must include the patient's name and identification number on all medical reports. It is critical to correctly spell the patient's name and accurately document the patient's birth date. Many facilities assign an identification number to every patient that is used every time the patient seeks care at the facility.

THE LOOK OF MEDICAL REPORTS

All medical reports include the title of the report (chart note, history and physical, x-ray, etc.), statistical data (patient's name, identification number, DOB, date of examination, physician's name, etc.), and signature line. In addition, chart notes, procedure reports, and diagnostic imaging reports contain sections or topics. History and physical examination reports contain headings, topics, and subtopics. However, in clinical practice, you may see a variety of formatting styles. Therefore you always should refer to your employer's own manual of style before transcribing medical reports.

Figure 2.1 shows models of three medical reports. More detailed illustrations are included later in this chapter.

Formatting Signature Lines. The formatting of statistical data varies among medical reports, but the formatting of signature lines is fairly consistent and applicable to all medical reports except letters. There are two common formats for the signature line. In Method 1, the physician's or dictator's name is followed by the initials of the transcriptionist on the third or fourth line below the last entry line. In Method 2, the physician's or dictator's initials are followed by the initials of the transcriptionist, the date of dictation, and date of transcription.

```
CHART NOTE (title)

PATIENT'S STATISTICAL DATA

SUBJECTIVE (section/topic)
OBJECTIVE (section/topic)
ASSESSMENT (section/topic)
PLAN (section/topic)


Potter T. Bucky MD
SIGNATURE LINE/xx
```

```
HISTORY AND PHYSICAL EXAMINATION (title)

PATIENT'S STATISTICAL DATA

HISTORY (heading)

CHIEF COMPLAINT (topic)
HISTORY OF PRESENT ILLNESS (topic)
PAST HISTORY (topic)
ALLERGIES (topic)
FAMILY HISTORY (topic)
SOCIAL HISTORY (topic)
REVIEW OF SYSTEMS (topic)

PHYSICAL (heading)

GENERAL (topic)
HEENT (topic)
GENITOURINARY (topic)
NECK (topic)
CHEST (topic)
HEART (topic)
LUNGS (topic)
ABDOMEN (topic)
PELVIC (topic)
EXTREMITIES (topic)
NEUROLOGIC (topic)

LABORATORY (when available)
DIAGNOSTIC TESTS (when available)

IMPRESSION (topic)
PLAN (topic)


Potter T. Bucky MD
SIGNATURE LINE/xx
```

```
X-RAY REPORT (title)

PATIENT'S STATISTICAL DATA

HISTORY (section/topic)
FINDINGS (section/topic)
IMPRESSION (section/topic)


Potter T. Bucky MD
SIGNATURE LINE/xx
```

FIGURE 2.1 Medical report models.

Physicians should not use rubber stamps or initials to sign dictation because it is difficult to prove legal authenticity without a complete signature. Rubber stamps can be stolen, and initials can be forged.

Method 1:

Potter T. Bucky MD
Potter T. Bucky, MD/cd

Method 2:

Potter T. Bucky MD
Potter T. Bucky, MD
ptb:XX
D: 11/20/xx (date the report was dictated)
T: 11/21/xx (date the report was transcribed)

OUTPATIENT MEDICAL DOCUMENTS

As a novice medical transcriptionist, you will probably begin your career in a private or group physician practice. For this reason, this textbook will devote its content to developing your transcription skills by familiarizing you with the medical documents commonly found in the private or group physician practice. Each component of the transcription process will be explained step by step. An emphasis on developing fundamental transcription skills and not requiring you to discern between multiple formatting and guideline rules that exist in current practice should simplify the learning process for a beginning medical transcriptionist. To assist you in this learning process, you will be asked to follow a specific format for each report presented in this chapter.

Chart Notes

The chart note (also called *progress note* or *follow-up note*) is dictated by the physician after talking, examining, or meeting with the patient. Remember, speaking with a physician over the phone still involves the patient's healthcare, and as such, this information needs to be documented in the medical record. The physician also must sign the report.

The chart note contains a precise description of the patient's major presenting problem (chief complaint), physical findings, and the physician's plan of treatment. It also may include the results of laboratory and x-ray tests. Chart notes can vary in length from a mere sentence or two to several pages, with the average length being two to four paragraphs. The items dictated into a chart note will vary depending on the severity of the patient's problem and brevity of the dictator.

Abbreviations and phrases are used often in a chart note to save space. It is imperative that all abbreviations are correctly transcribed and no ambiguity exists as to their exact meaning. An example would be *Ca*, which could be interpreted as *calcium* or *cancer*. When in doubt, spell out the word and verify its meaning with the dictator. Many healthcare facilities have an approved list of abbreviations with clearly defined definitions that are acceptable to all practitioners of the organization, whereas other facilities may not allow the use of abbreviations. Healthcare facilities owned by hospital organizations are required to follow JCAHO rules and regulations, including having an approved abbreviation list on site.

THE LOOK OF CHART NOTES

Over the years, a patient's medical record can become quite bulky, especially in a family physician practice. To conserve space, the transcriptionist is often directed to format chart notes using narrow margins (0.5 inches), single spacing, and no blank lines separating the topics. Because the physician often is in a hurry or between patients, the dictation is full of phrases and abbreviations. The transcript should reflect this effort to conserve space by using approved or accepted abbreviations and phrases within the document. As with all medical records, be sure that the patient's name is spelled correctly and the document is dated with the month, day, and year of the visit. Your ability to produce accurate and error-free medical documents will determine your success as a medical transcriptionist.

For the purpose of this textbook, you will be asked to format chart notes and other medical documents in block style using 1-inch margins, single spacing, and blank lines separating the topics, which are capitalized. Using this format style will enable you and your instructor to read and evaluate transcripts more easily than the compressed style typically found in clinical practice.

Formatting Statistical Data on Chart Notes. Chart notes, like other medical reports, require the patient's statistical data on the first and succeeding pages. The patient's statistical data on the first page include the patient's full name, date of birth, and examination visit. The same information is included on the document if it extends beyond one page. The patient's full name, date of birth, and page number appear on continuation sheets as shown:

Statistical data for the first page:
  Patient Name: Doe, Jane
  Date of Birth: December 21, 1952
  Examination Date: April 1, 20xx

Statistical data for continuation pages:
  Patient Name: Doe, Jane
  Date of Birth: December 21, 1952
  Page 2

CHART NOTES USING THE SOAP FORMAT

A common chart note format is the SOAP method, which is an acronym for *subjective, objective, assessment, plan.* The SOAP format is illustrated in Figure 2.2. Each topic has a distinctive meaning.

S: Subjective findings are typically associated with what prompted the patient to seek medical care. A patient will describe feelings and symptoms to the physician.
For example: My head and throat hurt, and I have been throwing up all day.

O: Objective finding are measurable findings discovered by the physician or by the results of diagnostic studies or laboratory tests.
For example: Temperature is 103.2° F, and throat culture is positive.

A: Assessment is the physician's diagnosis or diagnoses of the patient's disease or condition,

↕ top margin 1" (line 6)

CHART NOTE
↕ **double space**
Patient Name: Felter, Michael
↕ **double space**
Date of Birth: July 3, 1954
↕ **double space**
Examination Date: *current date*
↕ **double space**
SUBJECTIVE: Patient complains of right elbow pain for past three months. He has been playing tennis once a week over the summer with gradually worsening pain.
↕ **double space**
OBJECTIVE: Tenderness over right medial epicondyle. Pain radiates to the forearm and back of the hand with flexion and supination.
↕ **double space**
ASSESSMENT: Epicondylitis.
↕ **double space**
PLAN: Advised patient to stop playing tennis for three weeks and rest elbow until inflammation subsides. Prescribed Motrin 200 mg p.o. q.i.d. Urged the patient to wear an elastic strap for support, when playing tennis in the future.
↕ **quadruple space**

Harry A. Medulla MD
Harry A. Medulla, MD/xx

←→ **left margin 1"**

FIGURE 2.2   Formatting a sample chart note using the SOAP note style.

based on subjective and objective findings.
For example: Strep throat.

P: Plan is the treatment plan developed by the physician relative to the findings of the subjective and objective assessment of the patient.
For example:
Amoxicillin 250 mg t.i.d. × 10 days.

When physicians are dictating chart notes using the SOAP format, they may say the topics or just give the first letter. Whether the topic is spelled out or only the first letter is typed depends on your employer's formatting guidelines. In such cases, a physician may dictate one of the following:

"Subjective: Patient complains of shortness of breath on exertion, with occasional pain radiating down left arm."

"S: Patient complains of shortness of breath on exertion, with occasional pain radiating down left arm."

In some medical practices, the physician dictates neither the letter nor the topic but requires the transcriptionist to know and apply the appropriate topic based on the facility's transcription guidelines. Exercises provided later will help you identify dictated sentences and their topics.

CHART NOTES USING THE HISTORY AND PHYSICAL FORMAT

Some physicians follow a history and physical (H&P) format when dictating a chart note (Figure 2.3). This format involves different topic names. The dictator may include the patient's chief complaint, history of present illness, past medical history, findings on the physical exam, and a treatment plan.

Here are two typical outlines of the H&P chart note format. There are variations on this style. These abbreviations are sometimes used in dictation. Depending on the dictator, some, all, or different combinations of the topics described are used.

Typical format 1
History of present illness (abbreviated *HPI*)
Past medical history (abbreviated *PMH*)
Physical exam (abbreviated *PX, PE,* or *CPX*)
Impression (abbreviated *IMP*)
Plan (abbreviated *RX*)

Typical format 2
Chief complaint (abbreviated *CC*)
Past medical history
Physical exam
Laboratory
X-ray
Diagnosis (abbreviated *DX*)
Treatment (abbreviated *TX*)

↔left margin 1" CHART NOTE
             ↕**double space**
Patient Name: Schaeffer, Carolyn
             ↕**double space**
Date of Birth: April 18, 19xx
             ↕**double space**
Examination Date: *current date*
             ↕**double space**
CHIEF COMPLAINT: Chest pain
             ↕**double space**
HISTORY OF PRESENT ILLNESS: Carolyn is a 52-year-old white female who experienced chest pressure, palpitations, heart racing, numbness and weakness in her right arm while at church services this morning. This episode lasted approximately four minutes. She also felt somewhat nauseated and clammy. Patient cardiac risk factors include tobacco abuse, hyperlipidemia, and obesity. She is currently under therapy for hyperthyroidism.
             ↕**double space**
PAST MEDICAL HISTORY:
1. Vaginal hysterectomy in 1975 for excessive bleeding.
2. Hyperlipidemia with triglycerides in the 350 range and cholesterol over 300. While taking Lopid, cholesterol fell to approximately 252 and triglycerides were 183.
3. Obesity.
4. Tobacco abuse.
5. Hypothyroidism.
             ↕**double space**
PHYSICAL EXAMINATION
             ↕**double space**
GENERAL: She is a very pleasant and cooperative patient in no acute distress.
             ↕**double space**
HEENT: She is wearing corrective lenses. Sclerae anicteric, tympanic membranes clear. Nose clear. Throat normal. She has a normal gag reflex. She has multiple filled caries.
             ↕**double space**
NECK: Supple without thyromegaly or lymphadenopathy. Carotids 2+ bilaterally without bruits.
             ↕**double space**
CHEST: Clear to auscultation anteriorly and posteriorly.
             ↕**double space**
continued

FIGURE 2.3 Formatting a sample chart note using the history and physical style.

History and Physical Examination Reports

The dictation style of history and physical examination reports contains recurrent phrases and terms. It also contains more negative than positive statements. The major topics do not vary much and are used repeatedly in almost every report, as illustrated in Box 2.1. However, sometimes not all topics are needed, and the standard format is modified according to the dictator's needs.

A characteristic of both the H&P report and the chart note is the tendency to condense and abbreviate whenever possible. Students who are first encountering chart notes or H&P reports often become frustrated because of the short, cryptic style of dictation. Clipped sentences, which often lack a subject or verb, are a common and acceptable dic-

tating style. When you are listening to such dictation, you will find that words may be omitted or a subject or verb may not be included, yet the meaning of the sentence will be clear to you even though some words are unspoken. The following are some examples of clipped sentence structure:

CHEST: Clear to percussion and auscultation. Heart regular rate and rhythm.
ABDOMEN: Flat, soft, nontender, nondistended, normoactive bowel sounds.
RECTAL: No masses. Guaiac negative.
This means: The chest was clear to percussion and auscultation. The heart rate and rhythm were regular. The abdomen was soft, nontender, was not distended, and had normal bowel sounds. The rectal exam was negative in that no masses

↕top margin 1" (line 6)

↔left margin 1"   Patient Name: Schaeffer, Carolyn
Date of Birth: April 18, 19xx
Page 2
↕double space
HEART: Regular rate and rhythm with a grade I/VI systolic murmur heard best at the aortic region.
↕double space
ABDOMEN: Mildly obese. Normoactive bowel sounds. Nontender, no organomegaly.
↕double space
BREASTS/PELVIC/RECTAL: Deferred as these were done at the office one month ago and were normal.
↕double space
EXTREMITIES: Without clubbing, cyanosis, or edema. Pulses 2+ in the upper and lower extremities.
↕double space
NEUROLOGICAL: No focal neurologic deficits.
↕double space
ASSESSMENT:
1. Chest pain.
2. Hypothyroidism.
3. Obesity.
4. Tobacco abuse.
↕double space
PLAN:
1. Obtain serial EKGs and cardiac enzymes to rule out myocardial infarction.
2. Obtain echocardiogram and stress thallium test.
3. Use nitroglycerin paste to the chest wall. Avoid any other cardiac medications unless there is an indication for them. Her symptoms are not clearly cardiac in nature.
↕quadruple space

Adam Valence MD
Adam Valence, MD/xx

FIGURE 2.3—CONT'D Formatting a sample chart note using the history and physical style.

were found, and the guaiac test found no occult blood in the feces.

FORMATTING STATISTICAL DATA ON HISTORY AND PHYSICAL EXAMINATION REPORTS

In this textbook, H&P reports, like chart notes, are formatted in block style using 1-inch margins, single spacing, and blank lines separating the topics, which are capitalized as illustrated in Figure 2.4. The patient's statistical data is required on the first and continuation pages and include the patient's full name, identification number, date of birth, examination date, and physician's name. The employer's transcription guidelines may expand the requirements to suit the needs of the individual facility and its staff members.

Statistical data for the first page:
Patient Name: Doe, Jane
File Number: 00912
Date of Birth: December 21, 1952
Examination Date: April 1, 20xx
Physician: Potter T. Bucky

Statistical data for continuation pages:
Patient Name: Doe, Jane
File Number: 00912
Date of Birth: December 21, 1952
Examination Date: April 1, 20xx
Physician: Potter T. Bucky
Page 2

Formatting Signature Lines on History and Physical Examination Reports. Formatting signature lines for all medical reports is discussed in "The Look of Medical Reports."

TOPICS INCLUDED IN THE "HISTORY" HEADING OF A HISTORY AND PHYSICAL EXAMINATION REPORT

The physical examination of a patient is an exact and involved process. As such the topics found in a H&P report are more numerous than on chart notes. It is divided into two headings: "History" and "Physical."

Virtually every "History" heading contains the same major topics and follows a specific format. In

BOX 2.1   HISTORY AND PHYSICAL EXAMINATION REPORT TOPICS

History
   Chief complaint
   History of present illness (or present illness)
   Past medical history
   Allergies
   Medications
   Family history
   Social history
   Habits
   Review of systems
Physical Examination
   General (this includes vital signs)
   HEENT (head, eyes, ears, nose, throat)
   Neck
   Chest (includes thorax, breasts, and axillae)
   Heart
   Lungs
   Abdomen
   Pelvic (sometimes listed as *genitalia*)
   Rectal
   Extremities
   Neurological (includes mental status)
Laboratory tests (when available)
Diagnostic tests (when available)
Impression
Plan (or recommendation)

this textbook, topic headings are formatted in all capital letters. These major topics are as follows:

- *Chief complaint* is the specific reason for which the patient sought medical care, stated in the most concise terms or sometimes quoted in the patient's own words.
- *History of present illness* contains all historical information that was given by the patient concerning the illness. This information includes all relevant symptoms and their duration and any remedies that have been attempted. Depending on the illness, this information may be stated in a concise sentence, or it may occupy a page or more of information if the problem is the culmination of weeks or even months of a chronic evolving illness.
- *Past medical history* includes information about previous illness, injuries, surgeries, and chronic conditions a patient may have had, along with any allergies to medications. This topic also may include immunizations.

- *Allergies* is a list of the patient's allergies. Allergies are keyed in either all capitals, boldfaced, or underlined to call attention to their importance. The format varies by facility. Medications may be included in this section or under a separate heading.
- *Medications* is a list of medications that the patient is currently taking. Sometimes this information is not listed as a separate topic but included under "Past Medical History" or "Allergies."
- *Family history* consists of information about any hereditary or familial diseases.
- *Social history* is included if the physician believes this information is pertinent to the patient's treatment plan. This topic may include lifestyle habits such as smoking and drinking, as well as the patient's occupation, hobbies, family structure, and living arrangements.
- *Review of systems* (ROS) includes a brief review of any relevant information about each major body system. Depending on the patient's problem, this topic can be very comprehensive and divided into subtopics such as HEENT, cardiovascular, respiratory, gastrointestinal, genitourinary, gynecologic, neuropsychiatric, and musculoskeletal, or it may be combined into one paragraph or simply be a brief statement such as "noncontributory" when all systems are negative.

TOPICS INCLUDED IN THE "PHYSICAL EXAMINATION" HEADING OF A HISTORY AND PHYSICAL EXAMINATION REPORT

The "Physical Examination" heading of the report is exactly what its name implies. The physician completes a physical examination of the patient, and the findings are transcribed under the pertinent topic. The major topics for the physical examination of the report include the following:

- The *general* section discusses the appearance of the patient such as pallor, gait, mood, and personal hygiene. It also includes a statement of the patient's vital signs (blood pressure, temperature, pulse, and respiration).
- *HEENT* is an abbreviation for the head, eyes, ears, nose, and throat.
- The *neck* is palpated for enlargement of the lymph nodes or thyroid gland, assessment of the carotid pulses, and any distention of the jugular veins.

↕top margin 1" (line 6)

↔left margin 1" HISTORY AND PHYSICAL EXAMINATION REPORT
↕double space
Patient Name: Rouf, Andrea
↕double space
File Number: 2348901
↕double space
Date of Birth: April 10, 19xx
↕double space
Examination Date: *current date*
↕double space
Physician: Gwenn Maltese, MD
↕double space
HISTORY
↕double space
CHIEF COMPLAINT: Abdominal pain, RLQ for three days.
↕double space
HISTORY OF PRESENT ILLNESS: The patient is a 27-year-old legal secretary, who first noted the onset of colicky lower abdominal pain situated slightly to the right of midline, below the umbilicus and above the pubic bone three days ago. The pain has been getting worse and is associated for the past 36 hours with anorexia and nausea. She has vomited 4-5 times in the past 24 hours, mostly a bile-colored, watery liquid. The pain is not affected by positional change or ingestion of food. There is no radiation of pain. She denies fever, chills, hematemesis or change in bowel habits.
↕double space
PAST HISTORY: The patient had varicella at age 2 and the mumps at age 4. She had a tonsillectomy and adenoidectomy at age 11. There is no family history of diabetes.
↕double space
REVIEW OF SYSTEMS:
↕double space
HEENT: Mild upper respiratory infection two weeks prior to present illness manifested by rhinitis and sore throat.
↕double space
GENITOURINARY: Gravida II, para II, ab 0. No frequency, hematuria, or nocturia.
↕double space
continued

FIGURE 2.4 Formatting a sample history and physical examination report.

- The *chest* also includes the thorax, breasts, and axilla areas.
- The *lungs* are evaluated by auscultation, during which the physician listens with a stethoscope to air moving in and out of the lungs. Diseases or injury can produce abnormal changes in the quality and volume or loudness in breath sounds. The physician also may perform the percussion (tapping) maneuver.
- The *heart* is evaluated with a stethoscope for any abnormal sounds, such as murmurs or bruits (sound or murmur heard in auscultation), clicks (brief, sharp sounds, especially any of the short, dry clicking heart sounds during systole), rubs (sounds caused by rubbing together of two serous surfaces), thrills (vibrations), and gallops (disordered heart rhythm).
- The *abdomen* is assessed by auscultation, in which the physician listens for any abnormal bowel sounds, and percussion, in which the physician palpates the abdomen for tenderness, guarding, and masses.
- The *pelvic* region or genitalia are examined. Women may undergo a bimanual pelvic exam and Papanicolaou (Pap) smear.
- The *rectal* exam involves a digital evaluation of the rectum for deformity or masses. The physician also may comment on the results of a guaiac test (for occult blood) or colonoscopy (fiberoptic instrument) in this topic of the report. Men may undergo a digital rectal examination of the prostate. Digital palpation is a useful method for detection of early prostatic carcinoma.
- The *extremities* are examined for developmental or traumatic deformities, muscle wasting, and stiffness. The bones, joints, and muscles of all extremities are evaluated.

↕ top margin 1" (line 6)

←→ left margin 1"   HISTORY AND PHYSICAL EXAMINATION REPORT
Patient Name: Rouf, Andrea
File Number: 2348901
Date of Birth: April 10, 19xx
Examination Date: *current date*
Physician: Gwenn Maltese, MD
Page 2
↕ double space
PHYSICAL EXAMINATION
↕ double space
GENERAL: The patient is alert, oriented and in moderate distress. BP 120/80, pulse 106 and regular, temperature 37.2 C, respirations 14/min.
↕ double space
LUNGS: Clear to P&A.
↕ double space
HEART: Normal sinus rhythm, no cardiomegaly, no murmurs, gallops, or thrills.
↕ double space
ABDOMEN: Flat. Tenderness with muscle guarding in right lower quadrant. Rebound tenderness was present. Bowel sounds are normal. No organomegaly.
↕ double space
PELVIC: Bartholins, urethral, and Skene's gland normal. Adnexa normal. Uterus not enlarged.
↕ double space
EXTREMITIES: Within normal limits. No edema. Good range of motion.
↕ double space
NEUROLOGICAL: Grossly intact.
↕ double space
IMPRESSION:
1. Acute appendicitis.
2. Rule out ureteral calculus.
↕ double space
PLAN:
1. Refer to John Smithson, MD for surgical consult.
2. Patient to be admitted to General Hospital.
3. WBC an IVP ordered upon admission.
↕ quadruple space

Gwenn Maltese MD
Gwenn Maltese, MD/xx

FIGURE 2.4—CONT'D   Formatting a sample history and physical examination report.

- The *neurological* examination is a systematic evaluation of the nervous system, including mental status, functioning of the cranial nerves and reflexes, and sensory and neuromuscular function. The Babinski reflex and deep tendon reflexes (DTRs) are usually checked.
- *Laboratory data* include laboratory test results, such as complete blood count (CBC), white blood cell count (WBC), and urinalysis (UA).
- The *impression* is the physician's diagnosis or diagnoses of the patient's clinical condition or disease based on the findings of the physical examination and diagnostic tests.
- The *plan of treatment* is developed by the physician based on the findings of the physical examination and diagnostic tests.

Diagnostic Imaging Reports and Letters

Diagnostic imaging reports typically include clinical radiology (x-ray), ultrasonography (US) or sonography, computerized tomography (CT), nuclear medicine (NM), and magnetic resonance imaging (MRI). Each area is classified as a separate imaging modality because each uses a different type of energy and recording device to image the body.

A computer is involved in the imaging process of almost all differing modalities. Hence the image can be displayed on a video monitor and then digitally stored or printed on traditional x-ray film. All modalities except diagnostic x-ray have cross-sectional image recording capabilities. Each modality has its own unique features and capabilities for anatomic imaging. A certain body structure is imaged better with one modality than with the other. It is up to the physician to choose the best, most effective imaging modality to evaluate the anatomy of interest.

Diagnostic x-rays use low levels of radiation to record images of the body on x-ray film. Newer methods sometimes allow the image to be digitized and stored in a computer.

Ultrasound or sonography uses high-frequency sound waves to image the body. It is unique in that it does not expose patients to ionizing radiation and therefore is the modality of choice to evaluate maternal or fetal anatomy in pregnant women.

In nuclear medicine the energy source is a radioactive isotope that is injected into the patient's body, and then specialized computers and cameras record and store the image.

Computerized tomography uses a combination of radiation and computerized imaging techniques to record and display an individual's anatomy. It is sometimes referred to as a *CAT scan* (computerized axial tomography). This term is technically incorrect because today's CT scanners can image the body in more than just the axial plane.

Magnetic resonance imaging is a very sophisticated machine that uses a magnetic field and radio-frequency waves to generate an image. It does not use ionizing radiation and often produces sharper soft-tissue images than other modalities.

THE LOOK OF DIAGNOSTIC IMAGING REPORTS AND LETTERS

Medical imaging reports look very different from SOAP notes, consultation letters, or H&P reports. The title of the report reflects the imaging modality chosen and the anatomy of interest. The report often includes a statement about various anatomic projections. To best visualize an anatomic part, the patient is imaged in many different positions, which are called *projections.*

A minimum of two perpendicular projections are taken during a medical imaging procedure. Because the human body is three-dimensional and most imaging techniques are one-dimensional, multiple projections are required to thoroughly evaluate the anatomy of interest. For example, multiple views of the lumbar spine are routinely taken in diagnostic x-ray. If the patient is supine, the resulting projection is termed an *anteroposterior* or *AP projection.* If

the patient is imaged when lying on the left side, the projections are termed a *left lateral projection.* And if the patient is rotated 45 degrees toward the left when in the supine position, this is termed a *left posterior oblique projection* or *LPO.*

The body of the medical imaging report uses this positioning terminology because the physician, typically a radiologist, interprets the film. Your success in this area will result largely from a firm grasp of medical terminology, along with a solid understanding of positional terms, body planes, and basic radiologic science terminology.

Patients are typically referred to imaging centers by physicians in the community. The transcribed report is sent back to the referring physician in a letter format. Hospital reports usually are not converted to letter format.

Formatting Statistical Data on Diagnostic Imaging Reports. In this textbook, diagnostic imaging reports are formatted in block style using 1-inch margins, single spacing, and blank lines separating the topics, which are capitalized as illustrated in Figure 2.5. The statistical data on the first page should include the patient's full name, identification or file number, date of birth, examination date, ordering physician, and type of examination. The employer's transcription guidelines may expand the requirements to suit the needs of the facility and staff members.

Statistical data for the <u>first page</u>:
Patient Name: Doe, Jane
File Number: 45231
Date of Birth: December 21, 1952
Examination Date: April 1, 20xx
Ordering Physician: Izzy Sertoli, MD
Examination: MAMMOGRAM

Statistical data for <u>continuation pages</u>:
Patient Name: Doe, Jane
File Number: 45321
Date of Birth: December 21, 1952
Examination Date: April 1, 20xx
Ordering Physician: Izzy Sertoli, MD
Page 2

The diagnostic imaging letter is formatted as illustrated in Figure 2.6. The patient's statistical data are also included in the reference line of the diagnostic imaging letter.

↔left margin 1"   X-RAY REPORT
↕double space
Patient Name: Farley, Cassandra
↕double space
File Number: 5690341
↕double space
Date of Birth: February 1, 19xx
↕double space
Examination Date: *current date*
↕double space
Ordering Physician: Izzy Sertoli, MD
↕double space
Examination: PA AND LATERAL CHEST X-RAY
↕double space
HISTORY: This is a 57-year-old female with a history of lung cancer and increased shortness of breath for one week.
↕double space
FINDINGS
↕double space
CHEST: There is mild fibrotic change at both lung bases, over the left lung apex, and along the left chest wall laterally. There is some deformity to the left rib cage, apparently reflecting several old, healed rib fractures. There are some increased markings at the left lung base.
↕double space
IMPRESSION: Early pneumonia, superimposed upon the underlying fibrotic changes. The heart size is normal.
↕quadruple space

Adam Valence MD
Adam Valence, MD/xx

FIGURE 2.5   Formatting a sample x-ray report.

FORMATTING SIGNATURE LINES ON DIAGNOSTIC IMAGING REPORTS

Formatting signature lines for medical reports was discussed in "The Look of Medical Reports."

Topics Included on Diagnostic Imaging Reports. *History* comprises the technologist's observations and remarks concerning the chief complaint. These findings provide clinical information helpful to the radiologist in interpreting the films. This is a relatively new topic of the report and may not be included. Use of computerized medical records necessitates that the radiologist dictate this information into the report.

The *findings* are the physician's interpretation in regard to the disorder and disease processes shown on the hard-copy film or monitor.

The *impression* is the physician's assessment of the patient's health status as determined by the diagnostic images. This is usually a brief summary of the findings.

Procedure Reports

With today's sophisticated computerized medical technology, many procedures once performed exclusively in the hospital setting are now routinely performed in the medical office environment. Compact, low-cost, and technologically sophisticated medical machines are common diagnostic tools in ambulatory medical practices. Hence transcriptionists employed in medical offices often find procedure reports, such as EKGs, sigmoidoscopy, and colposcopy, as standard components of a dictation.

The format and heading used for these reports is very similar to those used in diagnostic imaging reports as illustrated in Figure 2.7. Identification of headings such as the patient name and identification data (usually date of birth, file number, or SSN), date of procedure, ordering physician, and name of procedure will accurately associate the physician's findings with the correct patient.

FORMATTING STATISTICAL DATA ON PROCEDURE REPORTS

In this textbook, procedure reports are formatted in block style using 1-inch margins, single spacing, and blank lines separating the topics, which are capitalized. Statistical data on the first page should include the patient's full name, date of birth (along

FedDes Wellness Center
Diagnostic Imaging Division, Suite 157
101 Wellness Way Drive
New York, NY 10036

←→left margin 1"   *current date*
                          ↕ **quadruple space**

Charles P. Davis, MD
FedDes Wellness Center
Family Practice Division, Suite 300
101 Wellness Way Drive
New York, NY 10036
                          ↕ **double space**
Re: Betty McWilliams
      Date of Birth: February 2, 1949
      Examination: RIGHT BREAST SONOGRAM
                          ↕ **double space**
Dear Dr. Davis
                          ↕ **double space**
Comparison is made to the prior mammogram dated January 25, 20xx. An
18 x 8 x 20 mm well-demarcated simple cyst is demonstrated within the central
12 o'clock position of the right breast corresponding to the well-demarcated
density noted on mammography in this region. The cyst exhibits posterior wall
enhancement and sound through transmission.
                          ↕ **double space**
A second cyst measuring 6.1 x 7.1 x 4.4 mm is present in the approximate
10 o'clock position of the breast projecting 6-7 mm from the nipple corresponding
to the density noted on mammography in this region.
                          ↕ **double space**
No additional lesions are identified.
                          ↕ **double space**
IMPRESSION: The two densities noted in the right breast on the recent
mammogram correspond to simple cysts as described.
                          ↕ **double space**
Thank you for the opportunity to participate in the care of this patient.
                          ↕ **double space**
Sincerely yours
                          ↕ **quadruple space**

Potter T. Bucky MD
Potter T. Bucky, MD
                          ↕ **double space**
xx

FIGURE 2.6 Formatting a sample diagnostic imaging letter with typical letterhead style. Diagnostic imaging letters are usually typed on letterhead.

with SSN or practice-specific file number), examination visit, ordering physician, and type of procedure. The employer's transcription guidelines may expand the requirements to suit the needs of the facility and staff members.

Statistical data for the <u>first page</u>:
Patient Name: Kleine, Ann
File Number: 186-00-6810
Date of Birth: March 7, 19xx
Examination Date: January 1, 20xx
Ordering Physician: Izzy Sertoli, MD
Procedure: EXERCISE STRESS TEST

Statistical data for <u>continuation pages</u>:
Patient Name: Kleine, Ann
File Number: 186-00-6810
Date of Birth: March 7, 19xx
Examination Date: January 1, 20xx
Ordering Physician: Izzy Sertoli, MD
Page 2

FORMATTING SIGNATURE LINES ON PROCEDURE REPORTS

Formatting signature lines for medical reports was discussed in "The Look of Medical Reports."

↕top margin 1" (line 6)

↔left margin 1"   PROCEDURE REPORT
↕double space
Patient Name: Shauback, Ann
↕double space
File Number: 200-00-2000
↕double space
Date of Birth: July 3,1955
↕double space
Examination Date: *current date*
↕double space
Ordering Physician: Charles P. Davis, MD
↕double space
Procedure: EXERCISE STRESS TEST
↕double space
Baseline electrocardiogram, normal sinus rhythm, normal active intervals, no
baseline ST segment abnormalities.
↕double space
The patient was exercised according to standard Bruce protocol, exercised for
nine minutes, achieving 10 mets. Reached a maximum heart rate of 186 which
was 101% of predicted. Reached a peak blood pressure of 140/110. There was
no chest pain with exercise. There were no arrhythmia observed.
↕double space
IMPRESSION:
1. Negative for ECG evidence for ischemia.
2. No chest pain with exercise.
3. No hypertensive response to exercise.
4. No arrhythmia with exercise.
5. Normal functional aerobic capacity.
↕quadruple space

Potter T. Bucky MD
Potter T. Bucky, MD/xx

FIGURE 2.7   Formatting a sample procedure report.

Operative Reports

Operative reports are very detailed and descriptive and allow the reader to visualize the operation. The operative reports here are of relatively simple operations. The preoperative and postoperative diagnoses are dictated in the report and may be the same, but it is not acceptable to type *same* under the postoperative topic. The transcriptionist must key the diagnostic statement. Abbreviations should be avoided.

FORMATTING STATISTICAL DATA ON OPERATIVE REPORTS

The format of this report is similar to procedure and diagnostic imaging reports. The differences are two additional headings in the statistical section (Figure 2.8).

Statistical data for the first page:
Patient Name: Mason, Charles
File Number: 00123
Date of Birth: March 27, 19xx
Examination Date: February 1, 20xx
Preoperative Diagnosis: Hematuria
Postoperative Diagnosis: Normal cystoscopy
Operation: CYSTOSCOPY

Statistical data for continuation pages:
Patient Name: Mason, Charles
File Number: 00123
Date of Birth: March 27, 19xx
Examination Date: February 1, 20xx
Preoperative Diagnosis: Hematuria
Postoperative Diagnosis: Normal cystoscopy
Operation: CYSTOSCOPY
Page 2

FORMATTING SIGNATURE LINES ON OPERATIVE REPORTS

Formatting signature lines for medical reports was discussed in "The Look of Medical Reports."

← left margin 1"   OPERATIVE REPORT
♦ double space
Patient Name: Samuelson, Jack
♦ double space
File Number: 203798
♦ double space
Date of Birth: July 13,1946
♦ double space
Examination Date: *current date*
♦ double space
Preoperative Diagnosis: Microscopic hematuria
♦ double space
Postoperative Diagnosis: Normal cystoscopy
♦ double space
Operation: CYSTOSCOPY
♦ double space
PROCEDURE: The patient was placed in the supine position and draped in the usual fashion. The penis was prepped with Betadine. A local anesthetic of 10 cc of 2% lidocaine jelly was injected into the urethra.
♦ double space
The flexible cystourethroscope was advanced through the urethra to the level of the verumontanum. No strictures were noted within the urethra. The prostate was not obstructed. Once entrance was obtained into the bladder, the mucosa was examined in a circumferential fashion and found normal. The orifices were normal. The scope was removed.
♦ double space
The patient tolerated the procedure well. There were no complications.
♦ double space
IMPRESSION: Normal examination.
♦ quadruple space

Theodore Trigone MD
Theodore Trigone, MD/xx

FIGURE 2.8   Formatting a sample operative report.

Consultation Reports

The consultation report advises the referring physician of the status of a patient who has been referred to a specialist. Because the patient usually returns to the primary care physician, documentation of the patient's assessment, care, and progress must be sent within a short period of time. The consultation report format uses topics associated with the history and physical examination (Figure 2.9).

FORMATTING STATISTICAL DATA ON CONSULTATION REPORTS

In this textbook, consultation reports are formatted in the same manner as other medical reports, in block style using 1-inch margins, single spacing, and blank lines separating the topics, which are capitalized. Statistical data on the first page should include the patient's full name and date of birth, along with SSN or practice-specific file number, examination visit, and requesting physician. The employer's transcription guidelines may expand the requirements to suit the needs of the facility and staff members.

Statistical data for the <u>first page</u>:
Patient Name: Kleine, Ann
File Number: 186-00-6810
Date of Birth: March 7, 19xx
Examination Date: May 1, 20xx
Requesting Physician: Izzy Sertoli, MD

Statistical data for <u>continuation pages</u>:
Patient Name: Kleine, Ann
File Number: 186-00-6810
Date of Birth: March 7, 19xx
Examination Date: May 1, 20xx
Requesting Physician: Izzy Sertoli, MD
Page 2

FORMATTING SIGNATURE LINES ON CONSULTATION REPORTS

Formatting signature lines for all medical reports was discussed in "The Look of Medical Reports."

‡top margin 1" (line 6)

←→left margin 1"   CONSULTATION REPORT
                    ‡double space
                 Patient Name: McWilliams, Betty
                    ‡double space
                 File Number: 5678123
                    ‡double space
                 Date of Birth: February 2, 1949
                    ‡double space
                 Examination Date: *current date*
                    ‡double space
                 Requesting Physician: Charles P. Davis, MD
                    ‡double space
                 HISTORY OF PRESENT ILLNESS: Ms. McWilliams appears to be more stable
                 with the supportive measures already instituted. The respiratory rate is still rapid,
                 but her color is better. There are no signs of congestive heart failure.
                    ‡double space
                 IMPRESSION/RECOMMENDATIONS: Review of the clinical picture, chest
                 x-ray, and lung scan point definitely toward a pulmonary embolus. I would
                 recommend checking the blood gases, maintaining the oxygen and supportive
                 measures, and starting her on anticoagulation with heparin. She should be
                 maintained on the EKG monitor.
                    ‡double space
                 I feel she also has evidence of thrombophlebitis of the left leg and should be
                 treated with elevation and soaks to this extremity. Thank you. I will follow.
                    ‡quadruple space

                 Adam Valence MD
                 Adam Valence, MD/xx
                    ‡double space
                 c June Davis, MD

FIGURE 2.9   Formatting a sample consultation report (informal style with headings).

Business and Consultation Letters

Both business letters and consultation letters are written in formal style. The consultation report can be presented in a letter format (Figure 2.10). The business letter is usually used for nonpatient correspondence such as supply orders, collection reminders, requests for information, and making travel arrangements.

The two common formats for letters are the block format and modified block format. In the block format, all information begins at the left margin. This textbook will present and provide exercises using the block format.

All letters are keyed on 8.5 × 11-inch paper and contain most, if not all, of the following components:

- *Dateline:* The dateline is positioned approximately 2.5 inches from the top of the page to allow for a printed letterhead. The dateline includes the month (no abbreviations), date, and year.
For example: December 21, 20xx.

- *Inside address:* The inside address is comprised of the addressee's name, title, street address, city, state (two-letter state abbreviation), and zip code.
For example: Adam Valence, MD
FedDes Wellness Center
Cardiology Division, Suite 413
101 Wellness Way Drive
New York, NY 10036

- *Reference line:* The reference line is commonly used in medical correspondence. It saves time by giving the addressee a specific named reference. It also is very helpful when filing the document. The reference line is introduced by the abbreviation *Re* and followed by a colon. *Note:* The reference line is double spaced and placed above the salutation line in a business letter. However, in a consultation letter, the reference line is sometimes double spaced and placed below the salutation line. You should refer to a manual of style or your practice's office manual for the preferred placement of this line.

FedDes Wellness Center
Diagnostic Imaging Division, Suite 157
101 Wellness Way Drive
New York, NY 10036

←→left margin 1"   *current date*
                          ↕ **quadruple space**

Charles P. Davis, MD
FedDes Wellness Center
Family Practice Division, Suite 300
101 Wellness Way Drive
New York, NY 10036
        ↕ **double space**
Re: Betty McWilliams
     Date of Birth: February 2, 1949
        ↕ **double space**
Dear Dr. Davis
        ↕ **double space**
Ms. McWilliams appears to be more stable with the supportive measures already
instituted. The respiratory rate is still rapid, but her color is better. There are no
signs of congestive heart failure.
        ↕ **double space**
Review of the clinical picture, chest x-ray, and lung scan point definitely toward a
pulmonary embolus. I would recommend checking the blood gases, maintaining
the oxygen and supportive measures, and starting her on anticoagulation with
heparin. She should be maintained on the EKG monitor.
        ↕ **double space**
I feel she also has evidence of thrombophlebitis of the left leg and should be
treated with elevation and soaks to this extremity. Thank you. I will follow.
        ↕ **double space**
Sincerely yours
        ↕ **quadruple space**

Adam Valence MD
Adam Valence, MD
        ↕ **double space**
xx
        ↕ **double space**
c June Davis, MD

FIGURE 2.10   Formatting a sample consultation letter (formal style without headings).

For example: Re: Betty McWilliams
                Date of Birth: February 2, 1949
- *Salutation:* The salutation line is the greeting line for all correspondence and begins with the word *Dear*. The recipient's last name is used only in the salutation. A colon (mixed punctuation) or no punctuation mark (open punctuation) follows the name. In some geographic locations, the title *Dr.* is spelled out.
Example of <u>mixed punctuation</u>: Dear Dr. Valence:

Example of <u>open punctuation</u>: Dear Dr. Valence
- *Body:* Business and consultation may be one or more pages. Paragraphs are single spaced.

Double spacing is used to separate paragraphs.
- *Closing line:* The complimentary close is the closing line for all correspondence and begins with words as "Sincerely, "Sincerely yours," or "Very truly yours." Only the first word of the closing line begins with a capital letter. A comma (mixed punctuation) or no punctuation (open punctuation) follows the last word of the closing.

Example of <u>mixed punctuation</u>: Sincerely yours,

Example of <u>open punctuation</u>: Sincerely yours

FedDes Wellness Center
Diagnostic Imaging Division, Suite 157
101 Wellness Way Drive
New York, NY 10036

↔left margin 1"   *current date*
                    ↕**quadruple space**

Mr. James McCleary
Savory Supplied Inc.
467 Montgomery Street
New York, NY 10013
        ↕**double space**
Re: Invoice No. 7231
        ↕**double space**
Dear Mr. McCleary
        ↕**double space**
Today I received the twenty boxes of latex gloves that I ordered last week.
        ↕**double space**
On your Invoice No. 7231, which I am enclosing, I notice that you have charged
me $12.50 per box for these gloves. This charge must be a mistake. I have your
price list, which gives the price as $10.50 per box.
        ↕**double space**
Please send me a corrected invoice.
        ↕**double space**
Sincerely yours
        ↕**quadruple space**

Adam Valence MD
Adam Valence, MD
        ↕**double space**
xx
        ↕**double space**
Enclosure

FIGURE 2.11 Formatting a sample business letter.

- *Signature line:* The signature line is composed of the writer's full name and title (if applicable). A handwritten signature would appear above the typed signature line. Physicians should not use rubber stamp signature pads. *For example:*

  Potter T. Bucky MD
  Potter T. Bucky, MD
  Diagnostic Imaging Division

- *Reference initials:* The reference initials identify the typist or transcriptionist. *For example:* fmf

- *Enclosure line:* This line alerts the addressee that items are enclosed with the letter. *For example:* Enclosure

- *Copy line:* This line informs the addressee that a copy of the correspondence will be sent to someone else. Use the abbreviation *c,* followed by the complete name of the recipient. The abbreviation *cc* (carbon copy) is no longer used. *For example:* c John Smith

- *Continuation sheet:* If the letter is longer than one page, a heading must appear on the succeeding pages. The heading is placed 1 inch from the top of the page. The heading includes the addressee's name, page number, and date. Example of <u>style 1</u>:
  Adam Valence, MD   2   December 21, 20xx

  Example of <u>style 2</u>:   Adam Valence, MD
                                Page 2
                                December 21, 20xx

The placement of the letter parts in a consultation and business letter is illustrated in Figure 2.10 and Figure 2.11.

Using Templates in Medical Transcription

To increase production speed, some transcriptionists will make a template or macro of a standard chart note, history and physical examination report, and diagnostic imaging report, and then add or delete the topics as needed. Another advantage to using a template is that along with the presented outline, the page margins and tab stops are established. Because transcriptionists' pay may be based on word count or line count, it becomes even more important to use templates. Selected activities in this textbook require the creation and use of templates.

There are a variety of standard headings, topics, and subtopics found on the different medical documents. You may find certain topics are more applicable to one specialty than another and that these topics can be easily added or modified to the template.

A template is a document file that allows customized formats, content, and features. Templates can contain a host of customized features, such as text, graphics, styles, macros, abbreviations, toolbars and menu bars. Templates are usually identified with the *.dot* file extension.

To create a template, follow these simple steps:

1. Launch your word processing software package.
2. Click *File, New, Options* (WordPerfect) or *Create* (Word), and *Template.*
3. Create the template as you would any other medical document, formatting the desired page margins, tab stops, headings, and topics. For example, when creating a template for a history and physical examination report, type the headings and topics.
4. To save the template, click *File* and *Save As.*
5. Type a description to display in the template list.
6. Type a name for the template. Include the extension (*.dot*) to identify the file as a template.
7. Click *Save* and then *Close.*
8. Open the template file when needed.
9. After you finish keying in the document, save the file under a new name.

Chapter 2 Activities

Activity 1 / Understanding Medical Documents

Understanding the contents of medical documents is the first step to becoming an accomplished transcriptionist. Assess your knowledge of medical document content by completing two worksheets.

Textbook Users
Select the best answer for each question or statement concerning medical reports.

Software Users
Click on *Chapter 2, Activity 1: Understanding Medical Documents.*
Key the appropriate answer to each question or statement concerning medical reports.
A pop-up screen will reveal your score.
Follow the same process and complete *Chapter 2, Activity 2: Understanding Medical Documents.*

ACTIVITY 1 / UNDERSTANDING MEDICAL DOCUMENTS

Directions: Select the best answer for each question or statement concerning medical reports.

1. T or F   Medical reports dictated in office practices differ from those dictated in hospital settings.

2. T or F   The most common medical reports found in inpatient facilities are chart notes, consultation letters, history and physical examinations, diagnostic imaging reports, and procedure reports.

3. T or F   The medical report must include patient identification information.

4. T or F   The assessment of the Babinski reflex is found under the "HEENT" topic.

5. T or F   Most beginning medical transcriptionists obtain employment at hospitals.

6. T or F   A chart note can also be referred to as a *follow-up note.*

7. T or F   TX is the abbreviation for *treatment.*

8. T or F   Abbreviations and phrases are not used in chart notes.

9. T or F   Medical reports require the patient's statistical data to appear on the first page but not on succeeding pages.

10. T or F   The assessment of the thorax is found under the "Chest" topic.

11. T or F   The letter *O* in the acronym *SOAP* stands for *objective.*

12. T or F   HPI is the abbreviation for *history of present illness.*

13. T or F   The history and physical format of a chart note contains no variations in topics.

14. T or F   DX is the abbreviation for *diagnosis.*

15. T or F   The dictation style of a history and physical examination report contains more negative than positive statements.

16. T or F   PMH is the abbreviation for *premenstrual history.*

17. T or F   Topics found on the H&P are more numerous than on chart notes.

18. T or F   All of the patient's relevant symptoms and their duration are found under the "Past Medical History" topic.

19. T or F   The patient's information about previous illness, injuries, and surgeries are found under the "Past Medical History" topic.

20. T or F   The patient's medication history can be found under the "Past Medical History" topic.

21. T or F   The assessment of the carotid pulses is found under the "Neck" topic.

22. T or F   The assessment of the deep tendon reflexes is found under the "Neurological" topic.

23. T or F   Consultation findings can be dictated in letter and report style.

ACTIVITY 1 / UNDERSTANDING MEDICAL DOCUMENTS *continued*

24. T or F   Abbreviations are acceptable in the dateline of a letter.

25. T or F   The salutation line is the greeting line for all correspondence.

26. In a chart note, the dictated word *epicondylitis* would be found under which topic?
    (a) Subjective
    (b) Objective
    (c) Assessment
    (d) Plan

27. In a chart note, the dictated sentence, "Prescribe Motrin 200 mg q.i.d.," would be found under which topic?
    (a) Subjective
    (b) Objective
    (c) Assessment
    (d) Plan

28. The dictated sentence, "Severe pain in the second and third fingers on the right hand," would be found under which topic?
    (a) Review of systems
    (b) Chief complaint
    (c) General
    (d) Extremities

29. The dictated sentence, "BP 120/80, pulse 106 and regular, temperature 37.2° C, respirations 14/min," would be found under which topic?
    (a) General
    (b) Genitourinary
    (c) Lungs
    (d) Heart

30. The dictated sentence, "Gavida II, para II," would be found under which topic?
    (a) HEENT
    (b) Genitourinary
    (c) Lungs
    (d) Heart

31. The dictated sentence, "Clear to P&A," would be found under which topic?
    (a) HEENT
    (b) Genitourinary
    (c) Lungs
    (d) Heart

32. The dictated sentence, "No frequency, hematuria, or nocturia," would be found under which topic?
    (a) HEENT
    (b) Genitourinary
    (c) Lungs
    (d) Heart

33. The dictated sentence, "Uterus not enlarged," would be found under which topic?
    (a) HEENT
    (b) Genitourinary
    (c) Pelvic
    (d) Heart

34. The dictated sentence, "She is currently under therapy for hyperthyroidism," would be found under which topic?
    (a) HEENT
    (b) Genitourinary
    (c) Pelvic
    (d) History of present illness

35. The dictated sentence, "She has multiple filled caries," would be found under which topic?
    (a) HEENT
    (b) Genitourinary
    (c) Pelvic
    (d) History of present illness

ACTIVITY 2 / UNDERSTANDING MEDICAL DOCUMENTS

Directions: Select the best answer for each question or statement concerning medical reports.

1. T or F   The letter *S* in the acronym *SOAP* stands for *symptoms.*

2. T or F   The number of topics found on the H&P is less than found on chart notes.

3. T or F   The patient is imaged in numerous different positions called *projections.*

4. T or F   Topics in medical documents are typically keyed in all capital letters.

5. T or F   Double spacing is used to separate topics.

6. T or F   To increase production speed, transcriptionists rely on templates.

7. T or F   All imaging modalities have cross-sectional image recording capabilities.

8. T or F   Diagnostic x-rays use low levels of radiation to record images of the body on x-ray film.

9. T or F   Ultrasound uses low-frequency sound waves to image the body.

10. T or F   Computerized tomography uses a combination of radiation and computerized imaging techniques to record and display anatomy.

11. T or F   The physician always dictates the letters of the acronym *SOAP.*

12. T or F   Magnetic resonance imaging uses radiofrequency waves to generate an image.

13. T or F   Left lateral projection describes the patient with the left side closest to the film.

14. T or F   The physician specialist who typically interprets films is the radiologist.

15. T or F   The "History" topic is a relatively new topic found in diagnostic imaging reports.

16. T or F   Ultrasound uses high-frequency sound waves to image the body.

17. T or F   The H&P report is used in both outpatient and inpatient facilities.

18. T or F   Magnetic resonance images produces sharper soft-tissue images than other modalities.

19. T or F   Medical imaging reports are formatted similar to H&P reports.

20. T or F   *SNN* is the abbreviation for *social security number.*

21. T or F   The complimentary closing is the closing line for all correspondence.

22. T or F   The letter *A* in the acronym *SOAP* stands for *allergies.*

23. T or F   A template is a document file with customized format, content, and features.

24. T or F   *PX* is the abbreviation for *physical examination.*

ACTIVITY 2 / UNDERSTANDING MEDICAL DOCUMENTS *continued*

25. T or F   The assessment of the thorax is found under the "Neck" topic.

26. In a chart note, the dictated sentence, "BP 120/70, weight 150 lb, height 5 ft 7 in," would be found under which topic?
    (a) Subjective
    (b) Objective
    (c) Assessment
    (d) Plan

27. In a chart note, the dictated sentence, "Patient complains of left elbow pain for the past two weeks," would be found under which topic?
    (a) Subjective
    (b) Objective
    (c) Assessment
    (d) Plan

28. In a chart note, the dictated sentence, "Tenderness over right medial epicondyle," would be found under which topic?
    (a) Subjective
    (b) Objective
    (c) Assessment
    (d) Plan

29. The dictated sentence, "Supple without thyromegaly or lymphadenopathy," would be found under which topic?
    (a) HEENT
    (b) Genitourinary
    (c) Pelvic
    (d) Neck

30. The dictated sentence, "Clear to auscultation anteriorly and posteriorly," would be found under which topic?
    (a) Chest
    (b) Genitourinary
    (c) Pelvic
    (d) Neck

31. The dictated sentence, "Nontender, no hepatomegaly," would be found under which topic?
    (a) Chest
    (b) Neurological
    (c) Pelvic
    (d) None of the above

32. The dictated sentence, "She denies fever, chills, hematemesis, or change in bowel habits," would be found under which topic?
    (a) Lungs
    (b) Genitourinary
    (c) History of present illness
    (d) None of the above

33. Diagnostic imaging reports include which of the following?
    (a) Ultrasonography
    (b) Nuclear medicine
    (c) Magnetic resonance
    (d) All of the above

34. In a chart note, the dictated sentence, "She has vomited five times during the last 24 hours," would be found under which topic?
    (a) Subjective
    (b) Objective
    (c) Assessment
    (d) Plan

35. In a history and physical examination, the dictated sentence, "Gravida I, para I," would be found under which topic?
    (a) Physical examination
    (b) HEENT
    (c) Genitourinary
    (d) None of the above

Activities 3–5
Keyboarding Medical Documents

The ability to format medical documents is the second step to becoming an accomplished transcriptionist. You are to create a template for Figures 2.2, 2.4, and 2.6 and then type the documents.

Textbook Users
Launch your word processing package.
On the open screen, create a template for Figure 2.2.
Save the template on your student disk for further use throughout the text.
Follow the same process to create templates for Figures 2.4 and 2.6.
Using your created templates, type the model medical documents shown in Figures 2.2, 2.4, and 2.6.
Save each typed model document under a new file name on your student disk.

Software Users
Click on *Chapter 2, Activity 3: Keyboarding Medical Documents.*
Type the model medical document shown in Figure 2.2.
(Please note that you cannot use templates when using the software.)
Identify and correct all errors.
Click on *File*, then *Done*, and a pop-up window will appear.
Click on *Score Document* to reveal your score.
Click on *View Errors* to see the errors you made.
Save your work (with errors showing) on your student disk by clicking on *File*, then *Save As*.
Click on *File*, then *Exit*, to proceed.
Follow the same process to complete *Activity 4* (using Figure 2.4) and *Activity 5* (using Figure 2.6).

Check Your Progress

Let's pause a minute and see how well you have mastered the information in this chapter. This section will allow you to evaluate your understanding of medical documents and their contents.

Textbook Users
Select the best answer for each question or statement concerning medical reports.
If you score below 90%, you are recommended to redo the chapter activities.
If you score 90% or above, congratulations! You have mastered the material covered in this chapter.

Software Users
Click on *Chapter 2, Check Your Progress.*
Key the appropriate answer to each question or statement concerning medical reports.
When you are finished, click on *End Test*.
A pop-up screen will reveal your score.
If you score below 90%, you are recommended to redo the chapter activities.
If you score 90% or above, congratulations! You have mastered the material covered in this chapter.

CHECK YOUR PROGRESS

1. T or F   The left posterior oblique projection describes the patient in the supine position who is rotated 45 degrees toward the left.

2. T or F   The medical reports found in the office practice are chart notes, history and physical examinations, consultation letters, diagnostic imaging reports, and procedure reports.

3. T or F   Continuation sheets for letters and reports require a page number.

4. T or F   The assessment of the deep tendon reflexes can be found under the "Extremities" topic.

5. T or F   Creating templates is a difficult process.

6. T or F   The assessment of the Babinski reflex is found under the "Neurological" topic.

7. T or F   A computer is involved in the imaging process of almost all differing modalities.

8. T or F   *ROS* is the abbreviation for *review of systems.*

9. T or F   Many medical facilities assign the SSN as a patient identification number.

10. T or F   Medical imaging reports are formatted similar to chart notes.

11. T or F   AP projection describes a patient who is imaged in the supine position.

12. T or F   To conserve space, chart notes are formatted with wide margins.

13. T or F   Medical reports should end with a signature line.

14. T or F   The letter *P* in the acronym *SOAP* stands for *procedure.*

15. T or F   *RX* is the abbreviation for *plan.*

16. T or F   The dictation style of a history and physical examination report contains more positive than negative statements.

17. T or F   The dictation style of chart notes contains cryptic sentences.

18. T or F   The assessment of the carotid pulses is found under the "Chest" topic.

19. T or F   The reference line in a business letter appears after the salutation line.

20. T or F   The copy line appears above the enclosure line.

21. T or F   The abbreviation *TX* means *treatment.*

22. T or F   The abbreviation *DX* means *diagnosis.*

23. T or F   Topics are keyed in such a way as to indicate their importance.

24. T or F   Diagnostic x-rays use high levels of radiation to record images of the body on x-ray film.

25. T or F   The abbreviation *CC* means *chief complaint.*

CHECK YOUR PROGRESS *continued*

26. T or F   Ultrasound is the modality of choice to evaluate maternal anatomy.

27. T or F   In nuclear medicine, the energy source is a radioactive isotope that is injected into the patient's body.

28. T or F   Consultation letters are written in a formal style.

29. T or F   Pathology reports are one of the basic four medical reports.

30. T or F   Chart notes are also commonly referred to as *progress notes*.

31. T or F   There is more than one format style for a chart note.

32. T or F   The reference line is commonly used in consultation letters.

33. T or F   A chart note using the history and physical examination format may include diagnosis, laboratory, and treatment topics.

34. In a chart note, the dictated sentence, "Bobby vomited five times during the last 24 hours," would be found under which topic?
    (a) Subjective
    (b) Objective
    (c) Assessment
    (d) Plan

35. In a history and physical examination, the dictated sentence, "Gravida II, para II" would be found under which topic?
    (a) Physical examination
    (b) HEENT
    (c) Genitourinary
    (d) None of the above

36. In a history and physical examination, the dictated sentence, "BP 120/72, pulse 105 and regular, temperature 37.2° C," would be found under which topic?
    (a) Physical examination
    (b) HEENT
    (c) General
    (d) Heart

37. In a history and physical examination, the dictated sentence, "Acute appendicitis," would be found under which topic?
    (a) Physical examination
    (b) General
    (c) Impression
    (d) Plan

38. What are the basic four medical reports in medical offices?
    (a) Consultation letter, chart note, history and physical, and pathology
    (b) Chart note, history and physical, diagnostic, and consultation
    (c) Chart note, history and physical, SOAP, and consultation
    (d) Consultation letter, SOAP, history and physical, and pathology

39. What four topics are in the acronym *SOAP*?
    (a) Symptom, objective, assessment, progress
    (b) Symptom, objective, assessment, plan
    (c) Subjective, objective, assessment, plan
    (d) Subjective, objective, assessment, progress

40. In a history and physical examination, the dictated sentence, "Clear to P&A," would be found under which topic?
    (a) HEENT
    (b) General
    (c) Lungs
    (d) Heart

CHECK YOUR PROGRESS *continued*

41. In a history and physical examination, the dictated sentence, "No murmurs, gallop, or thrills," would be found under which topic?
    (a) Impression
    (b) Neurologic
    (c) Pelvis
    (d) Heart

42. In a history and physical examination, the dictated sentences, "Bowel sounds are normal. No organomegaly," would be found under which topic?
    (a) Impression
    (b) Abdomen
    (c) Rectal
    (d) None of the above

43. Medical reports are vital in which of the following?
    (a) Research
    (b) Compiling statistics
    (c) Evaluating our healthcare delivery system
    (d) All of the above

44. Reference initials must be included on which of the following?
    (a) Chart notes
    (b) History and physical examination reports
    (c) Consultation letters
    (d) All of the above

45. The findings of an EKG would be included in which of the following?
    (a) Diagnostic imaging report
    (b) Procedure report
    (c) Business letter
    (d) None of the above

46. The dictated sentence, "Discontinue use of perfumed body lotion," would be found in a chart note under which topic?
    (a) Subjective
    (b) Chief complaint
    (c) Plan
    (d) Assessment

47. The dictated sentence, "Smooth, erythematous rash over neck extending over trunk and back," would be found in a chart note under which topic?
    (a) Subjective
    (b) Objective
    (c) Assessment
    (d) None of the above

48. The dictated sentence, "My head and throat hurts," would be found in a chart note under which topic?
    (a) Subjective
    (b) Objective
    (c) Assessment
    (d) Symptom

49. The dictated sentence, "BP 120/82," would be found in a chart note under which topic?
    (a) Subjective
    (b) Objective
    (c) Assessment
    (d) Progress

50. The dictated sentence, "Acute otitis," would be found in a chart note under which topic?
    (a) Subjective
    (b) Objective
    (c) Assessment
    (d) Plan

Chapter 3

Proofreading

OBJECTIVES

At the completion of Chapter 3, you should be able to do the following:

1. Explain the importance of accurate proofreading in medical transcription.

2. Identify common errors found in medical documents.

3. Proofread from a computer screen.

4. Improve proficiency at creating and using templates in medical documents.

5. Reinforce spelling and keyboarding skills.

44

Pretest 1–3

Let's find out if you are able to type and proofread three medical documents that contain various errors by scoring 90% or better.

Textbook Users
Launch your word processing package.
Use the formatting guidelines established in Chapter 2.
On the open screen, type and proofread the medical documents shown in *Chapter 3, Pretests 1–3. Chapter 3: Pretest 1–3.*
Identify and correct all errors.
Save your work on your student disk.
After completing the Pretests, refer to the answer key.
Manually complete the error analysis chart for each document.
If you score below 90%, continue onto *Activities 1–3: Proofreading Worksheet Exercises.*
If you score 90% or above, congratulations! You have mastered the material covered in *Activities 1–3: Proofreading Worksheet Exercises.* If you wish, you can immediately move on to *Activities 4–6: Keyboarding and Proofreading Exercises.*

Software Users
Click on *Chapter 3, Pretest 1.*
On the open screen, type and proofread the medical document shown in *Pretest 1* of the textbook.
Identify and correct all errors.
Click on *File,* then *Done,* and a pop-up window will appear.
Click on *Score Document* to reveal your score.
Click on *View Errors* to see the errors you made.
Save your work (with errors showing) on your student disk by clicking on *File,* then *Save As.*
Click on *File,* then *Exit,* to proceed.
Follow the same process to complete *Chapter 3, Pretests 2* and *3.*
If you score below 90%, continue on to *Activities 1–3: Proofreading Worksheet Exercises.*
If you score 90% or above, congratulations! You have mastered the material covered in *Activities 1–3: Proofreading Worksheet Exercises.* If you wish, you can immediately move on to *Activities 4–6: Keyboarding and Proofreading Exercises.*

PRETEST 1

Directions: Type and proofread this medical document that contains multiple errors using full block, open punctuation, and all other formatting guidelines established in this textbook.

current date

Arthur Guttenberg, M.D.
5723 North Front Street
New York, New York 10010

RE: Martha Ultress
Date of birth: 6/19/59

Dear Dr. Cuttenberg

Thank you for seeing Mary for her right rotator cuff tendinitis. She has has intermittent pain of the right shoulder during the past 2 months. Over the passed few days the pain has gotten very severe. On examination she could barely abduct past thirty degrees. Thee x ray was notable for some calcific tendinitis. I injected the subacromial bursa with Steroids and obtained a rather dramatic improvement in her bursitis only to have it return again; one wk later. I started her on a physical-therapy program and would appreciate you evaluation concerning the continuing care and treatment of this patient.

Very Truly Yours,

Harry A. Medulla MD

PRETEST 2

Directions: Type and proofread this medical document that contains multiple errors using full block, open punctuation, and all other formatting guidelines established in this textbook.

CHART NOTE
Jose Ramirez
DOB: 5/23/xx
Allan Pore, MD
History of Present Illness, This fifteen year old male is seen for a follow-up on his acne. He has been using clearasil medicated astringent and oxy wash for about two months with no improvement. He is on no orale medications denies any alergies and is in good health.

Physical Esamination, Todays exam reveal inflammatory systic lesions along the jaw line and upper back. Some deep systs are palpable on the chin and over the right shoulder area.

Plan, She is to start E-Mycin two hundred fifty milligrams bid and ten percent Benzac topically hs after washing. He is to contine washing with oxy wash up to 3x a day as tolerated. He has been cautioned not to pick-at the lessions. We discussed the need to keep her hands away from his face as much as possible and to stop leaning on his elbow with his chin in his hand. It is a bad habit that only promotes the spread of bacteria and should be continued. He will be seen again in four to six weeks.

PRETEST 3

Directions: Type and proofread this medical document that contains multiple errors using full block, open punctuation, and all other formatting guidelines established in this textbook.

CHART NOTE
Linda Smithers
DOB: August 13, XX

Allan Pore, M.D

CHEIF COMPLANT Itching and a rash.

SUBJECTION The patient is a pleasant, 26 year old female who is quiet cooperative and in no a cute distress. She complains a rash that began about 2 week's ago. She's taken benadryl at bedtime with no relief. Upon questioning he admits to using a new perfumed body lotion after her shower.
OBJECTION Vital Signs: Temperature 98.6 blood pressure 136/72 weight 165 lbs height 5 3 pulse 74 respirations 22. Smooth erythematous rash over neck extending over trunk and back. On the upper extremities she has a erythematous rash extending to her wrists.
ASESMENT: Contact dermatits, secondary to allergy to perfume

PLAN:
1. Discontine use of perfumed body lotion.
2. Wash all clothing and bed linen that were exposed to the perfumed lotion.
3. Take benadryl twenty five milligrams q6hx3 days

To become an accomplished medical transcriptionist, proofreading is an essential skill. Too often, this skill is neglected in the learning process. As computer technology rapidly advances, the potential role of the medical transcriptionist may change to that of a document manager and editor. The shift to this role is foreseeable as voice technology takes a foothold in document preparation.

The Proofreading Process

The process of proofreading involves multiple steps that include reading, correcting, and revising a document to produce a final copy. Each document must be proofread word for word, figure for figure, and thought for thought.

Medical dictation can be highly technical and complex in nature, and the potential for transcribing errors is high. Certain skills are essential to good proofreading—spelling, knowledge of punctuation rules, and knowledge of grammar. You should proofread a document three times. The first step is reading for spelling, typographic errors, and repeated words. To obtain the fundamental skills in medical transcription, it is advisable to find the errors yourself and not rely on spell-check software. Professional medical transcriptionists use electronic medical dictionaries and spellers from numerous publishing companies, such as *Dorland's* and *Stedman's* electronic dictionaries, to increase their production speed and accuracy.

The second step in proofreading is looking for punctuation and grammar errors. Use your word processing software features to check your grammar.

The third step is reading the document for meaning. Does the sentence make sense within the content of the report? You need to learn the meaning of words, not just their spellings. In addition, you should be familiar with common English and medical sound-alike words. Play back the dictation at normal speed. Listen and follow along with the dictator as you check for errors. You should never change the meaning or intent of the dictation. As a novice transcriptionist, proofreading accuracy may require you to listen to the dictation more than once!

Proofreading requires excellent critical thinking skills. Paramount among these skills is the ability to know and use reference books. This process will be discussed in detail in the next chapter.

Guidelines to Proofreading Success

Do not proofread too quickly. Proofreading is not a haphazard event but a sequential, detailed process.

Proofread on the screen as you type. This is a good habit to develop now, because professional medical transcriptionists are under production deadlines. Check for typographic, spelling, grammar errors, and incongrueties in meaning or style. After correcting these errors, print a copy. It is easier to correct a document on paper than on a computer screen.

When in doubt, look it up. Use every available reference material to clarify the meaning or spelling or grammar rule in question. If your investigation is futile, leave a blank space that approximates the length of the misunderstood word. Then attach a flag (usually an adhesive note) that indicates where the problem is found within the transcription and includes its phonetic spelling. You should be able to grammatically defend every comma, period, hyphen, and so on, that you have placed on your document.

Let time elapse between when you complete the document and when you proofread it for the final time. Errors seem to stand out after a waiting period has elapsed. Another trick is to read the document backwards, which forces you to slow down and focus on each word. Also look for any illogical words and phrases, such as "The right hand was draped and prepped," when later in the report is the statement, "Sutures in left hand."

Error Analysis Chart

The error analysis chart was developed as a tool to categorize and track undetected errors. A transcription error analysis chart for each document will help you and your instructor prescribe a remedy for each error. Observing the occurrence of repeated mistakes through charting will improve your transcription skills.

The chart is divided into two major categories, Medical Language and English Language, as shown in Table 3.1. The medical language errors are weighted heavier. Because medication and allergy errors and incorrect patient identification adversely affect patient care, medical transcriptionists are heavily penalized if such errors are found during quality assurance audits. Some institutions strip in-

TABLE 3.1 ERROR ANALYSIS CHART

NAME _____   DOCUMENT NO. _____

TYPE OF ERROR	ERROR VALUE	NUMBER OF ERRORS	*TOTAL ERROR VALUE
Medical Language			
Add/omit word(s)			
Misspelled word(s)			
Incorrect date(s) or number(s)			
Total Medical Language Errors	3 ×	=	
English Language			
Add/omit word(s)			
Misspelled word(s)			
Grammatical error(s)			
Punctuation error(s)			
Total English Language Errors	1 ×	=	
Total Language Errors			

*To compute total error value, multiply the number of errors by error value (number of errors × error value = total error value).

TABLE 3.2 COMPLETED ERROR ANALYSIS CHART

NAME Mary Jones   DOCUMENT NO. 1

TYPE OF ERROR	ERROR VALUE	NUMBER OF ERRORS	*TOTAL ERROR VALUE
Medical Language			
Add/omit word(s)			
Misspelled word(s)		3	
Incorrect date(s) or number(s)			
Total Medical Language Errors	3 ×	3 =	9
English Language			
Add/omit word(s)			
Misspelled word(s)		2	
Grammatical error(s)			
Punctuation error(s)			
Total English Language Errors	1 ×	2 =	2
Total Language Errors			11

*To compute total error value, multiply the number of errors by error value (number of errors × error value = total error value).

centive pay regardless of when the error is discovered, even if it is weeks later. An error follows you!

ANALYZING ERRORS

Wrong Words. Failure to catch this type of error indicates the transcriptionist lacks knowledge of the terminology of the medical specialty. It is important that the sentence makes sense. Sound-alikes cause many of the wrong word errors. Any unfamiliar word should never be transcribed before it is referenced. Physicians may also dictate nonwords, especially by using an incorrect prefix or suffix, such as *nonavoidable* instead of *unavoidable.*

Added or Omitted Letters and Words. Errors in which letters are added or omitted at the end of a word are overlooked if the addition or omission does not make the typed word meaningless. Failure to catch this type of error indicates the copy is being read word by word rather than for meaning.

Misspelled Words. Failure to catch this type of error indicates the transcriptionist did not use the word processing software and reference materials effectively.

Grammatical Errors. Failure to catch this type of error indicates the transcriptionist did not use the word processing software effectively or failed to recognize common sentence errors, such as subject-verb agreement, pronoun-antecedent agreement, number usage, word division, and capitalization.

Punctuation Errors. Failure to catch this type of error indicates the transcriptionist did not use the word processing software effectively or failed to recognize the essential uses of all marks of punctuation. However, do not spend too much time pondering the proper placement of commas, semicolons, and so on.

Let's look at a completed error analysis chart in Table 3.2. Student Mary Jones has completed her transcript and proofread the document. Upon checking her work against the answer key, she finds three medical language errors and two English language errors. Because the errors are weighted differently, her total error value for her document is 11.

REVIEWING PROOFREADING MARKS

The standard proofreading marks that are used by copywriters to make corrections to various types of both medical and general documents are shown in Figure 3.1.

Basic English Usage Review

Because the medical language is a scientific language, you will encounter discrepancies in usage and punctuation between those rules found in an English grammar textbook and the rules found in a medical transcription manual of style. Discrepancies in usage and punctuation rules are also found in the various medical transcription manuals of style.

To avoid questions when medical transcription manuals of style contradict one another, as well as discrepancies found in your English grammar, word processing, or keyboarding textbooks, use the following guidelines for the activities presented in this textbook:

ABBREVIATIONS GUIDELINES

A-1
Abbreviations are used for all metric measurements with numbers.
Example: The kidneys each weigh 80 gm.

A-2
Abbreviations are used for chemical and mathematical compounds.
Example: Na (sodium), NaCl (sodium chloride), T4 (thyroxine)

A-3
Abbreviations are used for units of measurement. Units of measurements are typed in lowercase letters without periods and kept on the same line.
Example: A CBC showed 12,000 WBC per cc mm.

A-4
Latin abbreviations are typed in lowercase letters with periods.
Example: The medication was ordered b.i.d.

A-5
Abbreviations are used with laboratory test results that use metric measurements.
Example: The hemoglobin was 13.6 gm% and the hematocrit 42 vols%.

A-6
Abbreviations are used for many tests, such as CBC (complete blood count), RBC (red blood cell),

MARK	EXPLANATION	EXAMPLE	RESULT
(?)	is this correct?	I saw your patient Janée Brun.	I saw your patient Jean Brun.
𝒪 or —	delete	Jean Brun, your patient, came in.	Jean Brun came in.
\	delete or change	Jean Bruc, your patient, came in.	Jean Brun, your patient, came in.
#	space	JeanBrun, your patient, came in.	Jean Brun, your patient, came in.
tr ⁀	transpose	Jean Brun, your patient, came in.	Your patient, Jean Brun, came in.
◡	close up space	Jean Brun, your patient, came in.	Jean Brun, your patient, came in.
stet	let it alone	Jean Brun, your patient, came in.	Jean Brun, your patient, came in.
⊏	move left	Jean Brun, your patient, came in.	Jean Brun, your patient, came in.
⊐	move right	Jean Brun, your patient, came in.	Jean Brun, your patient, came in.
⌐	move up	Jean Brun, your patient, came in.	Jean Brun, your patient, came in.
⌎	move down	Jean Brun, your patient, came in.	Jean Brun, your patient, came in.
lc or /	use lower case	Jean Brun, your Patient, came in.	Jean Brun, your patient, came in.
𝒪	delete and close up	I can see it's surface now.	I can see its surface now.
(sp)	spell out	There were (2) patients to be...	There were two patients to be...
¶	paragraph	...high fever. On physical exam...	...high fever.
no ¶	no paragraph	On physical exam I found...	On physical exam I found a ...
⊙	change to period	...high fever, On physical exam...	...high fever. On physical exam...
∧	insert	Your patient came in to see me.	Your patient came in to see me.
⨀	insert semcolon	blood pressure: 130/90 temperature	blood pressure: 130/90; temperature
⌄	insert apostrophe	She doesnt remember asking for...	She doesn't remember asking for...
( )	insert parentheses	(1)Sterile field. (2)Suture materials.	(1) Sterile field. (2) Suture materials.
=	insert hyphen	She was seen in follow up exam on...	She was seen in the follow-up exam on...
∧	insert comma	Jean Brun your patient, came in.	Jean Brun, your patient,came in.
(:)	insert colon	Diagnosis Appendicitis	Diagnosis: Appendicitis
⌄	insert quotation marks	There has been some hurting in my...	There has been some"hurting" in my...
] [	center	]Physical Examination[	Physical Examination
cap ≡	use capital letters	Physical Examination	PHYSICAL EXAMINATION
	don't spell out	There was fifty-seven cents.	There was 57 cents.

FIGURE 3.1 Proofreader's marks. (From Fordney MT, Diehl MO; *Medical Transcription DO'S and DONT'S*, ed 2, Philadelphia, 1999, WB Saunders.)

and SGPT (serum glutamic-pyruoic transaminase). The plural is formed by adding the letter *s* only (no added commas).

Example: A CBC showed 12,000 WBC per cc mm. His WBCs were borderline high.

A-7

Abbreviations are used in vital signs.

Example: BP 136/86, pulse 76, and respirations 20/min.

A-8

Plural abbreviations are formed by adding the letter *s*, except in measurement.

Example: TMs are within normal limits, with no erythema noted.

BP 136/86, pulse 76, weight 178 lb, and height 6 ft
2 in.

A-9

The letter *x* is used to abbreviate *by* or *times* when
it precedes a number or another abbrevia-
tion.

Example: The lesion is 1.5 x 1 cm on her leg.

The patient was prescribed Augmentin 500 mg p.o.
t.i.d. x 2 weeks.

CAPITALIZATION GUIDELINES

C-1

Capitalization usually indicates importance.

C-2

Capitalize the first word of every sentence, the first-
person pronoun *I*, the first word of a salutation in a letter, any noun or title in the salutation, and the first word of a complimentary
closing.

Example: He responded to treatment.

Dear Dr. Smith

Sincerely yours

C-3

Capitalize the days of the week and months of the
year, but not the seasons.

Example: The tests were ordered for Monday,
May 8.

The doctor will attend the convention in the
spring.

C-4

Capitalize personal and business titles when they
precede a name.

Example: Dr. Smith will do the consultation.

The orthopaedic doctor will do the consultation.

C-5

Capitalize eponyms, which are surnames teamed
with a disease, instrument, or surgical procedure. The American Medical Association rec-
ommends an eponym not be used if a com-
parable medical term is available.

Example: The patient presents symptoms of Dreuw
syndrome.

The patient presents symptoms of alopecia parvi-
maculata syndrome.

C-6

Capitalize trade names, brand names of drugs,
and trademarked suture materials. Generic
drugs and suture materials are not capitalized.

Example: The patient was given Tylenol.

The patient was given acetaminophen.

C-7

Capitalize Roman numbers.

Example: The patient is a gravida II, para II, white
female.

Blood clotting is factor VI.

C-8

Capitalize the names of the genus but not the
names of the species that may follow it. The
genus also may be referred to by its first
initial only.

Example: The patient suffered with E. coli.

C-9

Capitalize acronyms.

Example: The patient was scheduled for an MRI
(magnetic resonance imaging).

C-10

Capitalize, underscore, or bold allergy information
to call attention to its importance.

Example: ALLERGIES: Codeine.

C-11

Capitalize the name of specific departments or sections in a hospital or institution.

Example: She presented to the University Hospital
Emergency Room yesterday evening.

C-12

Capital letters are used for electrocardiographic
leads, waves, and segments. Chest leads are
indicated with a *V* for the central terminal, an
Arabic number for the chest electrode, and a
letter for right or left arm or foot. The leads
are *V1* through *V6* and *aVL, aVR,* and *aVF.*
Waves include *P, Q, R, S, T,* and *U* and their
combinations.

Example: There is 1 mm of ST segment depression in
leads II, III, and aVF and approximately 1
mm of ST elevation in leads I, aVL.

NUMBER EXPRESSION GUIDELINES

Different disciplines have different rules for spelling out numbers instead of using figures (Arabic numbers). Figures are usually used in medical documents because they are easy to read and stand out in the sentence. Figures are used to express quantities accompanied by a unit of measure, patients' ages and other vital statistics, and laboratory values, as well as in any other instance when it is important to communicate the information quickly and easily.

N-1
Numbers are spelled out at the beginning of a sentence.
Example: Three tests were conducted on the woman.

N-2
Numbers one through and including ten are spelled out when they do not refer to technical items and the sentence does not contain numbers over ten.
Example: Mrs. Jones is widowed, but she resides with one of her three children.
Patient complains of right elbow pain for the past three weeks.

N-3
Figures are used to express the day of the month and the year.
Example: The patient underwent prostatic resection in 1998.

N-4
Figures are used in ranges and ratios
Example: The last time he vomited was 4-5 hours ago.
The solution was diluted 1:1000.

N-5
Figures are used for numbers over ten (unless mixing large numbers).
Example: The new clinic will cost $4.5 million.

N-6
If a sentence contains numbers under and over ten, use figures for all.
Example: She had an appendectomy done approximately 4 years ago and had her spleen removed when she was 24 years old.

N-7
Figures are used in lists.
Example: IMPRESSION:
1. Resolving cellulitis of the right side of abdomen and chest.
2. Right hip pain.
3. Questionable alcohol abuse vs. dementia.

N-8
Figures are used to indicate the patient's age, weight, height, blood pressure, pulse, and respiration.
Example: This is the second admission for this 2-year-old.
Her physical findings are: Weight 25 lb, height 21 in, BP 142/72, pulse 117, respirations 20/min.

N-9
Figures are used for temperature. Temperature also includes the degree symbol (°) or word *degree;* F (Fahrenheit); or C (Celsius).
Example: Her temperature was 98.6°F.
Her temperature was 98.6 degrees.
Her temperature was 98.6 Fahrenheit.

N-10
Figures are used to indicate the dosage and the number of times that the medicine needs to be taken.
Example: His medications include Naprosyn 30 mg t.i.d. x 2 weeks, Dyazide 40 mg q.d., and Synthroid 40 mg p.c.

N-11
Figures are used for suture materials. Suture materials range in size. The sizes can be transcribed as follows:
Using the pound symbol, figure, and zeros: #1-0, #2-0, #3-0, #4-0
Using figure and zeros: 1-0, 2-0, 3-0, 4-0
Using zeros only (no more than three zeros): 0, 00, 000
Example: The subcutaneous tissues were closed with interrupted #3-0 plain catgut.
The subcutaneous tissues were closed with interrupted 3-0 plain catgut.
The subcutaneous tissues were closed with interrupted 000 plain catgut.

N-12
Figures with capital letters refer to the vertebral column.
Example: The disk was herniated at L4-5.

N-13
Figures are used with electrocardiographic leads.
Example: The intrinsicord deflection was 0.08 sec. in V6.
Use chest leads V1 and V2.

N-14
Figures and capital letters are used to refer to the vertebral column and spinal nerves.
Example: There is left-sided point tenderness over the C5-C6 paraspinal areas.
There is evidence of degenerative arthritis involving the L3-4 and L5-S1 facet joints bilaterally.

N-15
Figures are used with the + or − symbols.
Example: Rigor mortis is 2+.

N-16
Figures are used with circular position.
Example: The incision was made at the 2 o'clock position.

N-17
Figures are used with drug names.
Example: The patient is taking Humulin 70/30.
The patient received Obetrol 20.

N-18
Figures are used when keying numbers containing decimal fractions. Convert fractions to decimals. Place a zero before a decimal that lacks a whole number.
Example: The physician injected 0.75% of medication in the arm.

Some common decimal equivalents are:
⅛ = 0.125; ¼ = 0.25; ½ = 0.5; ¾ = 0.75

N-19
Figures are used for measurements and Latin terms. No period follows metric abbreviations unless the abbreviation ends a sentence.
Example: The physician prescribed 80 mEq of potassium.

Some common metric abbreviations are:

cc	cubic centimeter
kg	kilogram
g or gm	gram
mg	milligram
mm	millimeter
mcg	microgram
mL or ml	milliliter
mEq	milliequivalent
cm	centimeter
dL	deciliter

Some common Latin abbreviations are:

a.c.	before meals
ad lib.	as needed
b.i.d.	twice a day
h.s.	at bedtime
n.p.o.	nothing by mouth
p.c.	after meals
p.o.	by mouth
p.r.n.	as needed
q.	every
q.d.	every day
q.h.	every hour
q.i.d.	four times a day
q.o.d.	every other day
q.2h.	every two hours
q.3h.	every three hours
q.4h.	every four hours
q.h.s.	every bedtime
t.i.d.	three times a day

N-20
Figures are used with symbols and abbreviations.
Example: The patient may take 1 q. 4-6 hours as needed for nausea.

N-21
Roman numerals are used to express class, cranial leads (EKG), cranial nerves, limb leads (ECG), factor (blood clotting), grade, phase, pregnancy and delivery, stage, and type.
Example: She was diagnosed with class II malignancy.
Blood clotting is factor VI.
Twenty participants completed phase II of the research project.
The patient is a gravida I, para II Hispanic female.
The patient had a stage II burn.

The patient's heart had regular rate and rhythm with a grade I/VI systolic murmur.

N-22
Roman numerals are used for standard leads and intercostal space positions.
Example: There is reciprocal depression in leads I and II.

N-23
Ordinal numbers are used to indicate order or succession.
Example: On the third day, the baby's temperature was normal.

N-24
The first through ninth ordinal numbers should be spelled out.
Example: He kicked a chair suffering an injury to the base of the fifth metatarsal of the right foot.
The best location for the liver biopsy was selected along the midaxillary line at approximately the 10th intercostal space.

N-25
Subscripts may be used in chemical elements, vitamin components, vertebral column, chest leads, heart sounds, and EEG electrodes.
Example: The medicine must be taken with a full glass of H_2O.
Use chest leads V_1-V_6.

N-26
Superscripts may be used in scientific notation.
Example: Cubic millimeters may be expressed as $mm.^3$

N-27
The use of subscripts and superscripts is often avoided because of the time involved in formatting them and the difficulty in reading them on single-spaced documents.

N-28
The plurals of numbers are formed by adding the letter *s*.
Example: The patient's blood pressure has been relatively well controlled with systolic pressures running 140-150s.

PUNCTUATION GUIDELINES
Punctuation marks such as periods, hyphens, commas, and colons signal the reader to stop, pause, hesitate, or anticipate what is to come.

Period
P-1
A period is used to end a sentence.
Example: The thyroid and adrenals are normal.

P-2
A period is used to separate a decimal fraction from the whole number.
Example: Her white blood count is 6.8.

P-3
A period is used to take the place of the word *point*.
Example: Her temperature was 98.6.

Hyphen
P-4
A hyphen is used when joining numbers or letters to form a word, phrase, or abbreviation.
Example: The woman is scheduled for a C-section.
The x-ray will be scheduled next week.
She attributes her improvement to B-12 injections.

P-5
A hyphen is used to join two or more words when used as an adjective that proceeds a noun.
Example: On follow-up examination, a lump was felt.
The patient will follow up with serology.

P-6
A hyphen is used when two or more words are viewed as a single word
Example: The well-behaved child was waiting patiently for his appointment.

P-7
A hyphen is used between numbers and *year old*.
Example: The patient was a 26-year-old female.
The patient is a 5 ½-year-old female with an ear infection.

P-8
A hyphen is used between two "like" vowels.
Example: We will see him again in three weeks for a re-evaluation.

P-9

A hyphen is used to take the place of the word *to* or *through* to identify ranges.

Example: The last time he vomited was 4-5 hours ago.

Use chest leads V1-V6.

P-10

A hyphen is used with words beginning with *ex* and *self*. Words beginning with *pre, re, post,* and *non* are generally not hyphenated. Words beginning with *co* and *vice* may or may not be hyphenated and should be researched in a dictionary.

Example: His abdomen is soft and nontender.

The patient is postinfarct dementia that requires persistent feeding through the PEG tube.

Patient returns today for a recheck of his left ankle pain.

No pretibial edema was noticed.

Comma

P-11

A comma is used to join independent clauses separated by the words, *and, but, or, for, nor, yet,* or *so*. Independent clauses can be written as individual sentences.

Example: The ducts appear to be somewhat congested, and there is marked fibrosis of the membranes of the glomeruli.

P-12

A comma is used after opening clauses that begin with the following words: *after, although, as, as if, because, before, for, how, if, once, since, so, so that, than, that, though, unless, when, whenever, where, whereas, whether,* and *while*.

Example: As noted above, she has had some nausea and vomiting.

P-13

A comma is used after an introductory element if it improves the clarity of the sentence.

Example: In cases involving diabetes, an endocrinologist may be consulted.

P-14

A comma is used to separate items in a series.

Example: The patient denies any hematuria, fever, chills, or dysuria.

P-15

A comma is used to set off nonessential or extraneous words, phrases, and clauses within a sentence.

Example: A diagnosis of a blood clot in the lung, pulmonary embolism, was made.

P-16

A comma is used to set off an appositive.

Example: The physician, Dr. Davis, recommended a follow-up visit.

P-17

A comma is used to set off words in a direct (spoken or written) address.

Example: Dr. Adams, I have your chart notes.

P-18

A comma is used to separate the parts of the date when the month, day, and year are given.

Example: She was scheduled for an appointment on Monday, May 1, 20xx.

P-19

A comma is used to separate vital signs.

Example: BP 130/80, pulse 112 and regular, and respirations 16/min.

P-20

A comma is used to separate city and state names used in the address of a letter.

Example: FedDes Wellness Center
101 Wellness Way Drive
New York, NY 10036

P-21

A comma is used to punctuate large numbers with five or more digits in units of three.

Example: One hundred boxes of latex gloves cost $1250.50.

The x-ray machine cost $25,000.

City Hospital services more than 1,250,000 patients a year.

Semicolon

P-22

A semicolon is used to join two sentences together that do not have a joining conjunction.

Example: The heart sounds were normal; there was no gallop.

P-23

A semicolon is used to separate items in a series when any of the items already contain commas.

Example: The college invited Potter T. Bucky, MD, radiologist; Benjamin Keytone, MD, urologist; Adam Valence, MD, cardiologist; and Allan Pore, MD, dermatologist, to the dedication of the new science lab.

Colon

P-24

A colon is used to set off headings, topics, and subtopics in medical documents.

Example: CHIEF COMPLAINT: Persistent right knee pain.

ALLERGIES: No known allergies.

P-25

A colon may be used in the salutation of a business letter.

Example: Dear Sir:

P-26

A colon is used in expressions of time.

Example: Her next scheduled appointment is at 2:30 p.m.

P-27

A colon is used to separate figures and ratios.

Example: The solution was diluted 1:1000.

Apostrophe

P-28

An apostrophe is used to form the possessive of singular and plural nouns.

Example: The patient's father is diabetic.

She experienced severe pain in the right side that radiated into the groin for approximately 8 hours' duration.

P-29

An apostrophe is used to form a contraction of words. However, contractions should be avoided in medical reports.

Example: It's the physician's recommendation to include regular exercise in her weight control program.

It is the physician's recommendation to include regular exercise in her weight control program.

Quotation Marks

P-30

Quotation marks are used to indicate a direct quote.

Example: The patient complained of food "getting caught in her throat when she eats."

Symbols

P-31

The diagonal (/) is used to indicate the words *per*, *to*, and *over*.

Example: BP 120/80, respirations 20/min.

His fasting blood sugar was 129 mg/dL.

P-32

The diagonal (/) is used to separate the indicators of visual acuity.

Example: Visual acuity is 20/30 both in the left and right eye but corrected 20/25.

P-33

The percent sign (%) is used with words and figures.

Example: The patient was injected with 2% Xylocaine.

Serum electrolytes were as follows: sodium 140 mg %, chloride 101 mg %, potassium 4.6 mg %, carbon dioxide 26 vols %.

P-34

The number or pound sign (#) is used to abbreviate the word *number* followed by a medical instrument or apparatus.

Example: The small piece of metal was removed with a #25 gauge needle.

P-35

The degree (°) sign is not used in describing temperature if the word *degree* is not dictated or represented on the keyboard.

Example: The findings were: Temperature 98.6, pulse 80.

There is no visible neck vein distension at 45 degrees.

Spacing Guidelines

S-1

Hit the space bar twice after end-of-sentence punctuation.

Example: The patient is a 45-year-old computer programmer.

S-2

Space twice after a colon, except when the colon is used to express time.

Example: The findings were: BP 120/80, respirations 20/min.

His next appointment was on Tuesday at 3:30 p.m.

S-3

Space once after a period that ends an abbreviation.

Example: Dr. Smith was called for the consultation.

S-4

Space once after a semicolon or comma.

Example: She denies associated fever, chills, or hematemesis.

Pupils are constricted and midline; they react to light.

S-5

No spaces are used after a period with an abbreviation.

Example: Her medication was ordered t.i.d. by her doctor.

S-6

No spaces are used before or after a hyphen, apostrophe, or diagonal.

Example: The patient was a well-developed, well-nourished 29-year-old in mild distress.

S-7

No spaces are used between symbol and referent.

Example: Her temperature was 98.6°.

Activities 1–3
Proofreading Worksheet Exercises

Being able to identify and correct errors in medical documents is a skill that qualifies an accomplished transcriptionist. Assess your proofreading skill by completing three worksheets.

Textbook Users

Proofread and correct errors in the medical documents shown in *Chapter 3, Activities 1–3: Proofreading Worksheet Exercises.*

After completing the activities, refer to the answer key.

Manually complete the error analysis chart for each document.

Software Users

Click on *Chapter 3, Activity 1: Proofreading Worksheet.*

Proofread and correct errors found in the medical document on screen.

Click on *File*, then *Done*, and a pop-up window will appear.

Click on *Score Document* to reveal your score.

Click on *View Errors* to see the errors you made.

Save your work (with errors showing) on your student disk by clicking on *File*, then *Save As*.

Click on *File*, then *Exit*, to proceed.

Follow the same process to complete *Chapter 3, Activities 2 and 3.*

ACTIVITY 1 / PROOFREADING WORKSHEET

Directions: Proofread this medical document that contains multiple errors using full block, open punctuation, and all other formatting guidelines established in this textbook.

CHART NOTE
Sue Bernshaw

Date of birth: 9/12/65

Examination Date: *current date*

SUBJECTION: Removal of sutures placed 10 days ago.

OBJECTION: The wound on the lateral expect of the left knee look well healed. The 00000 nylon sutures were removed without difficulty.

ASSESMENT: Laceration of right knee, well healed.

PLAN: Advised applying vitamin e to the area.

_____

Harry A. Medulla, MD

ACTIVITY 2 / PROOFREADING WORKSHEET

Directions: Proofread this medical document that contains multiple errors using full block, open punctuation, and all other formatting guidelines established in this textbook.

CHART NOTE
Gapolli, Rachi

Date of birth: 2/3/69

Examination Date: *current date*

SUBJECTIVE: Patient complains of sensitive pimplelike bump on right posterior shounder area.

OBJECTIVE: A mole, approximately one centimeter in diameter is visible. It is uniformly brown in color with know iregular borders. Patient denies pain or discharge all though she does amit that the area is quite sensitive for the passed 3 days.

TREATMENT: Nevus.
PLAN: I am referring the patient to a dermatologist for it's removal and biopsy.

_____

Charles Davis, MD/x

ACTIVITY 3 / PROOFREADING WORKSHEET

Directions: Proofread this medical document that contains multiple errors using full block, open punctuation, and all other formatting guidelines established in this textbook.

CHART NOTE
Heather Brodrick,

DOB: 4/19/89

Charles Davis M.D

OBJECTIVE: Patient complains of warks on palm of right-hand that is becoming bother some.

SUBJECTIVE: Examination of the of both hands reveals a three millimeter growth over the dorsum of the distal 4th and 5th matacarpal of the left hand.

PLAN: Verruca.

ASSESSEMNT: The warks were frosen with liquid Nitrogen without incident. Recheck in two three weeks if problem not resolved.

_____

Charles Davvis, MD/x

Activities 4–6
Keyboarding and Proofreading Exercises

Being able to type and proofread medical documents is a distinguishing characteristic of an accomplished transcriptionist. You are to create a template for a chart note using SOAP format, a history and physical examination report, and a consultation letter. Print a copy of the transcribed document after you have proofread and corrected any errors you have found on the computer screen. Once again, proofread the printed copy. It is not sufficient to just identify any errors, but you also must correct the errors you find. This systematic approach will reinforce your understanding of grammar, spelling, and punctuation rules.

Textbook Users
Launch your word processing package.
Use the formatting guidelines established in Chapter 2.
On the open screen, type and proofread the medical documents shown in *Chapter 3, Activities 4–6: Keyboarding and Proofreading Exercises.*
Identify and correct all errors.
Save your work on your student disk.
After completing the activities, refer to the answer key.
Manually complete the error analysis chart for each document.

Software Users
Click on *Chapter 3, Activity 4: Keyboarding and Proofreading.*
Use formatting guidelines established in Chapter 2.
On the open screen, type and proofread the medical document shown in *Activity 4* of the textbook.
Identify and correct all errors.
Click on *File*, then *Done*, and a pop-up window will appear.
Click on *Score Document* to reveal your score.
Click on *View Errors* to see the errors you made.
Save your work (with errors showing) on your student disk by clicking on *File*, then *Save As.*
Click on *File*, then *Exit*, to proceed.
Follow the same process to complete *Chapter 3, Activities 5* and *6.*

ACTIVITY 4 / KEYBOARDING AND PROOFREADING EXERCISE

Directions: Type and proofread this medical document that contains multiple errors using full block, open punctuation, and all other formatting guidelines established in this textbook.

CHART NOTE
Nathan Wright,

DOB: 11/30/83

Charles Davis, MD

SUBJECTION: Patient present with typical flu like symptoms of fever muscular ackes and pains shaking chills headacke and weakess.

OBJECTION: Bilateral tympanic membranes are clear. Orofarynx is not ejected. no neck nodes detected. Chest is clear to percussion and auscultation. Temperature 102. 3 F.

ASESMENT: Influencza.

PLAN: Symptomatic therapy. acetaminophen prn for fever and pain. Recheck in five to twelve days if not improving.

_____
Charles Davis MD

ACTIVITY 5 / KEYBOARDING AND PROOFREADING EXERCISE

Directions: Type and proofread this medical document that contains multiple errors using full block, open punctuation, and all other formatting guidelines established in this textbook.

HISTORY AND PHYSICAL EXAMINATION

Patient Name: Esther Monahan
File Number: 2348901

Date of birth: 9/10/xx

Harry A. Medulla, MD

HISTORY OF PRESENT ILLNESS: This 88 year old lady was admited to a nursing home with an intensive cellulitis involving the right side of the adbomen and the chest. She had been living at home with her daughter but had become increasingly unable to eat. He developed hyponatremia and dehydration along with the cellulitis. The cause of the cellultis was never clearly determined. It was felt ultimate to be dew too cracks in the skin from his poor condition and than a infection starting. She received six-days of ancef, was put on keflex for follow-up. There is some suggestion of possible aclohol use involved and he receive did receive same thiamine.

Past Medical History, Otherwise fairly benige. Dr. Peebody had provided most of her care.

Family History, As above

Social History, No pertinent data.

Review of System, Left hip has bothered him from a hip fracture twelve-years ago with pining.
Other medical problems include gi bleed which occured back in February. Decision was made by the daughter, and the patient not to investigate farther. Shd had been on Aspirin at the time and it was stoped. It sounds-slike a lower gi bled rather then an upper at that time.

PHYSICAL EXAMINATION:
General, Elder woman who is a little hard-of-hearing. Her vision is poor. Vital signs are good.

Heent, No jaudice. Mouth and farynx are un-remarkable.

Neck: Supply. Carotids are equal. No jvd.

Lungs, Clear to percussion and auscultation.
Heart, Regular rhythmn. No murmurs, no galops.

Breast, Atrophic.

ACTIVITY 5 / KEYBOARDING AND PROOFREADING EXERCISE *continued*

Adbomen, Soft with out organmegaly. The right side of the abdomen and chest particularly under neath the breast is still abit irritated and red but clearly much better then had been previously described.

Extemities, ankles show three plus edema up to the knee.

Impression
Resolving cellultis of the right side of adbomen and chest. Continue Antibiotics.
Ankle edema attributed to chf. Prescribed lotensin, five milligrams daily along with brief regimen of diuretics. Will monitor progress.
Right hip pain.
Questionable alcohol abuse vs. dementa.

_____

Harry A. Medulla M.D

ACTIVITY 6 / KEYBOARDING AND PROOFREADING EXERCISE

Directions: Type and proofread this medical document that contains multiple errors using full block, open punctuation, and all other formatting guidelines established in this textbook.

current date

Dr. Katherine Davis
Medical Practice Ltd.
312 Main Street
New York, New York 10010

Dear Mrs. Davis
RE: Kevin Schlitz, Date of birth: 10/29/36

I had the opportunity to examine Mr. Shlitz in my office on *(current date)* in regard too his slow healing ulceration of her right foot. The wond definitely looks emproved from the last time I saw it. He has been doing a good job at not bearingweight upon his left foot.
At this point I think it would be appropriate to place him in some extra depth shoes or boots with accommodative in soles to help reduce pressure in the four foot area. I am concerned that he has a very high potential for ulceration beneath the 3rd metatarsal dew too increased loading in this area.
I rote a prescription and sent her to an orthotic specialist four knew shoes and to have accommodative in soles constucted. I think the patient has an un-realistic out look in regards to what type of in soles will be in his shoes. He is currently waring a very rigid functional devise. This is not the appropriate devise to reduce pressure in the four foot area. The prosthesis I am recommending should help cushion, and distribute his weight evenly in the four foot area; as well as help maintain the rear foot in a better functioning position. Please feel free to contract me if you have any questions in regard to this matter.

Sincerely

Harry A. Medulla M.D

Check Your Progress, 1–3

Let's pause a minute and see how well you have mastered typing and proofreading medical documents. This section will allow you to evaluate your skills.

Textbook Users
Launch your word processing package.
Use the formatting guidelines established in Chapter 2.
On the open screen, type and proofread the medical documents shown in *Chapter 3, Check Your Progress 1–3*.
Identify and correct all errors.
Save your work on your student disk.
After completion, refer to the answer key.
Manually complete the error analysis chart for each document.
If you score below 90%, you are recommended to redo the chapter activities.
If you score 90% or above, congratulations. You have mastered the material in this chapter.

Software Users
Click on *Chapter 3, Check Your Progress 1*.
On the open screen, type and proofread the medical document shown in *Check Your Progress 1* of the textbook.
Identify and correct all errors.
Click on *File*, then *Done*, and a pop-up window will appear.
Click on *Score Document* to reveal your score.
Click on *View Errors* to see the errors you made.
Save your work (with errors showing) on your student disk by clicking on *File*, then *Save As*.
Click on *File*, then *Exit*, to proceed.
Follow the same process to complete *Chapter 3, Check Your Progress 2* and *3*.
If you score below 90%, you are recommended to redo the chapter activities.
If you score 90% or above, congratulations. You have mastered the material in this chapter.

CHECK YOUR PROGRESS 1

Directions: Type and proofread this medical document that contains multiple errors using full block, open punctuation, and all other formatting guidelines established in this textbook.

current date

Arthur Guttenberg, MD
5723 North Front Street
New York, New York 10010

RE: Martha Ultress
         Date of birth: 6/19/59
Dear Dr. Cuttenberg

Thank you for seeing Mary for her right rotator cuff tendinitis. She has has intermittent pain of the right shoulder during the past 2 months. Over the passed few days the pain has gotten very severe. On examination she could barely abduct past thirty degrees. Thee x ray was notable for some calcific tendinitis. I injected the subacromial bursa with Steroids and obtained a rather dramatic improvement in her bursitis only to have it return again; one wk later. I started her on a physical-therapy program and would appreciate you evaluation concerning the continuing care and treatment of this patient.

Very Truly Yours,

Harry A. Medulla, MD/xx

CHECK YOUR PROGRESS 2

Directions: Type and proofread this medical document that contains multiple errors using full block, open punctuation, and all other formatting guidelines established in this textbook.

CHART NOTE
Jose Ramirez
DOB: 5/23/xx
Allan Pore, MD
History of Present Illness, This fifteen year old male is seen for a follow-up on his acne. He has been using clearasil medicated astringent and oxy wash for about two months with no improvement. He is on no orale medications denies any alergies and is in good health.

Physical Esamination, Todays exam reveal inflammatory systic lesions along the jaw line and upper back. Some deep systs are palpable on the chin and over the right shoulder area.

Plan, She is to start E-Mycin two hundred fifty milligrams bid and ten percent Benzac topically hs after washing. He is to contine washing with oxy wash up to 3x a day as tolerated. He has been cautioned not to pick-at the lessions. We discussed the need to keep her hands away from his face as much as possible and to stop leaning on his elbow with his chin in his hand. It is a bad habit that only promotes the spread of bacteria and should be continued. He will be seen again in four to six weeks.

CHECK YOUR PROGRESS 3

Directions: Type and proofread this medical document that contains multiple errors using full block, open punctuation, and all other formatting guidelines established in this textbook.

CHART NOTE
Linda Smithers
DOB: August 13, XX
Examination Date: *current date*

Allan Pore, MD
CHEIF COMPLANT Itching and a rash.

SUBJECTION The patient is a pleasant, 26 year old female who is quiet cooperative and in no a cute distress. She complains a rash that began about 2 week's ago. She's taken benadryl at bedtime with no relief. Upon questioning he admits to using a new perfumed body lotion after her shower.
OBJECTION Vital Signs: Temperature 98.6 blood pressure 136/72 weight 165 lbs height 5 3 pulse 74 respirations 22. Smooth erythematous rash over neck extending over trunk and back. On the upper extremities she has a erythematous rash extending to her wrists.
ASESMENT: Contact dermatits, secondary to allergy to perfume

PLAN:
1. Discontine use of perfumed body lotion.
2. Wash all clothing and bed linen that were exposed to the perfumed lotion.
3. Take benadryl twenty five milligrams q6hx3 days

Chapter 4

Transcription Process

OBJECTIVES

At the completion of Chapter 4, you should be able to do the following:

1. Understand the transcription process.
2. Operate a transcriber.
3. Use reference materials proficiently.
4. Select the appropriate reference material with the medical term.

What's Ahead

72

Pretest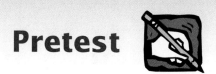

Let's find out if you can select the appropriate or best reference material to locate a particular medical term by scoring 90% or better.

Textbook Users

Select the best answer for each question or statement concerning reference materials.

Refer to the answer key for immediate feedback.

If you score below 90%, continue with *Activities 1–2: Word Search Worksheets.*

If you score 90% or above, congratulations. You have mastered the material covered in *Activities 1–2: Word Search Worksheets.* If you wish, you can immediately move on to *Activities 3–5: Transcribing Medical Documents.*

Software Users

Click on *Chapter 4, Pretest.*

Key the appropriate answer to each question or statement concerning reference materials.

When you are finished, click on *End Test.*

A pop-up screen will reveal your score.

If you score below 90%, continue with *Activities 1–2: Word Search.*

If you score 90% or above, congratulations. You have mastered the material covered in *Activities 1–2: Word Search Worksheets.* If you wish, you can immediately move on to *Activities 3–5: Transcribing Medical Document*s.

PRETEST

Directions: Select the best answer for each question or statement concerning reference materials.

1. T or F   The character is the preferred method of measuring productivity.

2. T or F   Document formats often vary from office to office.

3. T or F   Electronic medical dictionaries contain all information found in printed versions.

4. T or F   Electronic spellers can recognize homonyms.

5. T or F   Sources found on the Internet are rarely useful.

6. T or F   The telephone book can be a helpful resource material.

7. T or F   The letter *s* in the word *prednisone* has the sound of *z*.

8. T or F   The abbreviation *A&P* means *auscultation and percussion.*

9. T or F   It is not necessary to clean the earphones every day.

10. T or F   The center of the footpedal is the position to press for *play* on a three-position foot pedal.

11. T or F   A transcriber operates similar to your musical cassette player.

12. T or F   The handheld transcribers uses the $3^{15}/_{16}'' \times 2\frac{1}{2}''$ size standard cassette.

13. T or F   Medical dictation seems to have an incoherent style of dictation.

14. T or F   It is important to study and know the introductory pages in a medical dictionary.

15. T or F   Pronunciation guides are included in medical dictionaries.

16. T or F   Drug books are updated every 2 years.

17. T or F   Eponym word books often include definitions.

18. T or F   There is only one correct way to transcribe a sentence.

19. T or F   A transcriptionist does not need an English dictionary.

20. T or F   Medical words are listed in the same manner as in an English dictionary.

21. T or F   Word books include homonyms.

22. T or F   Anatomy and physiology textbooks are usually not helpful to a medical transcriptionist.

23. T or F   To a beginning transcription student, listening to medical dictation may sound like a foreign language.

24. T or F   Increasing the speed control on the transcriber will help the transcriptionist transcribe the material faster.

25. T or F   Word expanders are an example of a productivity tool.

PRETEST *continued*

Directions: Which reference book would you select to find the word or phrase to verify spelling, capitalization, punctuation, or definition?

26. Foley's catheter
    (a) eponym word book
    (b) English dictionary
    (c) manual of style
    (d) all of the above

27. *Discrete* or *discreet*
    (a) standard English dictionary
    (b) eponym word book
    (c) manual of style
    (d) a and c

28. Keflex
    (a) medical dictionary
    (b) anatomy and physiology textbook
    (c) drug book
    (d) none of the above

29. K wire
    (a) English dictionary
    (b) orthopaedic word book
    (c) abbreviation book
    (d) b and c

30. Transurethral resection
    (a) surgery word book
    (b) orthopaedic word book
    (c) cardiology word book
    (d) none of the above

31. I&D
    (a) cardiology word book
    (b) urology word book
    (c) abbreviation word book
    (d) radiology word book

32. Endoscopic retrograde cholangiopancreatography
    (a) drug book
    (b) radiology word book
    (c) eponym book
    (d) all of the above

33. *Follow up* or *follow-up*
    (a) manual of style
    (b) eponym book
    (c) neither a nor b
    (d) a and b

34. *Xanax* or *Zantac*
    (a) eponym book
    (b) surgical book
    (c) drug book
    (d) cardiology book

35. *Parental* or *parenteral*
    (a) homonym book
    (b) PDR
    (c) eponym book
    (d) all of the above

36. Tetracycline
    (a) PDR book
    (b) drug word book
    (c) neither a nor b
    (d) a and b

37. The plural form of *bronchus*
    (a) medical dictionary
    (b) surgical word book
    (c) eponym book
    (d) none of the above

PRETEST *continued*

38. Achilles heel
    (a) English dictionary
    (b) manual of style
    (c) eponym book
    (d) none of the above

39. *Fogarty catheter* or *Fogarty's catheter*
    (a) eponym book
    (b) manual of style
    (c) medical dictionary
    (d) all of the above

40. *e coli* or *E coli*
    (a) manual of style
    (b) eponym book
    (c) surgical book
    (d) cardiology book

Directions: Select the best word that completes the meaning of the sentence.

41. The patient who had _____ went to the dermatologist.
    (a) psoriasis
    (b) cirrhosis
    (c) anuresis
    (d) enuresis

42. The man was experiencing itching of the foreskin and _____.
    (a) ileum
    (b) glands
    (c) glans
    (d) ilium

43. Physical examination revealed erythematous _____ on the chin, just right of midline.
    (a) faucis
    (b) fauces
    (c) macula
    (d) macule

44. Examination of the skin revealed several _____ nodes.
    (a) shoddy
    (b) radical
    (c) shotty
    (d) radicle

45. The doctor felt the patient's _____ may be associated with his otosclerosis.
    (a) tinnitus
    (b) neither a nor c
    (c) tendinitis
    (d) all of the above

46. After the tenth day, the child finished his complete _____ of antibiotics.
    (a) coarse
    (b) course
    (c) dilation
    (d) dilution

PRETEST *continued*

47. The knife wound resulted in _____ bleeding.
    (a) serious
    (b) perfuse
    (c) cerious
    (d) serous

48. The young man was complaining of _____ after running 6 miles.
    (a) palpitation
    (b) profusion
    (c) perfusion
    (d) palpation

49. There was a green _____ discharge from the child's nose.
    (a) mucas
    (b) malleus
    (c) mucous
    (d) malleolus

50. The physician _____ many good reasons to quit smoking.
    (a) sighted
    (b) sited
    (c) cited
    (d) cighted

The transcription process is the integration of listening, keyboarding, and understanding the dictation. With practice, this skill can be mastered. Your goal is to synchronize your fingers, foot, and brain into one fluid motion. This chapter discusses various transcription tools and their usage.

Sound of Medical Transcription

Just like hearing French or German spoken, listening to medical dictation for the first time also may sound like a foreign language. Hearing all those newly learned medical terms dictated at a fast pace with liberal doses of clinical slang, abbreviations, and assorted acronyms sometimes intimidates even the most dedicated student. Fear not. We will test the waters one toe at a time! An awareness of the style and phrasing of medical dictation will make it easier to understand and therefore transcribe.

To the inexperienced ear, medical dictation seems to have an incoherent style of prose. The dictation has a terse, staccato sound, and the dictator has a tendency to abbreviate words and condense sentences wherever possible. Because of these challenges, transcriptionists must be familiar with and able to use the resources and standard reference materials of the industry. Knowledge of how to effectively use reference materials can increase productivity and perhaps your income. If your paycheck is tied to your productivity, knowing what reference materials to choose in a word search should increase your speed, which should boost your income.

Using Reference Materials

Reference materials are essential tools that increase productivity, save time, and ultimately increase production pay for the medical transcriptionist. A medical transcriptionist must have immediate access to a medical reference library that consists of a comprehensive medical dictionary, word books or spellers covering a variety of medical specialties, drug books, abbreviations and acronyms word books, style guides, textbooks in anatomy and physiology, and an English dictionary.

MEDICAL DICTIONARY

The medical dictionary holds a wealth of information to the knowledgeable transcriptionist who is familiar with its layout and understands its design. You should study the preface, front matter or introductory pages, color plates, and tables, as well as the appendices. Unlike an English dictionary, medical words are listed under the governing noun in a medical dictionary, with multiple word terms listed as subentries. Each entry includes the word origin, plural form, preferred spellings, cross reference, and pronunciation guides, as well as the definitions of the main entry and subentries. Two popular medical dictionaries are *Dorland's Illustrated Medical Dictionary* and *Stedman's Medical Dictionary*.

WORD BOOKS

Word books have become very popular in the last 15 years and are available in each major branch of medicine. Word books such as surgery, radiology, cardiology, and laboratory word books, are designed as alphabetic lists of medical words without definitions to make it easier and quicker to find the terms. These reference books often include the word division and pronunciation aids. However, because the book contains no definitions, a medical dictionary is still needed in conjunction with the word book to check the correct meaning of the term. The use of word books is invaluable, but you should be aware there is usually no indication that a word may have a sound-alike word or homophone, and word books do not differentiate between preferred and alternative acceptable spellings. This is where critical thinking and word discrimination skills come into practice. The "correct" medical term must make sense in the context of the report.

PHARMACEUTICAL REFERENCES

Drug books are specialized textbooks that contain an alphabetic indexing, a description of the drug, method of administration and dosage, classification, indications for use and contradiction, and the differentiation between generic and brand names. Leading drug books are updated monthly, quarterly, or annually. Three popular drug books are *The American Drug Book, The Physicians' Desk Reference* (PDR), and *Physicians' GenRx*. Various publishing companies offer drug handbooks whose compact size facilitates ease of handling and use, such as W.B. Saunders' *Nursing Drug Handbook* and *Merck Manual*.

ABBREVIATION BOOKS

Abbreviations and acronyms are commonly used and are found in their own word books. Eponyms, which are adjectives taken from a surname and used to describe diseases, instruments, procedures, and so on, can also be found in their own word book. The entries are listed alphabetically by the adjective, not the noun. For example, you would find *Valsalva maneuver* under *Valsalva* (adjective) rather than *maneuver* (noun). Eponym word books often include brief definitions of the terms.

STYLE GUIDES

The need for consistency, accuracy, and clarity in preparing medical documents has resulted in the development of many different, yet acceptable manuals of style that determine proper editing, punctuation, and grammar guidelines. This volatility makes learning transcription sometimes difficult. Often there is no one correct way of transcribing a sentence. The *AAMT Book of Style for Medical Transcription,* Fordney and Diehl's *Medical Transcription Guide Do's and Dont's* and the *American Medical Association Manual of Style* are all respected manuals of style in medical transcription. Yet even respected reference materials such as these differ and may offer varying guidelines among them. However, every good transcriptionist should be familiar with these reference materials and use them for guidance when technical questions arise. If the sentence is grammatically correct and the meaning of the sentence is not distorted, there are a variety of different acceptable formats.

ANATOMY AND PHYSIOLOGY TEXTBOOKS

Anatomy and physiology textbooks are useful reference materials that can help clarify your understanding of the content of the dictation. These textbooks discuss body structure and function in detail and may include disease processes and disorders.

ENGLISH DICTIONARY

Medical transcriptionists must possess a good command of the English language and know how to use an English dictionary. An English dictionary is helpful in finding synonyms, antonyms, grammar, spellings, pronunciations, hyphenations, and definitions.

ELECTRONIC REFERENCE MATERIALS

Two distinct electronic reference materials, medical dictionaries and medical spellers, are available for purchase. Both of these are compatible with popular word processing software packages.

Electronic medical dictionaries contain all information found in the printed version, but they have the ability to search the entire database of words in a matter of seconds. Many electronic dictionaries also contain a thesaurus, which displays a list of words similar to the selected term.

Electronic medical spellers have the capability of working with the existing spell checker and also can be customized to include troublesome medical terms. You should always use your speller and dictionary features of the word processing package when you proofread your transcription, but be aware of their limitations. Simply running the spell check will not determine if you have selected the correct word, only that all the words in the document are spelled correctly. Homonyms or sound-alike words are prime examples where the computer will not recognize the word as misspelled or suggest a substitute word.

Other available electronic reference software use macros, which are word processing files containing recorded commands for a series of tasks that will increase speed and accuracy by saving keystrokes and time. These packages incorporate productivity tools such as word expanders, abbreviation exploders, and other customized features. Once you become an experienced medical transcriptionist, you should investigate the benefits of such specialized software packages.

ONLINE RESOURCES

You can find a wealth of information through the Internet. By accessing the following online resources, you can obtain information on new medical techniques, procedures, drugs, transcription products, and so on. You also can enter a chat room with a medical transcriptionist. This enables you to obtain advice about word usage and spelling questions, which can be particularly helpful if you work out of your home. Using a web browser, you can key in the string, *medical transcription,* to obtain numerous entries. Box 4.1 shows some online resources that will get you started as you explore the Internet.

OTHER REFERENCE SOURCES

Other reference materials that may be helpful to you include telephone books, current magazines, the *American Hospital Association Guide to the Health Care Field,* and *American Medical Association Membership Directory.* Telephone books can be used to verify spelling of names, companies, schools, health care facilities, and so on. Keeping abreast of new developments in medicine and products can be achieved through periodical reading of current professional magazines, such as *Journal of the American Association for Medical Transcription* (JAAMT) and *Perspectives on the Medical Transcription Profession.*

Word Search

One of the most common frustrations shared by both inexperienced and experienced medical transcriptionists is the difficulty in finding a word in available reference materials. If earnest effort to decipher a word proves futile, you may be *hearing* the wrong word. Many letters sound alike or even share the same sound. Common sound-alike terms are found in Box 4.2. For example, the letter *m* may sound like an *n*. The *z* sound you hear in the prescription drug *prednisone* is actually an *s*. You may even miss the first letter of a word if you do not understand its meaning. The word *anomaly* (meaning a marked deviation from normal) may sound like *nomaly* but begins with the letter *a*. *Apposed* (being placed or fitted together) may be incorrectly transcribed as *opposed*. Be alert for medical terms that contain silent letters, such as *exogenous* or *psoas muscle.*

You should try to find a medical word under its main entry. Be aware that not all first words in a medical term are the main entry. Medical terms also may be searched under an alternative entry. Diseases may be searched under the category of syn-

dromes. Procedures may be searched under the category of operations. Occasionally, medical terms are formed by back formation, such as a noun used as a verb. Medical terms composed of a noun and adjective, such as eponyms (Valsalva maneuver, Foley catheter), are found under the noun.

In the work environment, if your own word search proves futile, you should ask a co-worker or supervisor, review pertinent medical chart, or flag the word and ask the dictator for clarification. It is not acceptable to simply guess at a word!

Transcription Process

As a novice, it is unrealistic to try to keep up with the dictating voice. This is not the time to be worried about speed. This is the time to concentrate on building your medical vocabulary. It is of no value if you have an excellent keyboarding speed but habitually omit some the dictated words or consistently misspell medical terms. As a beginning transcription student, now is the time to invest in learning the proper transcription techniques and procedures.

There is a natural tendency to want to immediately transcribe a medical document rather than take a few moments to listen to the dictation in its entirety. As a beginning medical transcriptionist, listening to the entire document for any instructions, corrections, and comments will familiarize you with its content and alert you to potentially challenging sections of the report. It is helpful to stop and start the cassette as often as desired. In this way, you will familiarize yourself with the pronunciation and the meaning of the various words. Take time now to learn the fundamentals of medical transcription. The

BOX 4.2   HOMONYMS AND SOUND-ALIKE MEDICAL TERMS

Afferent (n)—moving toward the center
Efferent (n)—moving away from the center

Anuresis (n)—retention of urine in the bladder
Enuresis (n)—involuntary discharge of urine

Atopic (adj)—displaced
Atrophic (adj)—decrease in the size of a normally developed organ or tissue
Ectopic (adj)—located away from normal position

Aural (adj)—pertaining to the ear
Oral (adj)—pertaining to the mouth

Basal (adj)—basic, elemental, forming the base
Basil (n)—herb used in cooking

Chorda (n)—a cord or sinew
Chordee (n)—downward deflection of the penis

Cirrhosis (n)—disease of the liver
Psoriasis (n)—chronic recurrent skin disease

Cite (v)—to quote
Site (n)—location in the body

Coarse (adj)—rough
Course (n)—duration of time

Colposcopy (n)—an examination of the vagina and cervix with an colposcope
Culdoscopy (n)—direct visual examination of the female viscera through an endoscope

Dilation (n)—expansion or an organ or vessel
Dilution (n)—reduction of a concentration of active substance by adding a neutral agent

Discreet (adj)—cautious
Discrete (adj)—make up of separated parts

Dysphagia (n)—difficulty in swallowing
Dysphasia (n)—difficulty in speaking

Elicit (v)—to bring out
Illicit (n)—illegal

Eminent (adj)—prominent, famous
Imminent (adj)—about to occur

Facial (adj)—pertaining to the face
Fascial (adj)—pertaining to the fibrous connective tissue

Faucial (adj)—pertaining to the passage from the mouth to the pharynx

Fissure (n)—a narrow slit or groove on the surface of an organ
Fistula (n)—any abnormal tubelike passage within body tissue

Fundal (adj)—pertaining to a fundus
Fungal (adj)—pertaining to a condition caused by a fungus

Fundus (n)—a general term for the bottom or base of an organ
Fungus (n)—a general term for a group of eukaryotic organisms

Generic (adj)—nonspecific, nontrademark
Genetic (adj)—hereditary

Glands (n)—organs or groups of cells that produce or secrete substances
Glans (n)—a small rounded mass

Hemostasis (n)—cessation of bleeding
Homeostasis (n)—maintain relative constant condition in the internal environment of the body

Ileum (n)—the last part of the small intestine between the jejunum and the large intestine
Ilium (n)—superior portion of the hipbone

In vitro (n)—in an artificial environment
In vivo (n)—within the living body

Macula (n)—spot discoloration or thickening of the skin
Macule (n)—small yellowish spot on the retina at the back of the eye

Malleolus (n)—a rounded bone on either side of the ankle
Malleus (n)—the largest of the three ossicles of the ear

Menorrhagia (n)—prolonged or heavy menses
Menorrhalgia (n)—pain during menstruation

Mucous (adj)—pertaining to or resembling mucus
Mucus (n)—sticky secretions of mucous membranes and glands

Continued

BOX 4.2 HOMONYMS AND SOUND-ALIKE MEDICAL TERMS—cont'd

Palpation (n)—examination by touching
Palpitation (n)—rapid or fluttering heartbeat

Parental (adj)—pertaining to a parent
Parenteral (adj)—pertaining to treatment other than through the digestive system

Patience (n)—ability to suppress restlessness
Patients (n)—recipients of a healthcare service
Patient's (adj)—possessive form of the noun *patient*

Perianal (adj)—pertaining to the area around the anus
Perineal (adj)—pertaining to the area between the genitals and rectum
Peroneal (adj)—pertaining to the fibula

Perfuse (v)—to force blood or other fluid to flow
Profuse (adj)—abundant
Perfusion (n)—amount of blood reaching a tissue
Profusion (n)—abundant

Pericardial (adj)—pertaining to the area surrounding the heart
Pericordial (adj)—pertaining to the area in front of the heart

Perineum (n)—pelvic floor
Peritoneum (n)—serous membrane lining the walls of the abdominal and pelvic cavities

Prostate (n)—male gland that surrounds the neck of the bladder and the urethra
Prostrate (adj)—lying face down

Radical (adj)—going to the root of the cause
Radicle (n)—one of the smallest branches of a vessel or nerve

Recession (n)—withdrawal of a part from its normal position
Resection (n)—the cutting out of a significant part of an organ or structure

Reflex (n)—involuntary reaction
Reflux (n)—an abnormal backward or return flow of a fluid

Serious (adj)—not joking
Serous (adj)—pertaining to serum

Shoddy (adj)—tattered; worn
Shotty (adj)—resembling pellets used in shotgun cartridges.

Tendinitis/tendonitis (n)—inflammation of a tendon
Tinnitus (n)—ringing in the ears

Ureteral (adj)—pertaining to the ureter
Urethral (adj)—pertaining to the urethra

Vesical (adj)—pertaining to the bladder
Vesicle (n)—blister

Viscous (adj)—sticky or glutinous
Viscus (n)—internal organ enclosed within a body cavity

more time you spend previewing the dictated material, the more productive you will be and less time will be needed for transcribing the material.

The transcription process is to listen to a block of dictation, stop, and then accurately transcribe what you have heard. Think about what you are transcribing. Concentration will avoid errors of wrong word choice and inconsistencies in text. When in doubt about a word, phonetically spell the word and either underscore or bold the word to remind you to verify its meaning. The dictator may repeat the words again, or you may get a clue from the content of the report.

The final step in the transcription process is to proofread the document, correct your errors, and print the final document. Because medical transcriptionists are compensated based on speed and accuracy, it may be helpful to retranscribe (not retype) difficult reports to strengthen your skills.

Getting Ready to Transcribe

Before you begin to transcribe, gather together all necessary materials and equipment at your desk. If you organize your materials and plan your work, you should encounter less frustration and be more productive. The following is a list of essential items along with a few troubleshooting ideas.

You will need the following:

1. A computer with a word processing software package installed. Word and WordPerfect are the two most common word processors.
2. Transcriber
3. Headset or earphones
4. Footpedal
5. Reference materials
6. Printer and paper
7. Audiocassette and/or CD-ROM with dictated material

Connecting your earphones to the transcriber allows you to hear the dictation. The three parts of an earphone are the chinband, cord, and connection tip. If you are having trouble hearing with your earphones, check the earphone connection; the tip may not be in tight contact with the transcriber. Another possible problem could be with the cord itself. It could be worn or cracked and may need replacement. Remember that earphones collect debris and wax and should be cleaned with rubbing alcohol after every use.

Make sure your footpedal is connected to the transcriber and the transcriber is turned on. The footpedal allows you to keep your hands free for keyboarding. A footpedal consists of two parts: the pedal and the cord. Pressing the footpedal causes the transcriber to play. As soon as you release the pedal with your foot, the machine stops. If you press on the footpedal and nothing happens, check the cord connection to make sure it is plugged firmly into the transcriber.

Footpedals are available in a variety of styles. With most models, the center of the footpedal is the position to press for play, fast forward is on the left, and rewind is on the right. Some footpedals have only two options: right for play and left for rewind (there is no fast forward). Check the directions of the model that you are using before you begin to transcribe a document.

THE TRANSCRIBER

The transcriber operates similar to your musical cassette player. Figure 4.1 shows the location of the common features that appear on the base control board on most portable and desktop models.

On/off or Power Button. This is used to turn the transcriber on and off and is indicated by a power light.

Index Counters. Some transcribers have an index counter that measures the length of dictation on a cassette. This is a useful tool for finding the correct dictation or scanning cassettes. As the tape is scanned, it is also rewound. At the end of every dictation series, you can hear a beep. At this point, the index counter lights up and marks where the dictation ends for each series on the control strip.

Auto Playback or Auto Rewind. The auto backspace button allows you to replay a word or a string of words. With a digital dictation system, this feature is adjusted by a computer system.

Speaker. Use the speaker button to listen aloud to dictation.

Eject. The eject button opens the cassette door. Press it to insert or remove a cassette.

Speed Control. You can increase or decrease the speed control knob while you are learning. Either extremes, whether too slow or too fast, will only distort the sound. Keep this in mind when you are trying to understand a garbled word. It sometimes helps to actually set the speed at a normal conversational level to more clearly understand the dictator.

Volume Control. You can increase or decrease the volume knob to compensate for a louder or softer voice.

Tone. This feature mutes or accentuates consonants (treble or bass) for nasal tones or a stuttering style of dictation.

Erase. This feature allows you to clear or erase tapes. Be careful with this button to make sure you do not erase dictation before it is transcribed.

Tapes. The most frequently used type of audiocassette transcriber, the standard cassette transcriber, uses $3^{15}/_{16} \times 2^{1}/_{2}$ inch standard audiocassettes. These cassettes are sold everywhere, ranging from supermarkets and department stores to music specialty stores.

The microcassette transcriber uses the smallest cassette tapes on the market today, the microsize audiocasette tapes ($2 \times 1^{1}/_{4}$ inches). The cassettes are frequently used by physicians' offices and clinics because of their easy use. The dictating machines that accommodate them are handheld, pocket-sized models. These cassettes are sold in supermarkets, department stores, and business supply stores.

The minicassette transcriber uses a cassette tape size whose use is almost exclusively limited to transcribing machines. These minisized audiotapes are $2^{3}/_{16} \times 1^{3}/_{8}$ inches. Minicassettes are frequently

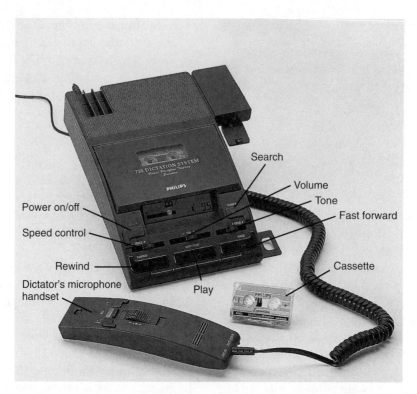

FIGURE 4.1 Features of the transcriber. (Courtesy Phillips Speech Processing, Atlanta, Georgia)

BOX 4.3 PRODUCTION FOR PAY SUMMARY	
Document No.	
Total Word Count	
Total Production Time	
Words per Minute (Total Word Count ÷ Total Production Time)	
Total Error Value (Error Analysis Chart)	
Net Production (Words per Minute − Total Error Value)	
Production for Pay ($.15 × Net Production)	

BOX 4.4 A COMPLETED PRODUCTION FOR PAY SUMMARY	
Document No.	1
Total Word Count	260
Total Production Time	13 minutes
Words per Minute (Total Word Count ÷ Total Production Time)	20
Total Error Value (Error Analysis Chart)	2
Net Production (Words per Minute − Total Error Value)	18
Production for Pay ($.15 × Net Production)	$2.70

used by physicians' offices that have been in practice for many years because the minicassette preceded the microcassette. Many physicians still continue to use minicassette dictating machines. Minicassettes are generally sold in dictation specialty stores.

Production for Pay Summary

In medical transcription the transcriber's salary is often based on the amount of work produced rather than a regular monthly salary. The character is the preferred method of measuring productivity and has been supported by several national allied health organizations. A character is any letter, number, symbol, or function key necessary for the final appearance and content of a document, including the space bar, enter key, underscore, bold, and any character contained within a macro, header, or footer. Typically, the industry calculates five characters as one word.

The following Production for Pay summary (Box 4.3) is an example of how a transcriber's wage is determined for documents transcribed in this textbook. The summary includes the total number of words produced, total production time, and total number of errors to compute the net production pay. A rate of $0.15 per minute per net production word is used as an arbitrary amount to compute wages. For example: You have just completed a 260-word history and physical examination report in 13 minutes with two uncorrected errors, as shown in Box 4.4. Completing the Production for Pay summary, you earned $2.70 for this report. If you transcribed at the same production rate for an hour, you would earn approximately $11!

Welcome to FedDes Wellness Center

Beginning in Unit 2, you will apply your knowledge of the transcription process as a medical transcriptionist employed at the fictitious medical office practice, FedDes Wellness Center. To make the process of learning transcription easier, the next sections will provide you with specific formatting guidelines, a physician's directory, and an audiocassette directory.

Document formats and dictation styles vary from office to office. Because of this diversity, each facility has its own format and guidelines for transcribing physician's dictation. In large institutions, medical committees develop their own manual of style that is followed by all transcriptionists throughout the facility. Healthcare facilities owned by hospital organizations must adhere to the Joint Commission on Accreditation of Healthcare Organizations' (JCAHO) rules and regulations regarding formatting medical reports. In single or small practices, the transcriptionist is given a little more freedom in style usage, as long as it conforms to known standards. Providing you with *FedDes Wellness Center's Transcription Guidelines* should enable you to focus on developing your transcription skills without the confusion of conflicting technical guidelines. After you understand and have practiced this formatting style, it will be easier to grasp alternative styles as you progress in your career.

FEDDES WELLNESS CENTER TRANSCRIPTION GUIDELINES

FedDes Wellness Center has its own format and guidelines for transcribing physician's dictation. All the rules and guidelines presented in Chapter 2 and Chapter 3, as well as those described in this section, apply to the medical documents that are transcribed at FedDes Wellness Center. To research extensive technical questions, FedDes Wellness Center complies with Fordney and Diehl's *Medical Transcription Guide Do's and Dont's*.

Formatting Guidelines
F-1

All medical reports and letters use the block style format with 1-inch margins. No tabulation appears in the document.

F-2

All medical reports and letters use open punctuation. No punctuation marks follow the salutation and complimentary closing.

F-3

The complete headings, topics, and subtopics are always used. These are keyed in all capital letters followed by a colon and separated by a blank line.

F-4

The dictated words *current date* must be transcribed as the actual month, day, and year.

F-5

Identifying statistical data must be included on medical reports. For consistency, FedDes Wellness Center uses the following format:

Chart notes using the SOAP or history and physical format styles require the patient's statistical data on the first and succeeding pages to include the patient's full name (surname, first name), date of birth, and examination date as shown:

For example: CHART NOTE
Patient Name: Felter, Michael
Date of Birth: July 3, 1954
Examination Date: *current date*

History and physical examination reports, diagnostic imaging reports, and procedure reports require the patient's statistical data for first and succeeding pages to include the patient's name, file number or social security number, date of birth, examination date, physician's name, and type of examination (keyed in all capital letters).

For example: HISTORY AND PHYSICAL EXAMINATION REPORT
Patient Name: Doe, Jane
File Number: 1235678
Date of Birth: January 3, 1950
Examination Date: Current date
Physician: Charles P. Davis, MD

For example: X-RAY REPORT
Patient Name: Doe, Jane
File Number: 1235678
Date of Birth: January 3, 1950
Examination Date: Current date
Ordering Physician: Izzy Sertoli, MD
Examination: MAMMOGRAM

For example: PROCEDURE REPORT
Patient Name: Doe, Jane
File Number: 1235678
Date of Birth: January 3, 1950
Examination Date: Current date
Ordering Physician: Izzy Sertoli, MD
Procedure: EXERCISE STRESS TEST

For example: CONSULTATION REPORT
Patient Name: Doe, Jane
File Number: 1235678

Date of Birth: January 3, 1950
Examination Date: Current date
Requesting Physician: Izzy Sertoli, MD

F-6

All medical documents formatted as a letter are transcribed on letterhead stationary. Shown below is an example of FedDes letterhead used with a letterhead template:

FedDes Wellness Center
Name of the Division, Suite No.
101 Wellness Way Drive
New York, NY 10036

F-7

All medical documents formatted as a letter should include a reference line above the salutation line, as shown:

Re: Betty Williams
Date of Birth: February 2, 1949
Examination: RIGHT BREAST SONOGRAM

Dear Dr. Davis

F-8

Continuation pages for all **medical reports** must include the patient's statistical data and page number beginning at the 1-inch top margin. The word *continued* appears at the left margin at the bottom of the previous page.

HISTORY AND PHYSICAL EXAMINATION
Patient Name: Doe, Jane
File Number: 1235678
Date of Birth: January 3, 1950
Examination Date: *current date*
Physician: Charles P. Davis, MD
Page 2

F-9

Continuation pages for **letters** must include a 3-line heading beginning at the 1-inch top margin, as shown:

Charles P. Davis, MD
Current date
Page 2

F-10

The signature line includes the physician's name followed by the transcriptionist's initials on the third or fourth line below the last entry, as shown:

For example: Charles P. Davis, MD/xx

Usage Guidelines

U-1

When the age of the patient is mentioned within the body of the transcript, the patient's year of birth is not provided, and the student will need to calculate this date.

U-2

All dates are spelled out in medical documents regardless of where the date appears on a report or letter.

For example: The patient was seen in this office on Monday, January 12, 20xx.

U-3

A comma separates each vital sign.

For example: BP108/72, pulse 78 and regular, respirations 20/min.

U-4

Drug allergies are underscored.

For example: Tetracycline

U-5

Drug dosages are expressed in Latin abbreviations and transcribed in lowercase letters with periods and no internal spaces.

For example: The patient was started on Keflex, 250 mg q.i.d.

U-6

Measurements of tumors are expressed in metric terms.

For example: The tumor measured 12 × 12 × 6 mm.

U-7

Fractions are converted to the decimal equivalent for metric measurements. Place a zero *before* a decimal that lacks a whole number.

For example: The lesion measured 0.75 × 1 cm.

U-8

Mixed numbers are transcribed in figures (Arabic numerals).

For example: The 5 ½-year-old female was seen at 1:00 p.m.

U-9

Numbers one through ten are spelled out when (1) they do not refer to technical items and (2) the sentence does not contain any numbers over ten.

For example: The patient will be seen again in three weeks.

U-10

Figures are used for numbers greater than ten.

For example: The diarrhea has been less frequent over the last 12 hours.

U-11

If a sentence contains numbers under and over ten, use figures for all.

For example: The patient smokes 2 packs per day and has done so for 24 years.

U-12

Figures are used in lists.

For example: IMPRESSION:

1. Acute appendicitis.
2. Rule out ureteral calculus.

U-13

Figures and the pound sign are used for suture materials.

For example: The subcutaneous tissues were closed with interrupted #3-0 plain catgut.

U-14

Figures are used for ranges and ratios.

For example: She has vomited 4-5 times in the past 24 hours, and the vomit is mostly a bile-colored, watery liquid.

U-15

Ordinal numbers are spelled out.

For example: He kicked a chair suffering an injury to the base of the fifth metatarsal of the right foot.

U-16

Do not use superscripts and subscripts when expressing electrocardiographic leads, vertebral columns, chemical compounds, and so on.

For example: The leads are V1 through V6.

We used distilled H2O.

U-17

Do not use the degree symbol when expressing temperature. The word *degree* is included only if dictated. Fahrenheit or Celsius is included only if dictated and expressed as a capital letter, *F* or *C*.

For example: Her temperature was 98.6 F.

U-18

The letter *x* is used to abbreviate *by* and *times* when it precedes a number or another abbreviation.

For example: The lesion is 1.5 x 1 cm on her leg.
The patient was prescribed
Augmentin 500 mg p.o. t.i.d. x 2 weeks.

U-19

A hyphen is used between numbers and *year old*.

For example: The patient was a 26-year-old female.

U-20

A hyphen is used between two "like" vowels.

For example: We will plan to see the patient in three weeks for re-evaluation.

U-21

A hyphen is used to take the place of the word *to* or *through* to identify ranges.

For example: The last time he vomited was 4-5 hours ago.

U-22

A diagonal (/) is used to indicate the word *per* in laboratory values and respirations or the word *over* in blood pressure.

For example: BP 120/80, pulse 106 and regular, temperature 37.2 C, respirations 14/min.

U-23

The number or pound (#) symbol is used to abbreviate the word *number* when followed by a medical instrument or apparatus.

For example: The small piece of metal was removed with a #25 gauge needle.

U-24

Specific departments or sections of a hospital such as Intensive Care are capitalized.

For example: After surgery, the patient was sent to City Hospital Intensive Care.

U-25

Nouns preceding Roman numbers are not capitalized unless the noun begins a sentence.

For example: The patient is gravida I, para I.

FEDDES WELLNESS CENTER APPROVED ABBREVIATION LIST

The following lists the approved abbreviations for the FedDes Wellness Center.

AB	abortion
ABG	arterial blood gas
ACTH	aderenocorticotropic hormone
A&D	ascending and descending
ADL	activities of daily living
AP	anteroposterior
A&P	auscultation and percussion
ARD	acute respiratory distress
ASAP	as soon as possible
ASCVD	atherosclerotic cardiovascular disease
AU	each ear, both ears
AV	atrioventricular
BCC	basal cell carcinoma
BE	barium enema
BLE	both lower extremities
BLT	bilateral tubal ligation
BM	bowel movement
BP	blood pressure
BPH	benign prostatic hypertrophy
BS	blood sugar, bowel sounds
BUN	blood urea nitrogen
BUS	Bartholin urethral and Skene (glands)
C&S	culture and sensitivity
CABG	coronary artery bypass graft surgery
CAD	coronary artery disease
CBC	complete blood count
CHF	congestive heart failure
CNS	central nervous system
COPD	chronic obstructive pulmonary disease
CPR	cardiopulmonary resuscitation
CR	cardiorespiratory
CVA	cerebrovascular accident
CT	computerized tomography
D&C	dilation and curettage
DJD	degenerative joint disease
DOE	dyspnea on exertion

DPT	diphtheria-pertussis-tetanus (vaccine)	PID	pelvic inflammatory disease
DTR	deep tendon reflexes	PIP	proximal interphalangeal
DVT	deep vein thrombosis	PSA	picryl sulfonic acid
EAC	external auditory canal	RBC	red blood cell count
ECG	electrocardiogram	RLQ	right lower quadrant
EGD	esophagogastroduodenoscopy	ROM	range of motion
EKG	electrocardiogram	RRR	regular rate and rhythm
EOM	extraocular movements	RUQ	right upper quadrant
EOMI	extraocular movements intact	SGOT	serum glutamic oxaloacetic transaminase
ER	emergency room	SOB	shortness of breath
ESR	erythrocyte sedimentation rate	STD	sexually transmitted disease
FB	foreign body	T&A	tonsillectomy and adenoidectomy
FBS	fasting blood sugar		
FUO	fever of unknown origin	TAB	therapeutic abortion
GB	gallbladder	TM	tympanic membrane
GI	gastrointestinal	TPR	temperature, pulse, respiration
GYN	gynecology/gynecologist	TUR	transurethral resection
HCG	human chorionic gonadotropin	TURP	transurethral resection of the prostate
H&P	history and physical		
HPI	history of present illness	UA	urinalysis
I&D	incision and drainage	URI	upper respiratory infection
IM	intramuscular	UTI	urinary tract infection
INR	International Normalized Ratio	UV	ultraviolet
IV	intravenous	VPB	ventricular premature beat
IVP	intravenous pyelogram	VS	vital signs
KUB	kidneys, ureters, bladder	V&T	volume and tension
L&A	light and accommodation	WBC	white blood cell count
LLQ	lower left quadrant	WF	white female
LMP	last menstrual period	WM	white male
LUQ	left upper quadrant	WNL	within normal limits
MI	myocardial infarction		
MM	mucous membrane		
NKA	no known allergies		
NOS	not otherwise specified		
NPH	no previous history		
NSAID	nonsteroidal anti-inflammatory drug		
NSR	normal sinus rhythm		
NTP	normal temperature and pressure		
OB-GYN	obstetrics and gynecology		
OS	left eye		
PA	posteroanterior		
P&A	percussion and auscultation		
PERL	pupils equal, reactive to light		
PERLA	pupils equal and reactive to light and accommodation		
PERRLA	pupils equal, round, reactive to light, and accommodation		

**FEDDES WELLNESS CENTER
PHYSICIAN'S DIRECTORY**

The center is at 101 Wellness Way Drive, New York, NY 10036. Providers on site include 24 physicians, a physical therapist, and a certified nurse practitioner.

Family Practice Division, Suite 300
Charles P. Davis, MD
J. Thomas Geiger, MD
Matthew D. Sponch, MD
Izzy Sertoli, MD
P. H. Waters, MD
Melissa A. Anconeus, MA, PT
Pamela S. Barthonin, MA, RN, CRNP

Orthopaedic Division, Suite 133
David Treppe, MD
James P. Osseous, MD
Harry A. Medulla, MD

Urology Division, Suite 237
Helen Loop, MD
Theodore Trigone, MD
Benjamin Keytone, MD

Pulmonary Medicine Division, Suite 451
Allan Bolus, MD
Neal Alveoli, MD
Douglas Sputum, MD

Gastroenterology Division, Suite 279
Gwenn Maltase, MD
Kate Cobalamin, MD
Anna Bolism, MD

Cardiology Division, Suite 413
Erica Purkinje, MD
Lucas Site, MD
A.B. Doner, MD
Adam Valence, MD

Diagnostic Imaging Division, Suite 157
William C. Roentgen, MD
Hounsfield T. Scanner, MD
Potter T. Bucky, MD
Scott E. Film, MD

Audiocassette Directory

There are six audiocassettes accompanying *Essentials of Medical Transcription,* as shown in Table 4.1.

TABLE 4.1   AUDIOCASSETTES TO ACCOMPANY *ESSENTIALS OF MEDICAL TRANSCRIPTION*

TAPE NUMBER	NUMBER OF DICTATIONS	CHAPTER NUMBER	CHAPTER TITLE
1	4T-1 through 4T-3, supplemental dictation	4	Transcription Guidelines
1, 2	5T-1 through 5T-23, supplemental dictation	5	Family Practice
2	6T-1 through 6T-19	6	Orthopaedics
3	7T-1 through 7T-15, supplemental dictation	7	Urology
4	8T-1 through 8T-12, supplemental dictation	8	Pulmonary Medicine
5, 6	9T-1 through 9T-15, supplemental dictation	9	Gastroenterology
7, 8	10T-1 through 10T-12, supplemental dictation	10	Cardiology
8	11T-1 through 11T-19, supplemental dictation	11	Diagnostic Imaging

Activities 1–2
Word Search Worksheets

Understanding the contents of medical documents is the first step to becoming an accomplished transcriptionist. Assess your knowledge of medical document content by completing two worksheets.

Textbook Users
Complete *Chapter 4, Activities 1–2: Word Search.*
Select the best answer for each question or statement concerning reference materials.
Refer to the answer key for immediate feedback.

Software Users
Click on *Chapter 4, Activity 1: Word Search.*
Key the appropriate answer to each question or statement concerning reference materials.
When you are finished, click on *End Test.*
A pop-up screen will reveal your score.
Follow the same directions for *Chapter 4, Activity 2: Word Search.*

WORD SEARCH WORKSHEET / ACTIVITY 1

Part I Directions: Which reference book would you select to find the word or phrase to verify spelling, capitalization, punctuation, or definition?

1. Parkinson's disease
   (a) eponym word book
   (b) English dictionary
   (c) manual of style
   (d) all of the above

2. *Afferent* or *efferent*
   (a) standard English dictionary
   (b) eponym word book
   (c) manual of style
   (d) a and c

3. Penicillin
   (a) medical dictionary
   (b) anatomy and physiology textbook
   (c) drug book
   (d) all of the above

4. CABG
   (a) English dictionary
   (b) cardiology word book
   (c) abbreviation book
   (d) b and c

5. Bypass graft
   (a) surgery word book
   (b) orthopaedic word book
   (c) urology word book
   (d) none of the above

6. LDH
   (a) pathology and lab word book
   (b) physician's drug reference book
   (c) abbreviation word book
   (d) a and c

7. Percutaneous transluminal angioplasty
   (a) drug book
   (b) radiology word book
   (c) eponym book
   (d) all of the above

8. *Check up* or *check-up*
   (a) manual of style
   (b) eponym book
   (c) neither a nor b
   (d) a and b

9. *Xanax* or *Zantac*
   (a) eponym book
   (b) surgical book
   (c) drug book
   (d) cardiology book

10. *Elicit* or *illicit*
    (a) homonym book
    (b) manual of style
    (c) standard English dictionary
    (d) all of the above

11. Retin-A
    (a) dermatology book
    (b) drug book
    (c) neither a nor b
    (d) a and b

12. The plural form of *vertebra*
    (a) medical dictionary
    (b) surgical word book
    (c) eponym book
    (d) none of the above

WORD SEARCH WORKSHEET / ACTIVITY 1 *continued*

13. Down's syndrome
    (a) English dictionary
    (b) manual of style
    (c) eponym book
    (d) a and c

14. *DeBakey clamp* or *DeBakey's clamp*
    (a) eponym book
    (b) manual of style
    (c) medical dictionary
    (d) all of the above

15. *H influenzae* or *h influenzae*
    (a) manual of style
    (b) orthopaedic word book
    (c) surgical book
    (d) cardiology book

16. *V1 and V2* or *V₁ or V₂*
    (a) dermatology
    (b) eponym book
    (c) manual of style
    (d) none of the above

17. McMurray's test
    (a) orthopaedic word book
    (b) eponym book
    (c) a and b
    (d) none of the above

18. San Antonio, TX
    (a) English dictionary
    (b) eponym word book
    (c) manual of style
    (d) abbreviation word book

19. Extirpative surgery
    (a) medical dictionary
    (b) English dictionary
    (c) surgical word book
    (d) all of the above

20. *Mucous* or *mucus*
    (a) medical dictionary
    (b) English dictionary
    (c) a and b
    (d) neither a nor b

Part II Directions: Select the best word that completes the meaning of the sentence.

21. The patient who had _____ went to the urologist.
    (a) psoriasis
    (b) cirrhosis
    (c) anuran
    (d) enuresis

22. His _____ was 20/40 uncorrected.
    (a) sight
    (b) cite
    (c) site
    (d) zite

23. The medical assistant tried to _____ the patient's complaints.
    (a) illicit
    (b) elicit
    (c) ilicit
    (d) ellicit

24. Mr. Thompson suffered from _____ as a result of a stroke, making eating solid foods difficult.
    (a) dysphagia
    (b) menorrhagia
    (c) dysphasia
    (d) menorrhalgia

WORD SEARCH WORKSHEET / ACTIVITY 1 *continued*

25. The physician examined the patient's breast by _____.
    (a) recession
    (b) palpation
    (c) resection
    (d) palpitation

26. The physician used eye drops for _____ in order to examine her eyes.
    (a) colposcopy
    (b) culdoscopy
    (c) dilation
    (d) dilution

27. The _____ was found to be normal on endoscopic examination.
    (a) ileum
    (b) illeum
    (c) ilium
    (d) illium

28. The boy denied any use of an _____ drug.
    (a) afferent
    (b) illicit
    (c) efferent
    (d) elicit

29. The examination revealed the man's _____ to be normal in size.
    (a) porcine
    (b) Bartholin's gland
    (c) prostate
    (d) prostrate

30. The stroke caused his left _____ weakness.
    (a) facial
    (b) faucial
    (c) fascial
    (d) fasucial

31. The patient underwent a _____ mastectomy due to cancer.
    (a) radicle
    (b) radical
    (c) vesical
    (d) visicle

32. The pharmacist asked if the _____ drug would be acceptable.
    (a) genic
    (b) genetic
    (c) generic
    (d) genetric

33. The little boy found his mother _____ on the kitchen floor.
    (a) perineum
    (b) peritoneum
    (c) prostate
    (d) prostrate

34. The pathology report concludes the lesion is a _____ cell carcinoma.
    (a) basal
    (b) chorda
    (c) basil
    (d) chordee

35. The _____ laboratory tests were normal.
    (a) patients
    (b) patience
    (c) patient's
    (d) patients'

WORD SEARCH WORKSHEET / ACTIVITY 2

Part I Directions: Which reference book would you select to find the word or phrase to verify spelling, capitalization, punctuation, or definition?

1. Hodgkin's disease
   (a) eponym word book
   (b) English dictionary
   (c) manual of style
   (d) all of the above

2. *Aural* or *oral*
   (a) standard English dictionary
   (b) eponym word book
   (c) manual of style
   (d) a and c

3. *gr3* or *grade 3*
   (a) ophthalmology word book
   (b) anatomy and physiology textbook
   (c) drug book
   (d) all of the above

4. HNP
   (a) English dictionary
   (b) orthopaedic word book
   (c) abbreviation book
   (d) b and c

5. Cholecystectomy
   (a) surgery word book
   (b) orthopaedic word book
   (c) cardiology word book
   (d) none of the above

6. BRAT
   (a) gastroenterology word book
   (b) urology word book
   (c) abbreviation word book
   (d) a and c

7. Cystoscopy
   (a) drug book
   (b) medical dictionary
   (c) eponym book
   (d) all of the above

8. *3 year old* or *3-year-old*
   (a) manual of style
   (b) eponym book
   (c) neither a nor b
   (d) a and b

9. *Xanax* or *Zantac*
   (a) eponym book
   (b) surgical book
   (c) English dictionary
   (d) cardiology book

10. *Shoddy* or *shotty*
    (a) homonym book
    (b) manual of style
    (c) eponym book
    (d) all of the above

11. Denorex
    (a) dermatology book
    (b) drug book
    (c) neither a nor b
    (d) a and b

12. The plural form of *diverticulum*
    (a) medical dictionary
    (b) surgical word book
    (c) eponym book
    (d) none of the above

WORD SEARCH WORKSHEET / ACTIVITY 2 *continued*

13. Tinel's sign
    (a) English dictionary
    (b) manual of style
    (c) eponym book
    (d) none of the above

14. *DeBakey clamp* or *DeBakey's clamp*
    (a) eponym book
    (b) English dictionary
    (c) surgical word book
    (d) a and c

15. *H influenzae* or *h influenzae*
    (a) manual of style
    (b) orthopaedic word book
    (c) surgical book
    (d) cardiology book

16. *L1 and L2* or L_1 and L_2
    (a) abbreviation book
    (b) eponym book
    (c) manual of style
    (d) none of the above

Part II Directions: Select the best word that completes the meaning of the sentence.

17. The smallest branch of a nerve is called a
    _____.
    (a) radicle
    (b) radical
    (c) vesical
    (d) visicle

18. The cutting out of a significant part of an organ or structure is referred to as
    _____.
    (a) recession
    (b) resection
    (c) reflex
    (d) reflux

19. Both great toenails were deformed by
    _____.
    (a) fundus
    (b) fungus
    (c) fungel
    (d) fundal

20. The rash was diagnosed as _____ dermatitis.
    (a) atopic
    (b) ectopic
    (c) atropic
    (d) topic

21. The child's feet were covered with small
    _____ from red ant bites.
    (a) fauces
    (b) viscous
    (c) vesicles
    (d) viscus

22. The fracture site was tender to
    _____.
    (a) palpitation
    (b) palpation
    (c) perfusion
    (d) profusion

23. It was concluded that the _____ was caused by prostatic hypertrophy.
    (a) anuresis
    (b) dysphagia
    (c) anuran
    (d) dysphasis

24. The patient was diagnosed with
    _____ of the liver.
    (a) cirrhosis
    (b) psoriasis
    (c) tinnitus
    (d) tendinitis

WORD SEARCH WORKSHEET / ACTIVITY 2 *continued*

25. The patient was diagnosed with severe gastroesophageal _____.
    (a) perfusion
    (b) reflex
    (c) profusion
    (d) reflux

26. The colonoscopy was performed all the way to the terminal _____.
    (a) ileum
    (b) illeum
    (c) ilium
    (d) illium

27. The patient was placed on _____ feedings after the gastrectomy.
    (a) perineal
    (b) parental
    (c) parenteral
    (d) peroneal

28. The _____ closure was accomplished with 0 silk after the hysterectomy.
    (a) parenteral
    (b) perineal
    (c) peroneal
    (d) parental

29. After the stroke, James had experienced _____ and was unable to communicate.
    (a) menorrhagia
    (b) dysphagia
    (c) menorrhalgia
    (d) dysphasis

30. The _____ lesions were found by examining the mouth.
    (a) oral
    (b) chorda
    (c) aural
    (d) chordee

31. The _____ physician had an article published in the *Journal of the American Medical Association.*
    (a) imminent
    (b) iminent
    (c) eminent
    (d) emminent

32. The Tay Saks disease was found to be _____.
    (a) generic
    (b) genetic
    (c) discreet
    (d) discrete

33. The examination of the female viscera through an endoscope is _____.
    (a) culdoscopy
    (b) resection
    (c) colposopy
    (d) recession

34. Mr. James complained of _____ and pain in his ears.
    (a) tinnitus
    (b) tendenitis
    (c) tendinitis
    (d) tinitus

35. Her favorite recipe included _____.
    (a) glands
    (b) glans
    (c) basal
    (d) basil

Activities 3–5
Transcribing Medical Documents

Being able to format and transcribe medical documents is the second step to becoming an accomplished transcriptionist. If you have not already done so, create a template for a chart note, history and physical examination, and letter and then transcribe the documents *4T-1*, *4T-2*, and *4T-3* from your audiocassette.

Textbook Users

Insert the appropriate audiocassette in your transcribing machine and find dictation *4T-1*.

Launch your word processing package.

On the open screen, transcribe and proofread dictation *4T-1*.

Identify and correct all errors.

Refer to the FedDes Physician Directory for the letterhead information.

Use the formatting guidelines established in Chapter 2.

Save your work on your student disk.

Follow the same process for dictations *4T-2* and *4T-3*.

After completing the transcriptions, refer to the answer keys.

Manually complete the error analysis chart for each document.

Manually complete the production for pay summary chart for each report.

Software Users

Click on *Chapter 4, Activity 3: Transcribing Medical Documents*.

Insert the appropriate audiocassette in your transcribing machine and find dictation *4T-1*.

(Please note that you cannot use templates when using the software.)

Refer to the FedDes Physician Directory for the letterhead information.

Click on *Start Watch*, then transcribe and proofread dictation *4T-1*.

Identify and correct all errors.

When you are finished, click on *Done*, then *Score Document*. A pop-up window will display your production for pay.

Click on *Display Error Analysis* to reveal your score.

Click on *View Errors* to see the errors you made.

Save your work (with errors showing) on your student disk by clicking on *File*, then *Save As*.

Follow the same process for dictations *4T-2* and *4T-3*.

Check Your Progress

Let's pause a minute and see how well you have mastered the information in this chapter. This section will allow you to evaluate your understanding of reference materials and how to use them.

Textbook Users

Select the best answer for each question or statement concerning reference materials.

Refer to the answer key for immediate feedback.

If you score below 90%, you are recommended to redo the chapter activities.

If you score 90% or above, congratulations. You have mastered the material covered in this chapter.

Software Users

Click on *Chapter 4, Check Your Progress.*

Key the appropriate answer to each question or statement concerning reference materials.

When you are finished, click on *End Test.*

A pop-up screen will reveal your score.

If you score below 90%, you are recommended to redo the chapter activities.

If you score 90% or above, congratulations. You have mastered the material covered in this chapter.

CHECK YOUR PROGRESS

Directions: Select the best answer for each question and/or statement.

1. T or F Ten characters are calculated to equal one word for production pay.

2. T or F Hospital medical committees may develop their own manuals of style as long as they comply with accreditation standards.

3. T or F Electronic medical spellers can be customized to include a transcriptionist's troublesome words.

4. T or F A *macro* is a word processing file that contains recorded commands for a series of tasks.

5. T or F Productivity tools increase speed and accuracy.

6. T or F Resources found on the Internet are helpful to a transcriptionist.

7. T or F Medical terms are sometimes formed by back formation.

8. T or F It is acceptable practice to guess at dictated words when all efforts have been exhausted to find the terms.

9. T or F When transcribing, it is realistic to keep pace with the dictating voice.

10. T or F As a beginning student transcriptionist, you must be concerned with speed.

11. T or F Before transcribing, it is important to have all materials available.

12. T or F Fast forward is located on the right side of a footpedal.

13. T or F Very fast or very slow speed extremes will distort the sound.

14. T or F The transcriptionist's salary is never based on a regular monthly salary.

15. T or F The transcription process is the integration of listening, keyboarding, and understanding the dictation.

16. T or F An awareness of the style and phrasing of medical dictation will make it easier to understand the dictation.

17. T or F Word books are only available in certain specialties.

18. T or F *Eponyms* are adjectives taken from a surname and used to describe a term.

19. T or F All manuals of style offer the same guidelines.

20. T or F Knowledge of how to effectively use reference materials will not increase productivity.

21. T or F Medical words are not listed in the same manner as words found in an English dictionary.

22. T or F Pronunciation guides are not included in word books.

23. T or F Drug books are updated annually.

24. T or F Electronic reference materials include dictionaries and spellers.

25. T or F Document formats remain consistent between medical facilities.

CHECK YOUR PROGRESS *continued*

Directions: Which reference book would you select to find the word or phrase to verify spelling, capitalization, punctuation, or definition?

26. TUR
    (a) urology word book
    (b) surgical word book
    (c) abbreviation word book
    (d) all of the above

27. *5 year old* or *5-year-old*
    (a) manual of style
    (b) eponym word book
    (c) English dictionary
    (d) none of the above

28. Foley's catheter
    (a) eponym word book
    (b) English dictionary
    (c) PDR
    (d) all of the above

29. *Patient* or *patience*
    (a) standard English dictionary
    (b) eponym word book
    (c) manual of style
    (d) a and c

30. Keflex
    (a) English dictionary
    (b) anatomy and physiology textbook
    (c) drug word book
    (d) all of the above

31. K wire
    (a) English dictionary
    (b) orthopaedic word book
    (c) abbreviation book
    (d) b and c

32. Circumcision
    (a) surgery word book
    (b) orthopaedic word book
    (c) cardiology word book
    (d) none of the above

33. D&C
    (a) drug book
    (b) cardiology word book
    (c) abbreviation word book
    (d) radiology word book

34. Diphenhydramine
    (a) drug book
    (b) laboratory word book
    (c) eponym book
    (d) all of the above

35. *X ray* or *x-ray*
    (a) manual of style
    (b) eponym book
    (c) neither a nor b
    (d) a and b

36. *Xanax* or *Zantac*
    (a) eponym book
    (b) surgical book
    (c) drug book
    (d) cardiology book

37. *Basal* or *basil*
    (a) homonym book
    (b) drug word book
    (c) eponym book
    (d) all of the above

CHECK YOUR PROGRESS *continued*

38. Cortaid
    (a) dermatology book
    (b) drug book
    (c) neither a nor b
    (d) a and b

39. The plural form of *thorax*
    (a) medical dictionary
    (b) surgical word book
    (c) eponym book
    (d) none of the above

Directions: Select the best word that completes the meaning of the sentence.

40. There was radiographic evidence of
    _____ esophagitis noted in the distal
    end of the patient's esophagus.
    (a) reflux
    (b) atopic
    (c) reflex
    (d) atropic

41. She denies the use of _____ drugs,
    including marijuana.
    (a) elicit
    (b) ellicit
    (c) illicit
    (d) ilicit

42. The physician diagnosed the patient with a
    distal left _____ obstruction due to
    calculi.
    (a) ureteral
    (b) urethral
    (c) atopic
    (d) atropic

43. The patient presented with pruritic red lesions
    on his face, leading the physician to a
    diagnosis of _____ dermatitis.
    (a) ureteral
    (b) urethral
    (c) atopic
    (d) atropic

44. The surgeon performed a deep
    _____ of the capsule throughout the
    bladder.
    (a) resection
    (b) dilation
    (c) recession
    (d) dilution

45. The radiologist's impression was that there
    was a soft tissue mass in the terminal.
    (a) ilium
    (b) ileum
    (c) illium
    (d) illeum

46. The patient's chronic liver diseases include
    _____.
    (a) cirrhosis
    (b) hemostasis
    (c) psoriasis
    (d) homeostasis

47. The neurologic examination showed the
    patient's _____ to be equal and
    active.
    (a) reflux
    (b) atopic
    (c) reflex
    (d) atropic

CHECK YOUR PROGRESS *continued*

48. The patient experienced cardiac
    _____ after strenuous exercise.
    (a) palpitation
    (b) palptation
    (c) palpation
    (d) palpaition

49. Mary complained of a burning and itching
    sensation of the _____ following an
    episiotomy.
    (a) parineal
    (b) peroneal
    (c) peritoneum
    (d) perineum

50. The surgeon removed the placenta from the
    incision side superior to the anterior
    _____.
    (a) fundal
    (b) fundus
    (c) fungal
    (d) fungus

UNIT II

Medical Transcription

Putting it all together

Chapter 5

Office Medical Transcription from the Family Practice

OBJECTIVES

At the completion of Chapter 5, you should be able to do the following:

1. Match medical terms associated with the family practice specialty with their definitions.

2. Spell medical terms associated with the family practice specialty with their definitions.

3. Transcribe medical terms in sentence structure.

4. Proofread, edit, and correct medical documents associated with the family practice specialty containing various errors.

5. Transcribe and proofread authentic medical documents associated with the family practice specialty.

What's Ahead

107

The Family Practice Rotation

The FedDes Wellness Center has five family practitioners, one physical therapist, one registered nurse, and one physician assistant on staff. The medical team treats the general health of the individual and the family. Pediatric patients are seen for well-baby care and infectious diseases, such as sore throats, gastroenteritis, and croup. Young adults are seen for infectious diseases and acute injuries, such as sprains, minor lacerations, and nondisplaced fractures. Older adults are seen for both acute and chronic illnesses, such as arthritis, hypertension, and diabetes mellitus. Patients requiring critical care are co-managed with the appropriate specialist. In addition, obstetrics and gynecology are incorporated into the practice, including pelvic examinations and Papanicolaou (Pap) smears.

The physicians in FedDes family practice division perform and interpret routine x-rays in their offices. More sophisticated imaging such as MRI, CT scans, and nuclear medicine studies are referred to an outside facility and interpreted by a radiologist.

In this unit, you assume the role of a medical transcriptionist employed at FedDes Wellness Center. **Please follow the guidelines pertaining to capitalization, numbers, punctuation, abbreviations, measurements, symbols, and use of templates to create medical reports at FedDes Wellness Center. Review of this material can be found in Unit 1.** A list of the patient's name and the type of report, as well as associated transcription tips, is included in this chapter.

You will work with the textbook, CD-ROM, and accompanying audiocassettes. Your mastery of family-practice transcription is assessed through worksheets, timed transcription exercises, the error analysis chart, and the production for pay summary.

All answer keys are found in the textbook and CD-ROM, providing immediate feedback. After transcribing a report, you will proofread your work and correct any errors. Then you will compare your proofread work against a master transcript, categorize all errors, and tabulate the errors on the error analysis chart. The production for pay summary correlates your production to the FedDes Wellness Center pay scale, which is based on industry compensation standards. The scale is also linked to your grade. This system allows you to assess your mastery of transcription skills in a real-world scenario.

Pretest

Let's find out if you can define and spell selected terminology and drugs of the family practice specialty that are included in this chapter by scoring 90% or better.

Textbook Users

Select the correctly spelled term that matches its definition.

Refer to the answer key for immediate feedback.

If you score below 90%, continue on to *Activities 1–3.*

If you score 90% or above, congratulations. You have mastered the material covered in Part I. If you wish, you can immediately move on to Part II.

Software Users

Click on *Chapter 1, Part I, Pretest.*

Key the correctly spelled term that matches its definition. When you are finished, click on *End Test.*

A pop-up screen will reveal your score.

If you score below 90%, continue on to *Activities 1–3.*

If you score 90% or above, congratulations. You have mastered the material covered in Part I. If you wish, you can immediately move on to Part II.

PART I / PRETEST

Directions: Select the correctly spelled term that matches its definition.

1. A benign tumor in which cells are derived
   from glandular epithelium:
   (a) adenoma
   (b) adnema
   (c) adnexa
   (d) adenxa

2. A body defense method to prevent movement
   of an injured part:
   (a) flank
   (b) garding
   (c) guarding
   (d) flenk

3. A generic name for a broad-spectrum
   antibiotic that is active against a wide range
   of gram-positive and gram-negative
   organisms:
   (a) doxycycline
   (b) pencillin
   (c) doxycyclene
   (d) penicillin

4. An abnormal sound heard on chest
   auscultation due to an obstructed airway:
   (a) nystagmus
   (b) rhonchus
   (c) rhinchus
   (d) nystigmus

5. An abnormal rhythm of the heart:
   (a) distal
   (b) destal
   (c) galop
   (d) gallop

6. An enlargement of the thyroid gland:
   (a) hepatosplenomegaly
   (b) hepatosplenmegaly
   (c) thyromegaly
   (d) thyramegaly

7. A knot or knotlike mass:
   (a) ganglion
   (b) ganlion
   (c) fundus
   (d) fundes

8. A reversed response occurring upon
   withdrawal of a stimulus:
   (a) reband
   (b) rebound
   (c) evert
   (d) revert

9. A small nodular, tumor, or growth:
   (a) buccal
   (b) bucca
   (c) granuloma
   (d) granduloma

10. A small soft structure hanging from the free
    edge of the soft palate:
    (a) vulva
    (b) vuvla
    (c) ulvula
    (d) uvula

11. A small tongue-shaped anatomic structure:
    (a) lingula
    (b) linula
    (c) lamina
    (d) lamena

12. A sound or murmur heard on auscultation:
    (a) bruit
    (b) palpitation
    (c) brut
    (d) palpation

PART I / PRETEST *continued*

13. A spasm of the orbicular muscle of the eyelid:
    (a) hyperlipidemia
    (b) blepharospasm
    (c) blefarospasm
    (d) hyprelipidemia

14. A thin, flat layer:
    (a) lingula
    (b) linula
    (c) lamina
    (d) lamena

15. A widespread genus of gram-negative, nonmotile bacteria:
    (a) chlamydia
    (b) chlamidia
    (c) myalgia
    (d) mialgia

16. A generic name for an opthalmic antibiotic:
    (a) sulfactamide
    (b) sulfacetamide
    (c) meclizine
    (d) meslicine

17. An antiemetic especially effective for control of nausea and vomiting of motion sickness:
    (a) sulfactamide
    (b) sulfacetamide
    (c) meclizine
    (d) meslicine

18. An endoscope for examining the peritoneal cavity:
    (a) laparoscope
    (b) sigmoidoscope
    (c) laproscopy
    (d) sigmoidscopy

19. An incision of the tympanic membrane:
    (a) adenopathy
    (b) adinopathy
    (c) myringomy
    (d) myringotomy

20. An opening, mouth, or bone:
    (a) oss
    (b) os
    (c) pruritus ani
    (d) puritus anis

21. An unusually rapid, strong, or irregular heartbeat:
    (a) bruit
    (b) palpitation
    (c) brut
    (d) palpation

22. Any of a large group of natural or semisynthetic antibacterial antibiotics:
    (a) doxycycline
    (b) pencillin
    (c) doxycyclene
    (d) penicillin

23. Around the rectum:
    (a) perrectal
    (b) prerectal
    (c) perirectal
    (d) parirectal

24. Coughing and spitting of blood:
    (a) sputum
    (b) sputim
    (c) hemoptysis
    (d) hemotysis

25. External genital organs in the female:
    (a) vulva
    (b) vuvla
    (c) ulvula
    (d) uvula

26. Accumulation of excess fluid in the tissues:
    (a) exdate
    (b) exudate
    (c) edema
    (d) exdema

PART I / PRETEST continued

27. Inflammation of the mucous membrane of the nose:
    (a) mucosa
    (b) mucos
    (c) rhinitis
    (d) rinitis

28. Intense chronic itching in the anal region:
    (a) pruritus ani
    (b) puritus ani
    (c) rhinitis
    (d) rinitis

29. Involuntary rapid rhythmic movement of the eyeball:
    (a) nystagmus
    (b) rhonchus
    (c) rhinchus
    (d) nystigmus

30. Labored or difficult breathing:
    (a) dysuria
    (b) dyspnia
    (c) rhinchus
    (d) dysurea

31. Muscular pain:
    (a) chlamydia
    (b) chlamidia
    (c) myalgia
    (d) mialgia

32. Painful menstruation:
    (a) amenorrhea
    (b) dysmenorrhea
    (c) amenorhea
    (d) dysmenorhea

33. Painful or difficult urination:
    (a) dysuria
    (b) dyspnia
    (c) dyspnea
    (d) dysurea

34. Pertains to the cheek:
    (a) buccal
    (b) bucca
    (c) granuloma
    (d) granduloma

35. Redness of the skin:
    (a) orthopnea
    (b) erthema
    (c) orthopea
    (d) erythema

36. Resembles a polyp:
    (a) polypiod
    (b) polypod
    (c) polypoid
    (d) polypide

37. The ability to breathe easily only in an upright position:
    (a) orthopnea
    (b) erthema
    (c) orthopea
    (d) erythema

38. The absence of the menses:
    (a) amenorrhea
    (b) dysmenorrhea
    (c) amenorhea
    (d) dysmenorhea

39. The accumulation of excess fluid in the tissues of the body:
    (a) exdate
    (b) exadate
    (c) edema
    (d) exdema

40. The state of lying down:
    (a) fundus
    (b) fundes
    (c) decubitus
    (d) decubitis

PART I / PRETEST *continued*

41. The bluish discoloration of the skin and mucous membranes due to excessive concentration of reduced hemoglobin in the blood:
    (a) labyrinthitis
    (b) cayonsis
    (c) labrinthitis
    (d) cyanosis

42. The bottom or base of an organ:
    (a) fundus
    (b) fundes
    (c) decubitus
    (d) decubitis

43. The elevated concentrations of any or all of the lipids in the plasma:
    (a) hyperlipidemia
    (b) blepharospasm
    (c) blefarospasm
    (d) hyprelipidemia

44. The enlargement of the glands, especially the lymph nodes:
    (a) hepatosplenomegaly
    (b) adenopathy
    (c) hepasplenomegaly
    (d) adenompathy

45. The enlargement of the liver and spleen:
    (a) hepatosplenomegaly
    (b) adenopathy
    (c) hepasplenomegaly
    (d) adenompathy

46. The escape of fluid from blood vessels because of rupture or seepage, usually into a body cavity:
    (a) aeration
    (b) effusion
    (c) eration
    (d) efusion

47. The examination of the interior of the sigmoid colon:
    (a) laparoscope
    (b) sigmoidscope
    (c) laproscopy
    (d) sigmoidoscopy

48. The exchange of carbon dioxide for oxygen by the blood in the lungs:
    (a) aeration
    (b) effusion
    (c) eration
    (d) efusion

49. The farthest from any point of reference; remote:
    (a) disal
    (b) galop
    (c) distal
    (d) gallop

50. The increase in the severity of a disease or its symptoms:
    (a) exaceration
    (b) exacerbation
    (c) auscultation
    (d) auscutation

51. The inflammation of the internal ear, otitis interna:
    (a) labyrinthitis
    (b) rhinitis
    (c) labrinthitis
    (d) rinitis

52. The act of listening for sounds produced within the body with the unaided ear or with a stethoscope:
    (a) palpitation
    (b) palpation
    (c) auscultation
    (d) auscutation

53. The mucous membrane:
    (a) mucoso
    (b) mucosa
    (c) mucousa
    (d) mucus

54. The mucous secretion from the lungs, bronchi, and trachea that is ejected through the mouth:
    (a) sputum
    (b) sputim
    (c) hemoptysis
    (d) hemotysis

55. The side of the body between the ribs and ilium:
    (a) flank
    (b) fundus
    (c) flanke
    (d) fundes

56. The tissues or body parts that are near or next to one another:
    (a) adenoma
    (b) adnema
    (c) adnexa
    (d) adenxa

57. To turn inside out:
    (a) reband
    (b) rebound
    (c) evert
    (d) revert

58. Used as an expectorant:
    (a) terpin
    (b) trepin
    (c) meclizine
    (d) mecilizine

59. Using both hands:
    (a) bimanaul
    (b) bimanual
    (c) bymanaul
    (d) bymanual

60. A blister:
    (a) blib
    (b) bleb
    (c) bleib
    (d) beb

61. Trade name for a corticosteroid:
    (a) Ortho-Tri-Cyclen
    (b) Ortho-Tri-Cyclin
    (c) Triamcinolone
    (d) Triamcinoline

62. Trade name for a corticosteroid for bronchial asthma; pocket inhaler:
    (a) Vancenase
    (b) Vancinase
    (c) Phenergan
    (d) Phenergin

63. Trade name for a powder for extraocular muscle injection:
    (a) Botex
    (b) Botox
    (c) Skelaxin
    (d) Skelaxen

64. Trade name for a preparation of amoxicillin, an antibiotic:
    (a) Co-Polymer
    (b) Copolymer
    (c) Amoxil
    (d) Amosil

65. Trade name for a preparation of amoxicillin, an antibiotic:
    (a) Klonopin
    (b) Augmenten
    (c) Klonpin
    (d) Augmentin

PART I / PRETEST *continued*

66. Trade name for a selective estrogen receptor modulator for the prevention of postmenopausal osteoporosis:
    (a) Paxil
    (b) Pasil
    (c) Evista
    (d) Evixta

67. Trade name for an antidepressant:
    (a) Paxil
    (b) Pasil
    (c) Evista
    (d) Evixta

68. Trade name for a skeletal muscle relaxant:
    (a) Botex
    (b) Botox
    (c) Skelaxin
    (d) Skelaxen

69. Trade name for a topical antibiotic:
    (a) Proctocreem HC
    (b) Proctocream HC
    (c) Neosporen
    (d) Neosporin

70. Trade name for a triphasic oral contraceptive:
    (a) Ortho-Tri-Cyclen
    (b) Ortho-Tri Cyclin
    (c) Triamcinolone
    (d) Triamcinoline

71. Trade name for an anticonvulsant:
    (a) Klonopin
    (b) Augmenten
    (c) Klonpin
    (d) Augmentin

72. Trade name for an antihistamine, antiemetic:
    (a) Vancenase
    (b) Vancinase
    (c) Phenergan
    (d) Phenergin

73. Trade name for an antihyperlipidemic that reduces cholesterol synthesis:
    (a) Lipitir
    (b) Lipitor
    (c) Lo-Ovral
    (d) Lo-Oral

74. Trade name for an oral contraceptive:
    (a) Lipitir
    (b) Lipitor
    (c) Lo-Ovral
    (d) Lo-Oral

75. Trade name for fixed combination preparation analgesic and antipyretic:
    (a) Darvoset
    (b) Darvocet
    (c) Melantonox
    (d) Melantonex

76. Trade name for preparations of lidocaine; classified as an antiarrhythmic, anesthetic:
    (a) Xylocaine
    (b) Ophthetic
    (c) Xylociane
    (d) Ophetic

77. Trade name for proparacaine hydrochloride, eye drops:
    (a) Xylocaine
    (b) Ophthetic
    (c) Xylociane
    (d) Ophetic

78. Trade name for topical corticosteroidal anti-inflammatory used as anorectal cream:
    (a) Proctocreem HC
    (b) Proctocream HC
    (c) Neosporen
    (d) Neosporin

PART I / PRETEST *continued*

79. Trade name for one of the immune modulating drugs:
    (a) Co-Polymer
    (b) Amoxil
    (c) Copolymer
    (d) Amosil

80. Trade name for a calcium channel blocker, antihypertensive:
    (a) Naprosyn
    (b) Naporsyn
    (c) Norvasc
    (d) Norvasic

81. Trade name for an antibiotic:
    (a) Claritin
    (b) Clariten
    (c) Baixin
    (d) Biaxin

82. Trade name for an antiplatelet agent:
    (a) Presantine
    (b) Persantine
    (c) Prilosec
    (d) Prelosec

83. Trade name for a drug used for the prevention of NSAID-induced gastric ulcers:
    (a) Cytotec
    (b) Cytotic
    (c) Ditropan
    (d) Ditropen

84. Trade name for an urinary antispasmodic.
    (a) Cytotec
    (b) Cytotic
    (c) Ditropan
    (d) Ditropen

85. Trade name for an antibiotic:
    (a) Indocen
    (b) Indocin
    (c) E.E.A.
    (d) E.E.S.

86. Trade name for a nonsteroidal anti-inflammatory drug, NSAID:
    (a) Indocen
    (b) Indocin
    (c) E.E.A.
    (d) E.E.S.

87. Trade name for a gastric acid secretion inhibitor:
    (a) Presantine
    (b) Persantine
    (c) Prilosec
    (d) Prelosec

88. Trade name for a sleep aid:
    (a) Melatonex
    (b) Melatonix
    (c) Darvocet
    (d) Darvocit

89. Trade name for a nonsedating antihistamine:
    (a) Claritin
    (b) Clariten
    (c) Baixin
    (d) Biaxin

90. Trade name for a calcium channel blocker, antihypertensive:
    (a) Naprosyn
    (b) Naporsyn
    (c) Norvasc
    (d) Norvasic

Part I / Activity 1
Keyboarding Medical Terms and Definitions

Let's learn to spell and define selected terminology and drugs of the family practice specialty that are included in this chapter. Keyboarding these terms is an innovative and fun way to improve your skills.

Textbook Users:
Launch your word processing package.
On the open screen, read and type each word and its definition as shown below.
Save your work on your student disk.

1. Adenoma (ad-ah-no-mah) is a benign tumor in which cells are derived from glandular epithelium.
2. Adenopathy (ad-ah-nop-ah-the) is the enlargement of the glands, especially the lymph nodes.
3. Adnexa (ad-nek-sa) are the tissues or body parts that are near or next to one another.
4. Aeration (aer-a-shun) is the exchange of carbon dioxide for oxygen by the blood in the lungs.
5. Amenorrhea (ah-men-o-re-ah) is the absence of the menses.
6. Auscultation (aw-skul-ta-shun) is the act of listening for sounds produced within the body with the unaided ear or with a stethoscope.
7. Bimanual (bi-man-u-al) is the use of both hands.
8. Bleb (bleb) is a bulla or blister.
9. Blepharospasm (blef-ah-ro-spazm) is a spasm of the orbicular muscle of the eyelid.
10. Bruit (broo-e) is a sound or murmur heard on auscultation.
11. Buccal (buk-al) pertains to the cheek.
12. Chlamydia (klah-mid-e-ah) is a widespread genus of gram-negative, nonmotile bacteria.
13. Cyanosis (si-ah-no-sis) is the bluish discoloration of the skin and mucous membranes due to excessive concentration of reduced hemoglobin in the blood.
14. Decubitus (de-ku-bi-tus) pertains to lying down.
15. Distal (dis-tal) is the farthest from any point of reference; remote.
16. Doxycycline (dok-se-si-klen) is a generic name for a broad-spectrum antibiotic that is active against a wide range of gram-positive and gram-negative organisms.
17. Dysmenorrhea (dis-men-o-re-ah) is painful menstruation.
18. Dyspnea (disp-ne-ah) is labored or difficult breathing.
19. Dysuria (dis-u-re-ah) is painful or difficult urination.
20. Edema (ed-ah-mah) is the accumulation of excess fluid in the tissues of the body.
21. Effusion (e-fu-zhun) is the escape of fluid from blood vessels because of rupture or seepage, usually into a body cavity.
22. Erythema (er-i-the-mah) is redness of the skin.
23. Evert (e-vert) is to turn inside out.
24. Exacerbation (eg-zas-er-ba-shun) is the increase in the severity of a disease or its symptoms.
25. Exudate (eks-u-date) is an accumulation of fluid in the tissues.
26. Flank (flangk) is the side of the body between the ribs and ilium.
27. Fundus (fun-dus) is the bottom or base of an organ.
28. Gallop (gal-op) is an abnormal rhythm of the heart.
29. Ganglion (gang-gle-on) is a knot or knotlike mass.
30. Granuloma (gran-u-lo-mah) is a small nodular, tumor, or growth.
31. Guarding (gahr-ding) is a body defense method to prevent movement of an injured part.
32. Hemoptysis (he-mop-ti-sis) is the coughing and spitting of blood.
33. Hepatosplenomegaly (hep-a-to-sple-no-meg-ah-le) is the enlargement of the liver and spleen.
34. Hyperlipidemia (hi-per-lip-i-de-me-ah) is the elevated concentration of any or all lipids in the plasma.
35. Labyrinthitis (lab-i-rin-thi-tis) is the inflammation of the internal ear, otitis interna.

36. Lamina (<u>lam</u>-i-nah) is a thin, flat layer.
37. Laparoscope (<u>lap</u>-ah-ro-skop) is an endoscope for examining the peritoneal cavity.
38. Lingula (<u>ling</u>-gu-lah) is a small tongue-shaped anatomic structure.
39. Meclizine (<u>mek</u>-li-zeen) is an antiemetic especially effective for control of nausea and vomiting for motion sickness.
40. Mucosa (mu-<u>ko</u>-sah) is the mucous membrane.
41. Myalgia (mi-<u>al</u>-je-ah) is muscular pain.
42. Myringotomy (mir-in-<u>got</u>-o-me) is an incision of the tympanic membrane.
43. Nystagmus (ni-<u>stag</u>-mus) is an involuntary rapid rhythmic movement of the eyeball.
44. Orthopnea (or-thop-<u>ne</u>-ah) is the ability to breathe easily only in an upright position.
45. Os (os) is an opening, mouth, or bone.
46. Palpitation (pal-pi-<u>ta</u>-shun) is an unusually rapid, strong, or irregular heartbeat.
47. Penicillin (pen-i-<u>sil</u>-in) is a natural or semisynthetic antibacterial antibiotic.
48. Perirectal (per-i-<u>rek</u>-tal) is around the rectum.
49. Polypoid (<u>pol</u>-y-poid) resembles a polyp.
50. Pruritus ani (proo-<u>ri</u>-tus a-ni) is the intense chronic itching in the anal region.
51. Rebound (<u>re</u>-bownd) is a reversed response occurring upon withdrawal of a stimulus.
52. Rhinitis (ri-<u>ni</u>-tis) is the inflammation of the mucous membrane of the nose.
53. Rhonchus (<u>rong</u>-kus) is an abnormal sound heard on chest auscultation due to an obstructed airway.
54. Sigmoidoscopy (sig-moi-<u>dos</u>-ko-pe) is the examination of the interior of the sigmoid colon.
55. Sputum (<u>spu</u>-tum) is the mucous secretion from the lungs, bronchi, and trachea that is ejected through the mouth.
56. Sulfacetamide (sul-fah-<u>set</u>-ah-mid) is a generic name for an ophthalmic antibiotic.
57. Terpin (<u>ter</u>-pin) is used as an expectorant.
58. Thyromegaly (thi-ro-<u>meg</u>-ah-le) is enlargement of the thyroid gland.
59. Uvula (<u>u</u>-vu-lah) is a small soft structure hanging from the free edge of the soft palate.
60. Vulva (<u>vul</u>-vah) is the external genital organs in the female.
61. Amoxil (ah-<u>moks</u>-il) is the trade name for a preparation of amoxicillin, an antibiotic.
62. Augmentin (awg-men-tin) is the trade name for a preparation of amoxicillin, an antibiotic.
63. Biaxin (bi-<u>ak</u>-sin) is the trade name for an antibiotic.
64. Botox (bo-<u>toks</u>) is the trade name for a powder for extraocular muscle injection.
65. Claritin (<u>klar</u>-i-tin) is the trade name for a nonsedating antihistamine.
66. Copolymer (ko-<u>pol</u>-i-mer) is the trade name for any of the group of immune-modulating drugs.
67. Cytotec (<u>si</u>-to-tek) is the trade name for a drug used for the prevention of NSAID-induced gastric ulcers.
68. Darvocet (<u>dar</u>-vo-set) is the trade name for fixed combination preparation analgesic and antipyretic.
69. Ditropan (<u>di</u>-tro-pan) is the trade name for an urinary antispasmodic.
70. E.E.S. (e-e-s) is the trade name for an antibiotic.
71. Evista (e-<u>vis</u>-ta) is the trade name for a selective estrogen receptor modulator (SERM) for the prevention of postmenopausal osteoporosis.
72. Indocin (<u>in</u>-do-sin) is the trade name for a nonsteroidal anti-inflammatory drug, NSAID.
73. Klonopin (<u>klon</u>-o-pin) is the trade name for an anticonvulsant.
74. Lipitor (<u>lip</u>-i-tor) is the trade name for an antihyperlipidemic, which reduces cholesterol synthesis.
75. Lo-Ovral (lo-<u>ov</u>-ral) is the trade name for an oral contraceptive.
76. Melatonex (mel-a-<u>to</u>-neks) is the trade name for a sleep aid.
77. Naprosyn (<u>na</u>-pro-sin) is the trade name for a nonsteroidal anti-inflammatory drug, NSAID.
78. Neosporin (ne-o-<u>spor</u>-in) is the trade name for a topical antibiotic.
79. Norvasc (<u>nor</u>-vask) is the trade name for a calcium channel blocker, antihypertensive.
80. Ophthetic (of-<u>the</u>-tik) is the trade name for proparacaine hydrochloride, eye drops.
81. Ortho-Tri-Cyclen (<u>or</u>-tho-tri-<u>si</u>-klen) is the trade name for a triphasic oral contraceptive.
82. Paxil (<u>paks</u>-il) is the trade name for an antidepressant.
83. Persantine (<u>per</u>-san-tin) is the trade name for an antiplatelet agent.
84. Phenergan (<u>fen</u>-er-gan) is the trade name for an antihistamine, antiemetic.
85. Prilosec (<u>pril</u>-o-sek) is the trade name for a gastric acid secretion inhibitor.

86. Proctocream HC (<u>prok</u>-to-kreem) is the trade name for topical corticosteroidal anti-inflammatory used as anorectal cream.
87. Skelaxin (skel-aks-in) is the trade name for a skeletal muscle relaxant.
88. Triamcinolone (tri-am-<u>sin</u>-o-lon) is the trade name for a corticosteroid.

89. Vancenase (van-kan-az) is the trade name for a corticosteroid for bronchial asthma, pocketin-haler.
90. Xylocaine (<u>zi</u>-lo-kan) is the trade name for preparations of lidocaine and is classified as an antiarrhythmic, anesthetic.

Part I / Activity 2
Spelling Medical Terms

Do you remember back in school when you had to write each spelling word 10 times? Because you had to physically write each word, your mind and body were focused on the assignment and the method worked! Let's follow this successful method by reinforcing the spelling of selected terms and drugs found in the family practice specialty through keyboarding drills.

Textbook Users
Launch your word processing package.
On the open screen, read, mentally spell, and type each word in its sequence.
Save your work on your student disk.

1. adenoma adenopathy adnexa adenoma adenopathy adnexa adenoma adenopathy adnexa
2. aeration amenorrhea auscultation aeration amenorrhea auscultation aeration amenorrhea
3. bimanual blepharospasm bruit bleb blepharospasm bruit bimanual blepharospasm bleb
4. buccal chlamydia buccal chlamydia buccal chlamydia buccal chlamydia buccal chlamydia
5. cyanosis decubitus distal cyanosis decubitus distal cyanosis decubitus distal cyanosis distal
6. dysmenorrhea dyspnea dysuria dysmenorrhea dyspnea dysuria dysmenorrhea dyspnea
7. edema effusion erythema edema effusion erythema edema effusion erythema edema effusion
8. evert exacerbation exudate evert exacerbation exudate evert exacerbation exudate evert
9. flank fundus gallop flank fundus gallop flank fundus gallop flank fundus gallop flank fundus
10. ganglion granuloma guarding ganglion granuloma guarding ganglion granuloma guarding
11. hemoptysis hepatosplenomegaly hemoptysis hepatosplenomegaly hemoptysis

12. hyperlipidemia labyrinthitis hyperlipidemia labyrinthitis hyperlipidemia labyrinthitis
13. lamina laparoscope lingula lamina laparoscope lingula lamina laparoscope lingula lamina
14. mucosa myalgia myringotomy mucosa myalgia myringotomy mucosa myalgia myringotomy
15. nystagmus orthopnea os nystagmus orthopnea os nystagmus orthopnea os nystagmus os
16. palpitation penicillin perirectal palpitation penicillin perirectal palpitation penicillin perirectal
17. polypoid pruritus ani rebound polypoid pruritus ani rebound polypoid pruritus ani rebound
18. rhinitis rhonchus sigmoidoscopy rhinitis rhonchus sigmoidoscopy rhinitis rhonchus rhinitis
19. sputum terpin thyromegaly sputum terpin thyromegaly sputum terpin thyromegaly sputum
20. doxycycline uvula vulva doxycycline uvula vulva doxycycline uvula vulva doxycycline
21. doxycycline meclizine doxycycline meclizine doxycycline meclizine doxycycline meclizine

22. Amoxil Augmentin Botox Amoxil Augmentin Botox Amoxil Augmentin Botox Amoxil
23. Biaxin Claritin Copolymer Biaxin Claritin Copolymer Biaxin Claritin Copolymer Biaxin
24. Cytotec Ditropan E.E.S. Cytotec Ditropan E.E.S. Cytotec Ditropan E.E.S. Cytotec Ditropan
25. Darvocet Evista Klonopin Darvocet Evista Klonopin Darvocet Evista Klonopin Darvocet
26. Indocin Melatonex Naprosyn Indocin Melatonex Naprosyn Indocin Melatonex Naprosyn

27. Lipitor Lo-Ovral Neosporin Lipitor Lo-Ovral Neosporin Lipitor Lo-Ovral Neosporin Lipitor
28. Norvasc Persantine Prilosec Norvasc Persantine Prilosec Norvasc Persantine Prilosec
29. Ophthetic Ortho-Tri-Cyclen Paxil Ophthetic Ortho-Tri-Cyclen Paxil Ophthetic Ortho-Tri-Cyclen
30. Phenergan Proctocream HC Skelaxin Phenergan Proctocream HC Skelaxin Phenergan
31. Triamcinolone Vancenase Xylocaine Triamcinolone Vancenase Xylocaine Triamcinolone

Part I / Activity 3
Transcribing Medical Sentences

Now you are ready to make the transition from keyboarding medical terms, a visual process, to transcribing medical terms, an aural process. You will use audiocassette tapes rather than printed material.

Textbook Users
Launch your word processing software.
Insert the appropriate audiocassette in your transcribing machine and find dictation *5T-1*.
You will be transcribing spelling words in sentence structure.
Listen carefully to each sentence on the audiocassette before transcribing.
Rewind and type (transcribe) the sentences.
Save your work on your student disk.
Refer to the answer key.

Part I / Check Your Progress

Let's pause a minute and see how well you are doing. This section will allow you to evaluate your mastery of keyboarding and spelling of selected terms and drugs found in the family practice specialty.

Textbook Users

Select the correctly spelled term that matches its definition.

Refer to the answer key for immediate feedback.

If you score below 90%, you are recommended to redo the Part I activities.

If you score 90% or above, congratulations. You have mastered the material covered in Part I. You can immediately move on to Part II.

Software Users

Click on *Chapter 5, Part I, Check Your Progress.*

Key the correctly spelled term that matches its definition.

When you are finished, click on *End Test.*

A pop-up screen will reveal your score.

If you score below 90%, you are recommended to redo the Part I activities.

If you score 90% or above, congratulations. You have mastered the material covered in Part I. You can immediately move on to Part II.

PART I / CHECK YOUR PROGRESS

Directions: Select the correctly spelled term that matches its definition.

1. Intense chronic itching in the anal region:
   (a) pruritus ani
   (b) puritus ani
   (c) rhinitis
   (d) rinitis

2. An abnormal sound heard on chest auscultation due to an obstructed airway:
   (a) nystagmus
   (b) rhonchus
   (c) rhinchus
   (d) nystigmus

3. A generic name for a broad-spectrum antibiotic that is active against a wide range of gram-positive and gram-negative organisms:
   (a) doxycycline
   (b) pencillin
   (c) doxycyclene
   (d) penicillin

4. A disorder in the rhythm of the heart:
   (a) distal
   (b) destal
   (c) galop
   (d) gallop

5. An enlargement of the thyroid gland:
   (a) hepatosplenomegaly
   (b) hepatosplenmegaly
   (c) thyromegaly
   (d) thyramegaly

6. A body defense method to prevent movement of an injured part:
   (a) flank
   (b) garding
   (c) guarding
   (d) flenk

7. A reversed response occurring upon withdrawal of a stimulus:
   (a) reband
   (b) rebound
   (c) evert
   (d) revert

8. A small nodular, tumor, or growth:
   (a) buccal
   (b) bucca
   (c) granuloma
   (d) granduloma

9. A knot or knotlike mass:
   (a) ganglion
   (b) ganlion
   (c) fundus
   (d) fundes

10. A small tongue-shaped anatomic structure:
    (a) lingula
    (b) linula
    (c) lamina
    (d) lamena

11. A sound or murmur heard on auscultation:
    (a) bruit
    (b) palpitation
    (c) brut
    (d) palpation

12. A spasm of the orbicular muscle of the eyelid:
    (a) hyperlipidemia
    (b) blepharospasm
    (c) blefarospasm
    (d) hyprelipidemia

PART I / CHECK YOUR PROGRESS continued

13. A small soft structure hanging from the free edge of the soft palate:
    (a) vulva
    (b) vuvla
    (c) ulvula
    (d) uvula

14. A widespread genus of gram-negative, nonmotile bacteria:
    (a) chlamydia
    (b) chlamidia
    (c) myalgia
    (d) mialgia

15. A generic name for an ophthalmic antibiotic:
    (a) sulfactamide
    (b) sulfacetamide
    (c) meclizine
    (d) meslicine

16. Coughing and spitting of blood:
    (a) sputum
    (b) sputim
    (c) hemoptysis
    (d) hemotysis

17. A thin, flat layer:
    (a) lingula
    (b) linula
    (c) lamina
    (d) lamena

18. An incision of the tympanic membrane:
    (a) adenopathy
    (b) adinopathy
    (c) myringomy
    (d) myringotomy

19. A benign tumor in which cells are derived from glandular epithelium:
    (a) adenoma
    (b) adnema
    (c) adnexa
    (d) adenxa

20. An unusually rapid, strong, or irregular heartbeat:
    (a) bruit
    (b) palpitation
    (c) brut
    (d) palpation

21. An endoscope for examining the peritoneal cavity:
    (a) laparoscope
    (b) sigmoidoscope
    (c) laproscopy
    (d) sigmoidscopy

22. Around the rectum:
    (a) perrectal
    (b) prerectal
    (c) perirectal
    (d) parirectal

23. An opening, mouth, or bone:
    (a) oss
    (b) os
    (c) pruritus ani
    (d) puritus anis

24. A generic name for any of a large group of natural or semisynthetic antibacterial antibiotics:
    (a) doxycycline
    (b) pencillin
    (c) doxycyclene
    (d) penicillin

25. An accumulation of fluid in the tissues:
    (a) exdate
    (b) exudate
    (c) edoma
    (d) exdem

PART I / CHECK YOUR PROGRESS *continued*

26. Inflammation of the mucous membrane of the nose:
    (a) mucosa
    (b) mucos
    (c) rhinitis
    (d) rinitis

27. An antiemetic especially effective for control of nausea and vomiting of motion sickness:
    (a) sulfactamide
    (b) sulfacetamide
    (c) meclizine
    (d) meslicine

28. Involuntary rapid rhythmic movement of the eyeball:
    (a) nystagmus
    (b) rhonchus
    (c) rhinchus
    (d) nystigmus

29. The bluish discoloration of the skin and mucous membranes due to excessive concentration of reduced hemoglobin in the blood:
    (a) labyrinthitis
    (b) cayonsis
    (c) labrinthitis
    (d) cyanosis

30. Muscular pain:
    (a) chlamydia
    (b) chlamidia
    (c) myalgia
    (d) mialgia

31. External genital organs in the female:
    (a) vulva
    (b) vuvla
    (c) ulvula
    (d) uvula

32. Painful or difficult urination:
    (a) dysuria
    (b) dyspnia
    (c) dyspnea
    (d) dysurea

33. Pertains to the cheek:
    (a) buccal
    (b) bucca
    (c) granuloma
    (d) granduloma

34. Redness of the skin:
    (a) orthopnea
    (b) erthema
    (c) orthopea
    (d) erythema

35. Painful menstruation:
    (a) amenorrhea
    (b) dysmenorrhea
    (c) amenorhea
    (d) dysmenorhea

36. The ability to breathe easily only in an upright position:
    (a) orthopnea
    (b) erthema
    (c) orthopea
    (d) erythema

37. The absence of the menses:
    (a) amenorrhea
    (b) dysmenorrhea
    (c) amenorhea
    (d) dysmenorhea

38. Labored or difficult breathing:
    (a) dysuria
    (b) dyspnia
    (c) dyspnea
    (d) dysurea

PART I / CHECK YOUR PROGRESS *continued*

39. The state of lying down:
    (a) fundus
    (b) fundes
    (c) decubitus
    (d) decubitis

40. Resembles a polyp:
    (a) polypiod
    (b) polypod
    (c) polypoid
    (d) polypide

41. The bottom or base of an organ:
    (a) fundus
    (b) fundes
    (c) decubitus
    (d) decubitis

42. The elevated concentrations of any or all
    lipids in the plasma:
    (a) hyperlipidemia
    (b) blepharospasm
    (c) blefarospasm
    (d) hyprelipidemia

43. The accumulation of excess fluid in a fluid
    compartment:
    (a) exdate
    (b) exadate
    (c) edema
    (d) exdema

44. The enlargement of the liver and spleen:
    (a) hepatosplenomegaly
    (b) adenopathy
    (c) hepasplenomegaly
    (d) adenompathy

45. The escape of fluid from blood vessels
    because of rupture or seepage, usually into a
    body cavity:
    (a) aeration
    (b) effusion
    (c) eration
    (d) efusion

46. The examination of the interior of the sigmoid
    colon:
    (a) laparoscope
    (b) sigmoidscope
    (c) laproscopy
    (d) sigmoidoscopy

47. The enlargement of the glands, especially the
    lymph nodes:
    (a) hepatosplenomegaly
    (b) adenopathy
    (c) hepasplenomegaly
    (d) adenompathy

48. The farthest from any point of reference;
    remote:
    (a) disal
    (b) galop
    (c) distal
    (d) gallop

49. The increase in the severity of a disease or its
    symptoms:
    (a) exaceration
    (b) exacerbation
    (c) auscultation
    (d) auscutation

50. The inflammation of the internal ear, otitis
    interna:
    (a) labyrinthitis
    (b) rhinitis
    (c) labrinthitis
    (d) rinitis

PART I / CHECK YOUR PROGRESS *continued*

51. The act of listening for sounds produced within the body with the unaided ear or with a stethoscope:
    (a) palpitation
    (b) palpation
    (c) auscultation
    (d) auscutation

52. The exchange of carbon dioxide for oxygen by the blood in the lungs:
    (a) aeration
    (b) effusion
    (c) eration
    (d) efusion

53. The mucous secretion from the lungs, bronchi, and trachea that is ejected through the mouth:
    (a) sputum
    (b) sputim
    (c) hemoptysis
    (d) hemotysis

54. The side of the body between the ribs and ilium:
    (a) flank
    (b) fundus
    (c) flanke
    (d) fundes

55. The tissues or body parts that are near or next to one another:
    (a) adenoma
    (b) adnema
    (c) adnexa
    (d) adenxa

56. The mucous membrane:
    (a) mucoso
    (b) mucosa
    (c) mucousa
    (d) mucus

57. Used as an expectorant:
    (a) terpin
    (b) trepin
    (c) meclizine
    (d) mecilizine

58. Using both hands:
    (a) bimanaul
    (b) bimanual
    (c) bymanaul
    (d) bymanual

59. To turn inside out:
    (a) reband
    (b) rebound
    (c) evert
    (d) revert

60. A blister:
    (a) blib
    (b) bleb
    (c) bleib
    (d) beb

61. Trade name for a corticosteroid for bronchial asthma; pocket inhaler:
    (a) Vancenase
    (b) Vancinase
    (c) Phenergan
    (d) Phenergin

62. Trade name for a powder for extraocular muscle injection:
    (a) Botex
    (b) Botox
    (c) Skelaxin
    (d) Skelaxen

63. Trade name for a corticosteroid:
    (a) Ortho-Tri-Cyclen
    (b) Ortho-Tricyclin
    (c) Triamcinolone
    (d) Triamcinoline

PART I / CHECK YOUR PROGRESS *continued*

64. Trade name for a preparation of amoxicillin, an antibiotic:
    (a) Klonopin
    (b) Augmenten
    (c) Klonpin
    (d) Augmentin

65. Trade name for an antidepressant:
    (a) Paxil
    (b) Pasil
    (c) Evista
    (d) Evixta

66. Trade name for a preparation of amoxicillin, an antimicrobial:
    (a) Co-Polymer
    (b) Copolymer
    (c) Amoxil
    (d) Amosil

67. Trade name for a skeletal muscle relaxant:
    (a) Botex
    (b) Botox
    (c) Skelaxin
    (d) Skelaxen

68. Trade name for a topical antibiotic:
    (a) Proctocreem HC
    (b) Proctocream HC
    (c) Neosporen
    (d) Neosporin

69. Trade name for an antidepressant:
    (a) Paxil
    (b) Pasil
    (c) Evista
    (d) Evixta

70. Trade name for an anticonvulsant:
    (a) Klonopin
    (b) Augmenten
    (c) Klonpin
    (d) Augmentin

71. Trade name for preparations of lidocaine; is classified as an antiarrhythmic, anesthetic:
    (a) Xylocaine
    (b) Ophthetic
    (c) Xylociane
    (d) Ophetic

72. Trade name for a triphasic oral contraceptive:
    (a) Ortho-Tri-Cyclen
    (b) Ortho-Tricyclin
    (c) Triamcinolone
    (d) Triamcinoline

73. Trade name for an oral contraceptive:
    (a) Lipitir
    (b) Lipitor
    (c) Lo-Ovral
    (d) Lo-Oral

74. Trade name for fixed combination preparation analgesic and antipyretic:
    (a) Darvoset
    (b) Darvocet
    (c) Melantonox
    (d) Melantonex

75. Trade name for an antihyperlipidemic that reduces cholesterol synthesis:
    (a) Lipitir
    (b) Lipitor
    (c) Lo-Ovral
    (d) Lo-Oral

76. Trade name for proparacaine hydrochloride, eye drops:
    (a) Xylocaine
    (b) Ophthetic
    (c) Xylociane
    (d) Ophetic

PART I / CHECK YOUR PROGRESS *continued*

77. Trade name for topical corticosteroidal anti-inflammatory used as anorectal cream:
    (a) Proctocreem HC
    (b) Proctocream HC
    (c) Neosporen
    (d) Neosporin

78. Trade name for an antihistamine, antiemetic:
    (a) Vancenase
    (b) Vancinase
    (c) Phenergan
    (d) Phenergin

79. Trade name for an immune modulator:
    (a) Co-Polymer
    (b) Amoxil
    (c) Copolymer
    (d) Amosil

80. Trade name for a nonsteroidial anti-inflammatory drug, NSAID:
    (a) Naprosyn
    (b) Naporsyn
    (c) Norvasc
    (d) Norvasic

81. Trade name for an antibiotic:
    (a) Claritin
    (b) Clariten
    (c) Baixin
    (d) Biaxin

82. Trade name for an antiplatelet agent:
    (a) Presantine
    (b) Persantine
    (c) Prilosec
    (d) Prelosec

83. Trade name for a drug used for the prevention of NSAID-induced gastric ulcers:
    (a) Cytotec
    (b) Cytotic
    (c) Ditropan
    (d) Ditropen

84. Trade name for an analgesic:
    (a) Melatonex
    (b) Melatonix
    (c) Darvocet
    (d) Darvocit

85. Trade name for an urinary antispasmodic:
    (a) Cytotec
    (b) Cytotic
    (c) Ditropan
    (d) Ditropen

86. Trade name for an antibiotic:
    (a) Indocen
    (b) Indocin
    (c) E.E.A.
    (d) E.E.S.

87. Trade name for a nonsteroidal anti-inflammatory drug, NSAID:
    (a) Indocen
    (b) Indocin
    (c) E.E.A.
    (d) E.E.S.

88. Trade name for a gastric acid secretion inhibitor:
    (a) Presantine
    (b) Persantine
    (c) Prilosec
    (d) Prelosec

89. Trade name for a sleep aid:
    (a) Melatonex
    (b) Melatonix
    (c) Darvocet
    (d) Darvocit

90. Trade name for a nonsedating antihistamine:
    (a) Claritin
    (b) Clariten
    (c) Baixin
    (d) Biaxin

Pretest (5T-2)

Professional transcriptionists proofread their own work. Can you? Scoring 90% or better proves it!

Textbook Users
Launch your word processing package.
Insert the appropriate audiocassette in your transcribing machine and find dictation *5T-2.*
On the open screen, transcribe and proofread dictation *5T-2.*
Identify and correct all errors.
Use formatting guidelines established in Chapter 2.
Save your work on your student disk.
After completing the transcription, refer to the answer key.
Manually complete the error analysis chart.
Manually complete the production for pay summary chart.
If you score below 90%, continue on to *Activities 4 and 5, Proofreading Worksheet Exercises* as well as *Activities 6 and 7, Proofreading Transcription Exercises.*
If you score 90% or above, congratulations. You have mastered the material covered in Part II. If you wish, you can immediately move on to Part III.

Software Users
Click on *Chapter 5, Part II, Pretest (5T-2).*
Insert the appropriate audiocassette in your transcribing machine and find dictation *5T-2.*
Click on *Start Watch,* the transcribe and proofread dictation *5T-2.*
Identify and correct all errors.
When you are finished, click on *Done,* then *Score Document:* a pop-up window will display your production for pay.
Click on *Display Error Analysis* to reveal your score.
Click on *View Errors* to see the errors you made.
Save your work (with errors showing) on your student disk by clicking on *File,* then *Save As.*
If you score below 90%, continue on to *Activities 4 and 5, Proofreading Worksheet Exercises* as well as *Activities 6 and 7, Proofreading Transcription Exercises.*
If you score 90% or above, congratulations. You have mastered the material covered in Part II. If you wish, you can immediately move on to Part III.

Part II / Activities 4–5
Proofreading Worksheet Exercises

Finding your own errors and correcting them is not easy, but it is an essential skill for your success as a medical transcriptionist. The two worksheets in this activity will help you develop your proofreading skills.

Textbook Users
Proofread and correct errors in the medical documents shown in *Activities 4–5*.
After completing the exercises, refer to the answer key.
Manually complete the error analysis chart for each document.

Software Users
Click on *Chapter 5, Part II, Activity 4.*
Proofread and correct errors found in the medical document.
Click on *File,* then *Done,* and a pop-up window will appear.
Click on *Score Document* to reveal your score.
Click on *View Errors* to see the errors you made.
Save your work (with errors showing) on your student disk by clicking on *File,* then *Save As.*
Click on *File,* the *Exit,* to proceed.
Follow the same process to complete *Activity 5.*

PART II / ACTIVITY 4
PROOFREADING WORKSHEET EXERCISE

Directions: Proofread this medical document that contains multiple errors using full block, open punctuation, and all other formatting guidelines established in this textbook.

CHART NOTE

Harris, Donna

Date of Birth: 10/21/50

Examination Date: *current date*

SUBJECT: Diane comes in today for follow-up. Her weight have fortunately stayed the same. She still feels weak. Her blood word looks good. X-ray demonstrates prominent markings in the R middle lobe and a questionable nodular density in the R apex.

Her appetite remains about the same. Her living situation is unchanged and despite our best efforts we have really not been able to help her significantly with this.

OBJECTIVE: Weight: 92 lbs BP 120/68. She has no cervical adenapathy. Lungs show decreased breathe sounds. Cardiac exam REGULAR IN RATE AND RHYTHM without murmurs, rubs or gallops appreciated. She has normal chest well excursion. Abdomen is soft. She has some tenderness in the right rib cage.

ASSESMENT: 1. Copd
               2. Weight loss which at this point has stabilized.

PLAN: I am planning to check apical lordotic views of this abnormality in her lung and have them compared to previous films. I will continue to follow her weight loss. I doubt that she has lung cancer , but, just to make sure, I will reevaluate that right upper lobe a little better. At this point I plan to follow her rib pain as well. I really wasn't able to elicit much information today.

Charles P. Davis, MD/xx

PART II / ACTIVITY 5
PROOFREADING WORKSHEET EXERCISE

Directions: Proofread this medical document that contains multiple errors using full block, open punctuation, and all other formatting guidelines established in this textbook.

FedDes Wellness Center
Diagnostic Imaging Division, Suite 157
101 Wellness Way Drive
New York, NY 10036

current date

J. Thomas Geiger, MD
Family Practice Division, Suite 300
101 Wellness Way Drive
New York, NY 10036
RE: Charlotte Mekola
        Date of birth: 10/19/58
        Examination: CHEST

Dear Dr. Gieger

There is a substantial area of alvelar infiltrate that involves the superior segment of the right lower lobe. I do not identify a mass or any definite hilar adenapathy. The lungs are otherwise clear. There is probably an element of Copd. The heart is mildly inlarged but the pulmonary vessels do not appear prominent. There is no efussion. The visualized bony thorax and soft tissues are remarkable for an acentuated kyphosis and probable osteoporosis.

IMPRESSION: Alveolar infiltrate in the superior segment of the left lower lobe. Simple pneumonia is the most likely diagnosis. A follow-up until clearing is reccommended.

Thank you for refering this patient to us.

Yours Truly,

Potter Bucky, MD/x

Part II / Activities 6–7
Proofreading Transcription Exercises (5T-3, 5T-4)

Now you are ready to make the transition from simply proofreading printed material to both transcribing and proofreading dictated material. This is the time to concentrate on building your medical vocabulary, which ultimately will improve your speed and accuracy. There are two activities in this section.

Textbook Users

Step 1: Launch your word processing package. Insert the appropriate audiocassette in your transcribing machine and find dictation *5T-3*. Listen to the entire dictation to gain an understanding of the medical concepts and terms involved in the report. Rewind the tape to the beginning of the dictation and transcribe what you hear. Do not worry about formatting, style, or speed. Simply type what you hear being dictated, using correct punctuation, capitalization, and spelling. Stop as needed to look up words you do not understand or cannot spell. Adjust the speed control of the transcriber to a comfortable level, starting slowly to assure no dictated words are missed, and then increase the speed as your accuracy improves.

Step 2: Rewind the tapes again and using your created template, transcribe dictation *5T-3* again, including correct spacing and formatting. Proofread the report. Identify and correct all errors. Save your work on your student disk. Refer to the answer key, and manually complete the error analysis and production for pay charts.

Repeat the same process for dictation *5T-4*.

Software Users

Click on *Chapter 5, Activity 6–Proofreading Transcription Exercise.*

Insert the appropriate audiocassette in your transcribing machine and find dictation *5T-3*.

Step 1: Listen to entire dictation to gain an understanding of the medical concepts and terms involved. Rewind the tape to the beginning of the dictation, click *Start Watch*, and transcribe what you hear. Do not worry about formatting, style, or speed. Simply type what you hear being dictated, using correct punctuation, capitalization, and spelling. Stop as needed to look up words you do not understand or cannot spell. Adjust the speed control of the transcriber to a comfortable level, starting slowly to assure no dictated words are missed, and then increase the speed as your accuracy improves. When you are finished, click on *Done*, then choose *Return to Main Menu*.

Step 2: Click on *Chapter 5, Activity 6* again. Rewind the tapes again, click on *Start Watch*, and transcribe dictation *5T-3* again, including correct spacing and formatting. Proofread the report. Identify and correct all errors. When you are finished, click on *Done*, then *Score Document* to display your production for pay. Click on *Display Error Analysis* to reveal your score and *View Errors* to see the errors you made. Save your work (with errors showing) on your student disk by clicking on *File*, then *Save As*.

Follow the same process for dictation *5T-4*.

Part II / Check Your Progress *(5T-2)*

Let's pause a minute and see how well you are doing. This section will allow you to evaluate your success at transcribing and proofreading reports.

Textbook Users

Launch your word processing package.

Insert the appropriate audiocassette in your transcribing machine and find dictation *5T-2.*

On the open screen transcribe and proofread dictation *5T-2.*

Identify and correct all errors.

After completing the transcription, refer to the answer key.

Manually complete the error analysis chart.

Manually complete the Production for Pay chart.

If you score below 90%, you are recommended to redo the Part II activities.

If you score 90% or above, congratulations. You have mastered the material covered in Part II. You can immediately move on to Part III.

Software Users

Click on *Chapter 5, Part II, Check Your Progress (5T-2).*

Insert the appropriate audiocassette in your transcribing machine and find dictation *5T-2.*

Click on *Start Watch*, then transcribe and proofread dictation *5T-2.*

Identify and correct all errors.

When you are finished, click on *Done*, then *Score Document*: a pop-up window will display your production for pay.

Click on *Display Error Analysis* to reveal your score.

Click on *View Errors* to see the errors you made.

Save your work (with errors showing) on your student disk by clicking on *File*, then *Save As.*

If you score below 90%, you are recommended to redo the Part II activities.

If you score 90% or above, congratulations. You have mastered the material covered in Part II. You can immediately move on to Part III.

Pretest (5T-5, 5T-6)

Professional transcriptionists can transcribe and proofread their own work. Can you? Scoring 90% or better proves it!

Textbook Users

Launch your word processing package.

Insert the appropriate audiocassette in your transcribing machine and find dictation *5T-5*.

On the open screen transcribe and proofread dictation *5T-5*.

Use formatting guidelines established in Chapter 2.

Save your work on your student disk.

Follow the same process for dictation *5T-6*.

Identify and correct all errors.

After completing the transcription, refer to the answer key.

Manually complete the error analysis chart for each document.

Manually complete the production for pay summary chart for each document.

If you score below 90%, continue with *Family Practice Transcription at FedDes Wellness Center.*

If you score 90% or above, congratulations. You have mastered the material covered in Part III. If you wish, you can immediately move on to the next chapter.

Software Users

Click on *Chapter 5, Part III, Pretest (5T-5).*

Insert the appropriate audiocassette in your transcribing machine and find dictation *5T-5*.

Click on *Start Watch,* then transcribe and proofread dictation *5T-5*.

Identify and correct all errors.

When you are finished, click on *Done,* then *Score Document:* a pop-up window will display your production for pay.

Click on *Display Error Analysis* to reveal your score.

Click on *View Errors* to see the errors you made.

Save your work (with errors showing) on your student disk by clicking on *File,* then *Save As.*

Follow the same process for dictation *5T-6*.

If you score below 90%, click on *Family Practice Transcription at FedDes Wellness Center.*

If you score 90% or above, congratulations. You have mastered the material covered in Part III. If you wish, you can immediately move on to the next chapter.

FAMILY PRACTICE TRANSCRIPTION
AT FEDDES WELLNESS CENTER

You finally made it! You have been hired as a transcriptionist at FedDes Wellness Center in the family practice division. Your supervisor has asked you to transcribe today's dictation.

Textbook Users

Launch your word processing package.

Insert the appropriate audiocassette in your transcribing machine and find dictation *5T-7*.

Create or use your existing templates for the six types of reports: chart note, chart note using history and physical format, history and physical examination report, x-ray report, procedure report, and consultation letter.

On the open screen, transcribe and proofread dictation *5T-7*.

Identify and correct all errors.

Use formatting guidelines established in Chapter 2.

Save your work on your student disk.

Follow the same process for dictations *5T-8* through *5T-23*.

After completing the transcriptions, refer to the answer key.

Manually complete the error analysis chart for each document.

Manually complete the production for pay summary chart for each document.

Software Users

Click on *Chapter 5, Part III, Family Practice Transcription at FedDes Wellness Center (5T-7)*.

Insert the appropriate audiocassette in your transcribing machine and find dictation *5T-7*.

(Please note that you cannot use templates when using the software.)

Click on *Start Watch*, then transcribe and proofread dictation *5T-7*.

Identify and correct all errors.

When you are finished, click on *Done*, then *Score Document*: a pop-up window will display your production for pay.

Click on *Display Error Analysis* to reveal your score.

Click on *View Errors* to see the errors you made.

Save your work (with errors showing) on your student disk by clicking on *File*, then *Save As*.

Follow the same process for dictations *5T-8* and *5T-9*.

NOTE: Continue with medical dictations *5T-10* through *5T-23* using your word processing package and manually complete the error analysis chart and production for pay summary sheet.

Index of Dictations and Associated Transcription Tips

Please remember to follow the guidelines pertaining to capitalization, numbers, punctuation, abbreviations, measurements, symbols, and use of templates to create medical reports at FedDes Wellness Center. Review of this material can be found in Unit 1.

5T-7
Chart Note Using SOAP Format
Patient's Name: Clark, Betrice
Physician: Charles P. Davis, MD

TRANSCRIPTION TIPS

- The expression *o'clock* is used to refer to points on a circular surface.
  You hear the dictator say: Three o'clock position.
  You should transcribe as: 3 o'clock position.

- The # symbol is used to abbreviate the word *number* followed by medical instrument or apparatus.
  You hear the dictator say: Number twenty-five gauge needle.
  You should transcribe as: #25 gauge needle.

- Figures are used for Latin abbreviations.
  You hear the dictator say: Place in eye two drops every two hours.
  You should transcribe as: Place in eye 2 drops q.2h.

- A hyphen is used to join two or more words when used as an adjective that proceeds a noun. The following word pair is dictated in this report: Metallic-looking.
  The word *follow up* in the next sentence is not hyphenated because it is a noun.
  You hear the dictator say: He will return tomorrow for a follow up.

- The following medication is dictated in this report:
  Ophthetic: the trade name for proparacaine hydrochloride, eye drops.

5T-8
Chart Note Using SOAP Format
Patient's Name: Meckonni, James
Physician: Charles P. Davis, MD

TRANSCRIPTION TIPS

- Vital signs are separated by commas and are transcribed as one sentence.
  You hear the dictator say: Temperature ninety-eight point four weight one hundred forty four pounds blood pressure one hundred twenty eight over seventy four pulse fifty six.
  You should transcribe as: Temperature 98.4, weight 144 lb, BP 128/74, pulse 56.

- Words beginning with *pre, re, post,* and *non* are generally not hyphenated: postnasal.

- The following medications are dictated in this report:
  Augmentin: the trade name for a preparation of amoxicillin, an antimibiotic.
  Vancenase: the trade name for a corticosteroid for bronchial asthma; pocket inhaler.

- The letter *x* is used to abbreviate the word *times* when it precedes a number.
  You hear the dictator say: Augmentin five hundred milligrams by mouth three times a day times two weeks.
  You should transcribe as:
  Augmentin 500 mg p.o. t.i.d. x 2 weeks.

5T-9
Chart Note Using SOAP Format
Patient's Name: Chesterfield, Fredrick
Physician: Charles P. Davis, MD

TRANSCRIPTION TIPS

- Words beginning with *pre, re, post,* and *non* are generally not hyphenated.
  For example: nonstop

- A hyphen is used to join two or more words when used as an adjective that proceeds a noun. The following word pair dictated in this report is hyphenated: over-the-counter.

- The following abbreviation is dictated in this report. Plural abbreviations are formed by adding the letter *s*.
  TM: tympanic membrane; TMs

- Capitalize trade names and brand names of drugs, not generic drugs. The following

medications are dictated in this report:
NyQuil: the trade name for an antitussive, decongestant, antihistamine
E.E.S.: the trade name for an antibiotic
Terpin hydrate with codeine: the generic name for an expectorant
Robitussin: trade name for an antitussive

- Figures are used in ranges.
  You will hear the dictator say: four to five times during the day.
  You should transcribe as: 4-5 times during the day.

5T-10
Chart Note Using SOAP Format
Patient's Name: Trepidor, Rodrigues
Physician: Charles P. Davis, MD

● **TRANSCRIPTION TIPS**
- A hyphen is used between numbers and *year old.*
  You will hear the dictator say: A thirty two year old white male.
  You should transcribe as: A 32-year-old white male.

- Words beginning with *pre, re, post,* and *non* are generally not hyphenated: nonproductive, nontoxic.

- The following abbreviation is dictated in this report:
  A&P: auscultation and percussion

- The following medication is dictated in this report:
  Amoxil: the trade name for a preparation of amoxicillin, an antimicrobial.

5T-11
Chart Note Using SOAP Format
Patient Name: Aswart, Sabine
Physician: Charles P. Davis, MD

● **TRANSCRIPTION TIPS**
- The following eponym is dictated:
  Romberg's sign: swaying or falling when standing with feet close together and eyes closed. If positive, the patient will sway and fall.

- Capitalize trade names and brand names of drugs, not generic drugs. The following medications are dictated in this report:
  Meclizine: a generic name for an antiemetic especially effective for control of nausea and vomiting of motion sickness
  Paxil: trade name for an antidepressant
  Klonopin: trade name for an anticonvulsant

- A hyphen is used when joining numbers or letters to form a word, phrase, or abbreviation.
  You will hear the dictator say: B twelve injections.
  You should transcribe as: B-12 injections.

- Words beginning with *pre, re, post,* and *non* are generally not hyphenated: nontender.

5T-12
Procedure Report, FLEXIBLE SIGMOIDOSCOPY WITH BIOPSY
Patient Name: Inshetski, Ann
Physician: Charles P. Davis, MD

5T-13
History and Physical Examination Report
Patient Name: Stephano, Jennifer
Physician: Charles P. Davis, MD

● **TRANSCRIPTION TIPS**
- The following abbreviations are dictated in this report:
  SOB: shortness of breath
  PERRLA: pupils equal, round, reactive to light, and accommodation
  EOM: extraocular movements
  P&A: percussion and auscultation
  ROM: range of motion
  DTR: deep tendon reflexes

- The diagonal (/) is used to separate the indicators of visual acuity.
  You will hear the dictator say: Visual acuity is twenty over thirty both in the left and right eye, but corrected twenty over twenty five.
  You should transcribe as: Visual acuity is 20/30 both in the left and right eye, but corrected 20/25.

- A hyphen joins two or more words when used as an adjective that proceeds a noun. The following word pair is not hyphenated because it is a noun: follow up.

- A hyphen is used when two or more words are viewed as a single word: well-child.

5T-14
Chart Note Using History and Physical Format
Patient Name: Smythers, Jane
Physician: P. H. Waters, MD

● **TRANSCRIPTION TIPS**
- The following abbreviations are dictated in this report:
  EAC: external auditory canal
  SOB: shortness of breath
  P&A: percussion and auscultation
  TM: tympanic membrane

- A hyphen is used to join two or more words when used as an adjective that proceeds a noun. The following word pairs are dictated in this report: over-the-counter, follow-up.

- The following laboratory test is dictated in this report:
  Rapid Strep test: a throat culture for a sore throat caused by a streptococcus

5T-15
Chart Note Using History and Physical Format
Patient Name: Mermain, Devon
Physician: Izzy Sertoli, MD

● **TRANSCRIPTION TIPS**
- The following words are not hyphenated because they end a sentence: check up, up to date.

- The hyphen is used to take the place of the word *to* or *through* to identify ranges.
  You will hear the dictator say: We should see him again in two to three years at his school.
  You should transcribe as: We should see him again in 2-3 years at his school.

5T-16
X-ray Report, PA AND LATERAL CHEST X-RAY
Patient Name: Holtzworth, Max
Physician: P. H. Waters, MD

● **TRANSCRIPTION TIPS**
- The following abbreviation is dictated in this report:
  COPD: chronic obstructive pulmonary disease

5T-17
Chart Note Using History and Physical Format
Patient Name: Margolis, Davy
Physician: P. H. Waters, MD

● **TRANSCRIPTION TIPS**
- The following abbreviations are dictated in this report:
  ASO: Antistreptolysin O is an antibody that inhibits streptolysin. Streptolysin is an oxygen-labile and antigenic hemolysin produced by most group A streptococcci that lyse red blood cells.
  ANA: Antinuclear antibody. The ANA test is used as a screen to detect autoimmune disease and/or systemic lupus erythematosus. It cannot identify the specifics of the disease; it only identifies the presence of antibodies of autoimmune disease.
  CBC: complete blood count
  ROM: range of motion

- The following medications are dictated in this report:
  Cytotec: the trade name for a drug used for the prevention of NSAID-induced gastric ulcers
  Indocin: the trade name for a nonsteroidal anti-inflammatory drug, NSAID
  Naprosyn: the trade name for a nonsteroidal anti-inflammatory drug, NSAID
  Lidocaine: the generic name for a topical local anesthetic

- Words beginning with *pre, re, post*, and *non* are generally not hyphenated.
  For example: recheck

- The # symbol is used to abbreviate the word *number* followed by medical instrument or apparatus.
  You hear the dictator say: number twenty two gauge needle.
  You should transcribe as: #22 gauge needle.

5T-18
Chart Note Using History and Physical Format
Patient Name: Duke, Marge
Physician: Gwenn Maltase, MD

● **TRANSCRIPTION TIP**
- A hyphen is used to join two or more words when used as an adjective that proceeds a noun. The following word pairs are dictated in this report: over-the-counter, follow-up.

5T-19
Chart Note Using History and Physical Format
Patient Name: Levy, Susan
Physician: Gwenn Maltase, MD

● **TRANSCRIPTION TIPS**
- Generic drugs are not capitalized.
  You will hear the dictator say: Will just treat with ibuprofen, rest, and fluids.
  You should transcribe as: Will just treat with ibuprofen, rest, and fluids.

- A hyphen is used to take the place of the word *to* or *through* to identify ranges.
  You will hear the dictator say: She will call if she is not improving over the next twenty four to forty eight hours.
  You should transcribe as: She will call if she is not improving over the next 24-48 hours.

5T-20
Consultation Letter
Inside address: Mr. Ben Over, Customer Services, Simon Seez Managed Care, Inc., 911 Dividend Drive, Cashflow, NY 10039
Reference line: Samuel Franklin, File Number 69024, Date of Birth January 1, 1986
Physician: J. Thomas Geiger, MD

● **TRANSCRIPTION TIPS**
- The following abbreviation is dictated in this report:
  HMO: health maintenance organization

- A hyphen is used to join two or more words when used as an adjective that proceeds a noun. The following word pair is dictated in this report: follow-up.

- The apostrophe is used to form the possessive of singular and plural nouns.
  You will hear the dictator say: Thank you for your timely assistance in Mr. Franklin's treatment plan.

- The following medication is dictated:
  Copolymer: the trade name for one of the immune-modulating drugs

5T-21
Physical Therapy Referral Letter
Inside address: David Treppe, MD, Orthopedic Division, Suite 133, FedDes Wellness Center, New York, NY 10036
Reference line: Betty Ross, File Number 51490, Date of Birth September 15, 19xx
Physical Therapist: Melissa A. Anconeus, MS, PT

● **TRANSCRIPTION TIPS**
- A hyphen is used to join two or more words when used as an adjective that proceeds a noun. The following word pairs are dictated in this report:
  30-foot
  right-sided
  left-sided
  pain-free
  part-time
  self-employed
  long-term

- A hyphen is used between two "like" vowels: anti-inflammatory, pre-existing.

- The percent sign (%) is used with words and figures.
  You will hear the dictator say: Cervical range of motion is restricted at seventy five percent of normal rotation.
  Transcribe as: Cervical range of motion is restricted at 75% of normal rotation.

You will hear the dictator say: treated with a one percent Xylocaine injection. Transcribe as: treated with a 1% Xylocaine injection.

- Figures with capital letters are used to refer to the vertebral column and spinal nerves.
The hyphen is used to take the place of the word *through* to identify ranges.
You will hear the dictator say: There is left-sided point tenderness over the C five through C six paraspinal areas.
You should transcribe as: There is left-sided point tenderness over the C5-C6 paraspinal areas.

- The words *palpation* and *palpitation* are often confused in dictation. Listen carefully! Palpation is an examination by touching. Palpitation is a rapid or fluttering heartbeat.
There is tenderness to palpation of the anterior glenohumeral capsule.
No chest pain, edema, palpitations, orthopnea, leg cramps, or exertional dyspnea was noted.

5T-22
Chart Note Using SOAP Format
Patient Name: Lee, My
Physician: Izzy Sertoli, MD

⬤ **TRANSCRIPTION TIPS**
- The following abbreviation is dictated in this report:
Pap: Papanicolaou test

- Capitalized Roman numerals are used to express class, cranial leads (EKG), cranial nerves, limb leads (ECG), factor (blood clotting), grade, phase, pregnancy and delivery, stage, and type.
For example: Gravida I, para I

- The following laboratory tests are dictated in this report:
Fasting Astra IV: a panel of four blood chemistry tests that require the patient to fast. The name of this test is linked to the manufacturer of the chemical analyzer, Astra.

TSH: to ascertain the thyroid stimulating hormone level
Erythrocyte sedimentation rate: The erythrocyte sedimentation rate test is helpful in identifying and monitoring disease activity in infectious, inflammatory, and neoplastic conditions.

- The following medication is dictated in this report:
Skelaxin: the trade name for a skeletal muscle relaxant

5T-23
History and Physical Examination Report
Patient Name: Feiffer, Madeline
Physician: Matthew Sponch, MD

⬤ **TRANSCRIPTION TIPS**
- A hyphen is used to join two or more words when used as an adjective that proceeds a noun. The following word pairs are dictated in this report: well-developed, well-nourished, 12-week.

- If a sentence contains numbers under and over ten, use figures for all numbers.
You will hear the dictator say: She is twelve weeks amenorrhea with complaints of vaginal spotting for the past three days.
You should transcribe as: She is 12-weeks amenorrhea with complaints of vaginal spotting for the past 3 days.

- The following abbreviation is dictated in this report:
HPI: history of present illness

- The hyphen is used to take the place of the word *to* or *through* to identify ranges.
You will hear the dictator say: The cervix is open one to two centimeters.
You should transcribe as: The cervix is open 1-2 cm.

- Words beginning with *pre, re, post,* and *non* are generally not hyphenated: noncontributory, nontender.

Part III / Check Your Progress

Professional transcriptionists can transcribe and proofread their own work with speed and accuracy. Have you mastered the family practice transcription rotation at FedDes Wellness Center?

Textbook Users

Launch your word processing package.

Insert the appropriate audiocassette in your transcribing machine and find dictation *5T-5*.

On the open screen, transcribe and proofread dictation *5T-5*.

Identify and correct all errors.

After completing the reports, refer to the answer key.

Use formatting guidelines established in Chapter 2.

Save your work on your student disk.

Follow the same process for dictation *5T-6*.

Manually complete the error analysis chart for each document.

Manually complete the Production for Pay summary chart for each document.

If you score below 90%, you are recommended to repeat Part III.

If you score 90% or above, congratulations. You have mastered the material presented in Part III.

Software Users

Click on *Chapter 5, Part III, Check Your Progress (5T-5)*.

Insert the appropriate audiocassette in your transcribing machine and find dictation *5T-5*.

Click on *Start Watch,* then transcribe and proofread dictation *5T-5*.

Identify and correct all errors.

When you are finished, click on *Done,* then *Score Document*: a pop-up window will display your production for pay.

Click on *Display Error Analysis* to reveal your score.

Click on *View Errors* to see the errors you made.

Save your work (with errors showing) on your student disk by clicking on *File,* then *Save As.*

Follow the same process for dictation *5T-6*.

If you score below 90%, you are recommended to repeat Part III.

If you score 90% or above, congratulations. You have mastered the material presented in Part III.

Chapter 6

Office Medical Transcription from the Orthopaedic Practice

OBJECTIVES

At the completion of Chapter 6, you should be able to do the following:

1. Match medical terms associated with the orthopaedic specialty with their definitions.

2. Spell medical terms associated with the orthopaedic specialty with their definitions.

3. Transcribe medical terms in sentence structure.

4. Proofread, edit, and correct medical documents associated with the orthopaedic specialty containing various errors.

5. Transcribe and proofread authentic medical documents associated with the orthopaedic specialty.

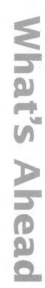

What's Ahead

143

The Orthopaedic Rotation

The FedDes Wellness Center has three *orthopedists*, or specialists in orthopaedic medicine, on staff. *Orthopaedics* is the field of medicine concerned with the diseases, injuries, and deformities of the musculoskeletal system. Patients who see an orthopedist may be suffering from a fracture, acute or chronic pain, inflammatory joint or stress injuries, osteoporosis, herniated intervertebral discs, or carpal tunnel syndrome.

During a physical examination by an orthopedist, the patient is first observed standing and walking. Posture, movement of the extremities, and any signs of pain are included in the observation. The examination includes full range of motion activities and strength assessment for each muscle group.

The physicians in FedDes orthopaedic division perform and interpret routine x-rays in their offices. More sophisticated imaging such as MRI, CT scans, and nuclear medicine studies are referred to an outside facility and interpreted by a radiologist.

In this unit, you assume the role of a medical transcriptionist employed at FedDes Wellness Center. **Please remember to follow the guidelines pertaining to capitalization, numbers, punctuation,** **abbreviations, measurements, symbols, and use of templates to create medical reports at FedDes Wellness Center. Review of this material is found in Unit 1.** A list of the patient's name and the type of report, as well as associated transcription tips, are included in this chapter.

You will work with the textbook, CD-ROM, and accompanying audiocassettes. Your mastery of orthopaedic transcription is assessed through worksheets, timed transcription exercises, the error analysis chart, and the Production for Pay summary.

All the answer keys are found in the textbook and CD-ROM, providing immediate feedback. After transcribing a report, you will proofread your work and correct any errors. Then you will compare your proofread work against a master transcript, categorize all errors, and tabulate the errors on the error analysis chart. The Production for Pay summary correlates your production to the FedDes Wellness Center pay scale, which is based on industry compensation standards. The scale is also linked to your grade. This system allows you to assess your mastery of transcription skills in a real-world scenario.

Pretest

Let's find out if you can define and spell selected terminology and drugs of the orthopaedic specialty that are included in this chapter by scoring 90% or better.

Textbook Users

Select the correctly spelled term that matches its definition.

Refer to the answer key for immediate feedback.

If you score below 90%, continue on to *Activities 1 through 3*.

If you score 90% or above, congratulations. You have mastered the material covered in Part I. If you wish, you can immediately move on to Part II.

Software Users

Click on *Chapter 6, Part I, Pretest*.

Key the correctly spelled term that matches its definition.

When you are finished, click on *End Test*.

A pop-up screen will reveal your score.

If you score below 90%, continue on to *Activities 1 through 3*.

If you score 90% or above, congratulations. You have mastered the material covered in Part I. If you wish, you can immediately move on to Part II.

PART I / PRETEST

Directions: Select the correctly spelled term that matches its definition.

1. A finger or toe:
   - (a) digit
   - (b) falanx
   - (c) fusiform
   - (d) degit

2. A fracture of the distal end of the radius with displacement of the hand backward and upward:
   - (a) Coles fracture
   - (b) Colles fracture
   - (c) Smith fracture
   - (d) Smythe fracture

3. A fracture of the lower end of the radius with forward displacement of the lower fragment:
   - (a) Coles fracture
   - (b) Colles fracture
   - (c) Smith fracture
   - (d) Smythe fracture

4. Frequent cause of shoulder pain thought to be due to pressure on the tendons of the shoulder:
   - (a) radiculitis
   - (b) rotator cuff tendenitis
   - (c) radeculitis
   - (d) rotater cuff tendinitis

5. Lubricating fluid of joints:
   - (a) apophysis
   - (b) apophyis
   - (c) synova
   - (d) synovia

6. A tearing away forcibly of a part or structure:
   - (a) avulsion
   - (b) crepitus
   - (c) avolsion
   - (d) creitus

7. Abnormal contact or pressure between two structures:
   - (a) impingement
   - (b) impingment
   - (c) debredment
   - (d) debridement

8. Abnormal, benign growth on the surface of a bone, also called *hyperostosis:*
   - (a) ecchymosis
   - (b) exostisis
   - (c) echymosis
   - (d) exostosis

9. Benign tumor composed mostly of fat cells:
   - (a) lymphedema
   - (b) lipoma
   - (c) lipima
   - (d) lymphodema

10. Affecting or relating to two sides:
    - (a) bilateril
    - (b) genu varum
    - (c) bilateral
    - (d) ganu varum

11. An attempt to forcibly exhale with the glottis, nose, and mouth closed:
    - (a) Valsalva maneuver
    - (b) Fabrey test
    - (c) Fabre test
    - (d) Valsava maneuver

12. An outgrowth of bone that is usually found around a joint:
    - (a) apophysis
    - (b) ostophyte
    - (c) osteophyte
    - (d) appophysis

PART I / PRETEST *continued*

13. Any outgrowth or swelling; a process or projection of a bone:
    (a) apophysis
    (b) ostophyte
    (c) osteophyte
    (d) appophysis

14. Between two joints:
    (a) bilateral
    (b) bilateril
    (c) intrarticuler
    (d) interarticular

15. Bowleg:
    (a) genu varum
    (b) gluteus medius
    (c) ganu varum
    (d) glutus medius

16. Commonly called a *bruise,* where there is trauma to the body part but there is no break in the skin surface:
    (a) contusion
    (b) volar
    (c) contrusion
    (d) volor

17. Containing pus:
    (a) pisiform
    (b) pesiform
    (c) purulence
    (d) prulence

18. Describes the pathway of the x-ray beam as it passes through anteriorly and exits posteriorly; anteroposterior x-ray:
    (a) NKA x-ray
    (b) PA x-ray
    (c) AP x-ray
    (d) KAN x-ray

19. Directional term, from posterior to medial:
    (a) postmedial
    (b) posteromedial
    (c) peripheral
    (d) peripharel

20. Black and blue appearance of the skin:
    (a) ecchymosis
    (b) exostisis
    (c) echymosis
    (d) exostosis

21. Draw in or out by suction:
    (a) turgor
    (b) asporate
    (c) turger
    (d) aspirate

22. Swelling due to obstruction of lymph vessels:
    (a) lymphedema
    (b) lipoma
    (c) lipima
    (d) lymphodema

23. Escape of fluid from blood vessels because of rupture or seepage, usually into a body cavity:
    (a) crepitus
    (b) effussion
    (c) effusion
    (d) creptus

24. Examination of the interior of a joint with an arthroscope:
    (a) arthroscopy
    (b) hypertrophy
    (c) arthriscopy
    (d) hyprotrophy

25. General term for any bone of a finger or toe:
    (a) fusiform
    (b) falanx
    (c) phalanx
    (d) degit

PART I / PRETEST *continued*

26. Grating sound of bone fragments rubbing together:
    (a) crepitus
    (b) effussion
    (c) effusion
    (d) creptus

27. Increase in the size of an organ or structure:
    (a) greater trochanter
    (b) hypertrophy
    (c) greater trichanter
    (d) hyprotrophy

28. Inflammation of a tendon:
    (a) tendinitis
    (b) radiculitis
    (c) tendenitus
    (d) radeculitis

29. Large projection at the proximal end of the femur:
    (a) greater trochanter
    (b) hypertrophy
    (c) greater trichanter
    (d) hyprotrophy

30. Movement by a joint that decreases the angle between the two adjoining bones; the bending of a joint:
    (a) abduction
    (b) flixion
    (c) flexion
    (d) abuction

31. Movement of an extremity away from midline:
    (a) abuction
    (b) aduction
    (c) abduction
    (d) adduction

32. Movement of an extremity toward the midline:
    (a) abuction
    (b) aduction
    (c) abduction
    (d) adduction

33. New growth of bony tissue surrounding the bone ends in a fracture; part of the repair process of a fractured bone:
    (a) plantar
    (b) callus
    (c) planter
    (d) calus

34. Normal resiliency of the skin:
    (a) turgor
    (b) trugor
    (c) volar
    (d) volor

35. Occurring away from the center:
    (a) postmedial
    (b) posteromedial
    (c) peripheral
    (d) peripharel

36. One of the three muscles that form the buttocks; acts to abduct and rotate the thigh:
    (a) genu varum
    (b) gluteus medius
    (c) ganu varum
    (d) glutus medius

37. Pea-shaped; smallest carpal bone:
    (a) pisiform
    (b) pesiform
    (c) purulence
    (d) prulence

PART I / PRETEST *continued*

38. Performed with patient supine, thigh and knee flexed; the ankle is placed over the patella of the opposite leg and then the knee is depressed.
    (a) Valsalva maneuver
    (b) Fabrey test
    (c) Fabre test
    (d) Valsava maneuver

39. A spinous projection off the scapula:
    (a) acromon
    (b) faciculations
    (c) acromion
    (d) fasciculations

40. Pertaining to the palm of the hand or sole of the foot:
    (a) turgor
    (b) trugor
    (c) volar
    (d) volor

41. Reconstruction surgery to repair or reshape a diseased joint:
    (a) arthroscopy
    (b) arthriscropy
    (c) arthroplasty
    (d) arthroplasy

42. Relating to the sole of the foot:
    (a) plantar
    (b) callus
    (c) planter
    (d) calus

43. Removal of dead or damaged tissue:
    (a) impingement
    (b) impingment
    (c) debredment
    (d) debridement

44. Situated or occurring between bone:
    (a) calcaneus
    (b) interosseous
    (c) clacaneus
    (d) intreosseous

45. Spindle shaped; structure that is tapered at both ends:
    (a) fusiform
    (b) fusform
    (c) pisiform
    (d) pesiform

46. Supporting one's own weight without assistance:
    (a) weightbearing
    (b) weightbaring
    (c) trapezius
    (d) trapeius

47. Surgical removal of a meniscus:
    (a) menisectomy
    (b) mellelus
    (c) melleolus
    (d) meniscectomy

48. Symptoms of a specific disease:
    (a) asympmatic
    (b) symptomatology
    (c) symptomology
    (d) asymptomatic

49. The movement of a finger is temporarily stopped in the extension or flexion position and then begins again with a jerk:
    (a) jerking finger
    (b) trigger finger
    (c) jerk finger
    (d) trig finger

PART I / PRETEST *continued*

50. The process by which energy travels through space or matter. In clinical medicine, it often refers to the divergence of pain from the site of injury to other areas of the body:
    (a) radiculitis
    (b) radaition
    (c) radiation
    (d) radiculation

51. Therapy program using simulated or real work tasks to gradually improve strength and endurance in anticipation of completing a full day's work:
    (a) workhardening
    (b) work hardening
    (c) workbearing
    (d) work bearing

52. To bend the joint toward the posterior aspect of the body:
    (a) dorsiflexion
    (b) flixion
    (c) abduction
    (d) dorsflexion

53. Uncontrolled twitching of a group of muscle fibers:
    (a) acromon
    (b) faciculations
    (c) acromion
    (d) fasciculations

54. Without symptoms:
    (a) asympmatic
    (b) symptomatology
    (c) symptomology
    (d) asymptomatic

55. The muscles of the back of the neck and shoulder:
    (a) metatarsus
    (b) trapezius
    (c) trapezsus
    (d) metatarus

56. The disease of the lymph nodes:
    (a) lymphadenopathy
    (b) lymphenopathy
    (c) lymphedema
    (d) lymphodema

57. Crescent-shaped fibrocartilage in the knee joint:
    (a) meniscus
    (b) malelus
    (c) menscus
    (d) malleolus

58. The long, medial bone of the forearm:
    (a) radius
    (b) radious
    (c) ulna
    (d) unla

59. Any of the five long bones of the foot between the ankle and toes:
    (a) metatarsus
    (b) trapezius
    (c) trapezsus
    (d) metatarus

60. Either of the two rounded projections on either side of the ankle joint:
    (a) meniscus
    (b) malelus
    (c) menscus
    (d) malleolus

61. The heel bone or os calcis:
    (a) colcaneus
    (b) calcaneus
    (c) ulna
    (d) unla

62. Inflammation of a spinal nerve root:
    (a) radiculitis
    (b) radaition
    (c) radiation
    (d) radiculation

PART I / PRETEST *continued*

63. Inflammation involving the folds of tissue surrounding the nail:
    (a) synovia
    (b) synomvia
    (c) parychia
    (d) paronychia

64. Trade name for as a beta-adrenergic blocker:
    (a) Lopressor
    (b) Percocet
    (c) Lopresor
    (d) Percoset

65. Trade name for an antibiotic:
    (a) tetrasysline
    (b) spironolactone
    (c) spironlactone
    (d) tetracycline

66. Trade name for an opioid analgesic:
    (a) Lopressor
    (b) Percocet
    (c) Lopresor
    (d) Percoset

67. Trade name for an antihyperlipidemic:
    (a) Linoxin
    (b) Lipitor
    (c) Lanoxin
    (d) Lippitor

68. Trade name for an antiarrhythmic cardiotonic:
    (a) Linoxin
    (b) Lipitor
    (c) Lanoxin
    (d) Lippitor

69. Generic name for an corticosteroid:
    (a) codeine
    (b) cortisone
    (c) codenine
    (d) cortisome

70. Generic name for an opioid analgesic:
    (a) codeine
    (b) cortisone
    (c) codenine
    (d) cortisome

71. Trade name for an antiarrhythmic; local anesthetic:
    (a) Xylocaine
    (b) Biaxin
    (c) Baixin
    (d) Xylacane

72. Generic name for a diuretic:
    (a) tetrasysline
    (b) spironolactone
    (c) spironlactone
    (d) tetracycline

73. Trade name for an antibiotic:
    (a) Xylocaine
    (b) Biaxin
    (c) Baixin
    (d) Xylacane

74. Trade name for a narcotic analgesic:
    (a) Keflex
    (b) Keplex
    (c) Vicoprofen
    (d) Vicoprophen

75. Trade name for an antibiotic:
    (a) Keflex
    (b) Keplex
    (c) Vicoprofen
    (d) Vicoprophen

76. Trade name for an anti-inflammatory:
    (a) Dolibid
    (b) Dolobid
    (c) Vicodin
    (d) Vicidin

77. Trade name for a narcotic analgesic:
    (a) Dolibid
    (b) Dolobid
    (c) Vicodin
    (d) Vicidin

78. Generic name for any of a large group of antibacterial antibiotics derived from the strains of fungi:
    (a) pencilin
    (b) pennicilin
    (c) penicilin
    (d) penicillin

Part I / Activity 1
Keyboarding Medical Terms and Definitions

Let's learn to spell and define some orthopaedic terms. Keyboarding these terms is an innovative and fun way to improve your skills.

Textbook Users
Launch your word processing package.
On the open screen, read and type each word and its definition as shown below.
Save your work on your student disk.

1. Abduction (ab-<u>duk</u>-shun) is the movement of an extremity away from the midline.
2. Acromion (ah-<u>kro</u>-me-on) is a spinous projection off the scapula.
3. Adduction (ad-<u>duk</u>-shun) is the movement of an extremity toward the midline.
4. Apophysis (ah-<u>pofi</u>-sis) is any outgrowth or swelling; a process or projection of a bone.
5. Arthroplasty (ar-<u>thro</u>-plas-te) is the reconstruction surgery to repair or reshape a diseased joint.
6. Arthroscopy (ar-<u>thros</u>-ko-pe) is the examination of the interior of a joint with an arthroscope.
7. Aspirate (as-<u>pi</u>-rat) is to draw in or out by suction.
8. Asymptomatic (a-<u>simp</u>-to-mat-ik) is without symptoms.
9. Avulsion (ah-<u>vul</u>-shun) is the tearing away forcibly of a part or structure.
10. Bilateral (bi-<u>lat</u>-er-al) is affecting or relating to two sides.
11. Calcaneus (kal-<u>kay</u>-nee-us) is the heel bone or os calcis.
12. Callus (<u>kal</u>-us) is the new growth of bony tissue surrounding the bone ends in a fracture; part of the repair process of a fractured bone.
13. Codeine (<u>ko</u>-den) is the generic name for an opioid analgesic.
14. Contusion (kon-<u>to</u>-shun) is commonly called a *bruise*, where there is trauma to the body part but there is no break in the skin surface.
15. Cortisone (<u>cor</u>-ti-son) is the generic name for a corticosteroid, used to treat inflammations.
16. Crepitus (<u>krep</u>-i-tus) is a grating sound of bone fragments rubbing together.
17. Debridement (da-<u>bred</u>-maw) is the removal of dead or damaged tissue.
18. Digit (<u>dij</u>-it) is a finger or toe.

19. Dorsiflexion (dor-si-<u>flek</u>-shun) is to bend the joint toward the posterior aspect of the body.
20. Ecchymosis (eki-<u>mo</u>-sis) is the black and blue appearance of the skin.
21. Effusion (e-<u>fu</u>-zhun) is the escape of fluid from blood vessels because of rupture or seepage, usually into a body cavity.
22. Exostosis (ek-sos-<u>to</u>-sis) is an abnormal, benign growth on the surface of a bone, also called *hyperostosis.*
23. Fasciculations (fa-sik-u-<u>la</u>-shun) are the uncontrolled twitchings of a group of muscle fibers.
24. Flexion (<u>flek</u>-shun) is the movement by a joint that decreases the angle between the two adjoining bones; the bending of a joint.
25. Fusiform (<u>fu</u>-zi-form) is a spindle-shaped structure that is tapered at both ends.
26. Genu varum (<u>je</u>-nu <u>va</u>-rum) is bowleg.
27. Gluteus medius ((<u>gloo</u>-te-us <u>me</u>-de-us) is one of the three muscles that form the buttocks; acts to abduct and rotate the thigh.
28. Greater trochanter (tro-<u>kan</u>-ter) is the large projection at the proximal end of the femur.
29. Hypertrophy (hi-<u>per</u>-tro-fe) is an increase in the size of an organ or structure.
30. Interarticular (in-ter-ar-<u>tik</u>-u-lar) is between two joints.
31. Interosseous (in-ter-<u>os</u>-e-us) is situated or occurring between bone.
32. Lipoma (li-<u>po</u>-mah) is a benign tumor composed mostly of fat cells.
33. Lymphadenopathy (lim-fad-e-<u>nop</u>-ah-the) is the disease of the lymph nodes.
34. Lymphedema (<u>lim</u>-fi-de-ma) is edema due to obstruction of lymph vessels.
35. Malleolus (mah-<u>lee</u>-o-lus) is either of the two rounded projections on either side of the ankle joint.
36. Meniscectomy (me-ni-<u>sek</u>-to-me) is the surgical removal of a meniscus.
37. Meniscus (me-<u>nis</u>-kus) is the crescent-shaped fibrocartilage in the knee joint.
38. Metatarsus (met-a-<u>tar</u>-sus) is any of the five long bones of the foot between the ankle and the toes.
39. Osteophyte (<u>os</u>-te-o-fit) is an outgrowth of bone that is usually found around a joint.
40. Paronychia (par-o-<u>nik</u>-e-ah) is the inflammation involving the folds of tissue surrounding the nail.
41. Penicillin (pen-I-<u>sil</u>-in) is the generic name for any of a large group of antibacterial antibiotics derived from strains of fungi of the genus *Pencillium.*
42. Peripheral (pe-<u>rif</u>-er-al) is occurring away from the center.
43. Phalanx (<u>fa</u>-langks) is the general term for any bone of a finger or toe.
44. Pisiform (<u>pi</u>-si-form) is pea-shaped; smallest carpal bone.
45. Plantar (<u>plan</u>-tar) is relating to the sole of the foot.
46. Purulence (<u>pu</u>-roo-lens) is containing pus.
47. Radiculitis (rah-dik-u-<u>li</u>-tis) is the inflammation of a spinal nerve root.
48. Spironolactone (sper-o-no-<u>lak</u>-ton) is the generic name for a diuretic.
49. Symptomatology (simp-to-mah-<u>tol</u>-o-je) is the symptoms of a specific disease.
50. Synovia (si-<u>no</u>-ve-ah) is the lubricating fluid of joints.
51. Tendinitis (ten-di-<u>ni</u>-tis) is the inflammation of a tendon, alt. Tendonitis.
52. Tetracycline (te-trah-<u>si</u>-klen) is the generic name for an antibiotic.
53. Trapezius (trah-pee-zee-us) is the muscles of the back of the neck and shoulder.
54. Turgor (<u>tur</u>-gor) is the normal resiliency of the skin.
55. Ulna (<u>ul</u>-nah) is the long, medial bone of the forearm.
56. Volar (<u>vo</u>-lar) pertaining to the palm of the hand or sole of the foot.
57. Biaxin (bi-<u>ak</u>-sin) is the trade name for an antibiotic.
58. Dolobid (<u>do</u>-lo-bid) is the trade name for an analgesic, anti-inflammatory.
59. Keflex (<u>kef</u>-leks) is the trade name for an antibiotic.
60. Lanoxin (lah-<u>nok</u>-sin) is the trade name for an antiarrhythmic, cardiotonic.
61. Lipitor is the trade name for an antihyperlipidemic.
62. Lopressor (lo-<u>pres</u>-or) is the trade name for a beta-adrenergic blocker.

63. Percocet (per-<u>ko</u>-set) is the trade name for an opioid analgesic (Schedule II).
64. Vicodin (vi-<u>co</u>-din) is the trade name for a narcotic analgesic.
65. Vicoprofen (vik-o-<u>pro</u>-fen) is the trade name for a narcotic analgesic.
66. Xylocaine (<u>zi</u>-lo-kan) is the trade name for an antiarrhythmic; local anesthetic.

Part I / Activity 2
Spelling Medical Terms

Do you remember back in school when you had to write each spelling word ten times? Because you had to physically write each word, your mind and body were focused on the assignment and the method worked! Let's follow this successful method by reinforcing the spelling of some orthopaedic terms through keyboarding drills.

Textbook Users
Launch your word processing package.
On the open screen, read, mentally spell, and type each word in its sequence.
Save your work on your student disk.

1. abduction acromial adduction abduction acromial adduction abduction acromial adduction
2. apophysis arthroplasty aspirate apophysis arthroplasty aspirate apophysis arthroplasty
3. arthroscopy asymptomatic avulsion arthroscopy asymptomatic avulsion arthroscopy avulsion
4. bilateral codeine cortisone bilateral codeine cortisone bilateral codeine cortisone codeine
5. calcaneus contusion crepitus calcaneus contusion crepitus calcaneus contusion crepitus
6. debridement digit dorsiflexion debridement digit dorsiflexion debridement digit dorsiflexion
7. ecchymosis effusion exostosis ecchymosis effusion exostosis ecchymosis effusion exostosis
8. fasciculations flexion fusiform fasciculations flexion fusiform fasciculations flexion fusiform
9. genu varum gluteus medius greater trochanter genu varum gluteus medius greater trochanter
10. hypertrophy interarticular interosseous hypertrophy interarticular interosseous hypertrophy
11. lipoma lymphadenopathy lymphedema lipoma lymphadenopathy lymphedema lipoma
12. malleolus meniscectomy meniscus malleolus meniscectomy meniscus malleolus meniscectomy
13. metatarsus osteophyte paronychia metatarsus osteophyte paronychia metatarsus osteophyte
14. peripheral phalanx pisiform peripheral phalanx pisiform peripheral phalanx pisiform phalanx
15. plantar purulence radiculitis plantar purulence radiculitis plantar purulence radiculitis plantar
16. symptomatology synovia tendinitis symptomatology synovia tendinitis symptomatology
17. trapezius turgor ulna volar trapezius turgor ulna volar trapezius turgor ulna volar trapezius
18. penicillin spironolactone tetracycline penicillin spironolactone tetracycline penicillin
19. Lanoxin Lipitor Lopressor Lanoxin Lipitor Lopressor Lanoxin Lipitor Lopressor Lanoxin
20. Biaxin Dolobid Keflex Biaxin Dolobid Keflex Biaxin Dolobid Keflex Biaxin Dolobid Keflex
21. Percocet Vicodin Vicoprofen Xylocaine Percocet Vicodin Vicoprofen Xylocaine Percocet

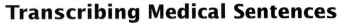

Part I / Activity 3
Transcribing Medical Sentences

Now you are ready to make the transition from keyboarding medical terms, which is a visual process, to transcribing medical terms, an aural process. You are going to use audiocassette tapes rather than printed material.

Textbook Users
Launch your word processing software.
Insert the appropriate audiocassette in your transcribing machine and find dictation *6T-1*.
You will be transcribing spelling words in sentence structure.
Listen carefully to each sentence on the audiocassette before transcribing.
Rewind and type (transcribe) the sentences.
Save your work on your student disk.
Refer to the answer key.

Part I / Check Your Progress

Let's pause a minute and see how well you are doing. This section will allow you to evaluate your mastery of keyboarding and spelling selected terms and drugs found in the orthopaedic specialty.

Textbook Users
Select the correctly spelled term that matches its definition.
Refer to the answer key for immediate feedback.
If you score below 90%, you are recommended to redo the Part I activities.
If you score 90% or above, congratulations. You have mastered the material covered in Part I. You can immediately move on to Part II.

Software Users
Click on *Chapter 6, Part I, Check Your Progress*.
Key the correctly spelled term that matches its definition.
When you are finished, click on *End Test*.
A pop-up screen will reveal your score.
If you score below 90%, you are recommended to redo the Part I activities.
If you score 90% or above, congratulations. You have mastered the material covered in Part I. You can immediately move on to Part II.

PART I / CHECK YOUR PROGRESS

Directions: Select the correctly spelled term that matches its definition.

1. A finger or toe:
   (a) digit
   (b) falanx
   (c) fusiform
   (d) degit

2. Lubricating fluid of joints:
   (a) apophysis
   (b) apophyis
   (c) synova
   (d) synovia

3. A tearing away forcibly of a part or structure:
   (a) avulsion
   (b) crepitus
   (c) avolsion
   (d) creitus

4. Abnormal, benign growth on the surface of a bone, also called *hyperostosis:*
   (a) ecchymosis
   (b) exostisis
   (c) echymosis
   (d) exostosis

5. Benign tumor composed mostly of fat cells:
   (a) lymphedema
   (b) lipoma
   (c) lipima
   (d) lymphodema

6. Affecting or relating to two sides:
   (a) bilateril
   (b) genu varum
   (c) bilateral
   (d) ganu varum

7. An outgrowth of bone that is usually found around a joint:
   (a) apophysis
   (b) ostophyte
   (c) osteophyte
   (d) appophysis

8. Any outgrowth or swelling; a process or projection of a bone:
   (a) apophysis
   (b) ostophyte
   (c) osteophyte
   (d) appophysis

9. Between two joints:
   (a) bilateral
   (b) bilateril
   (c) interarticuler
   (d) interarticular

10. Bowleg:
    (a) genu varum
    (b) gluteus medius
    (c) ganu varum
    (d) glutus medius

11. Commonly called a *bruise,* where there is trauma to the body part but there is no break in the skin surface:
    (a) contusion
    (b) volar
    (c) contrusion
    (d) volor

12. Containing pus:
    (a) pisiform
    (b) pesiform
    (c) purulence
    (d) prulence

PART I / CHECK YOUR PROGRESS continued

13. Black and blue appearance of the skin:
    (a) ecchymosis
    (b) exostisis
    (c) echymosis
    (d) exostosis

14. Draw in or out by suction:
    (a) turgor
    (b) asporate
    (c) turger
    (d) aspirate

15. Swelling due to obstruction of lymph vessels:
    (a) lymphedema
    (b) lipoma
    (c) lipima
    (d) lymphodema

16. Escape of fluid from rupture or seepage of blood vessels, usually into a body cavity:
    (a) crepitus
    (b) effussion
    (c) effusion
    (d) creptus

17. Examination of the interior of a joint with an arthroscope:
    (a) arthroscopy
    (b) hypertrophy
    (c) arthriscopy
    (d) hyprotrophy

18. General term for any bone of a finger or toe:
    (a) digit
    (b) falanx
    (c) phalanx
    (d) degit

19. Grating sound of bone fragments rubbing together:
    (a) crepitus
    (b) effussion
    (c) effusion
    (d) creptus

20. Increase in the size of an organ or structure:
    (a) greater trochanter
    (b) hypertrophy
    (c) greater trichanter
    (d) hyprotrophy

21. Large projection at the proximal end of the femur:
    (a) greater trochanter
    (b) hypertrophy
    (c) greater trichanter
    (d) hyprotrophy

22. Movement by a joint that decreases the angle between the two adjoining bones; the bending of a joint:
    (a) abduction
    (b) flixion
    (c) flexion
    (d) abuction

23. Movement of an extremity away from midline:
    (a) abuction
    (b) aduction
    (c) abduction
    (d) adduction

24. Movement of an extremity toward the midline:
    (a) abuction
    (b) aduction
    (c) abduction
    (d) adduction

25. New growth of bony tissue surrounding the bone ends in a fracture; part of the repair process of a fractured bone:
    (a) plantar
    (b) callus
    (c) planter
    (d) calus

PART I / CHECK YOUR PROGRESS *continued*

26. Normal resiliency of the skin:
    (a) turgor
    (b) trugor
    (c) volar
    (d) volor

27. One of the three muscles that form the buttocks; acts to abduct and rotate the thigh:
    (a) genu varum
    (b) gluteus medius
    (c) ganu varum
    (d) glutus medius

28. Pea-shaped; smallest carpal bone:
    (a) pisiform
    (b) pesiform
    (c) purulence
    (d) prulence

29. A spinous projection off the scapula:
    (a) acromon
    (b) faciculations
    (c) acromion
    (d) fasciculations

30. Pertaining to the palm of the hand or sole of the foot:
    (a) turgor
    (b) trugor
    (c) volar
    (d) volor

31. Reconstruction surgery to repair or reshape a diseased joint:
    (a) arthroscopy
    (b) arthriscropy
    (c) arthroplasty
    (d) arthroplasy

32. Relating to the sole of the foot:
    (a) plantar
    (b) callus
    (c) planter
    (d) calus

33. Situated or occurring between bone:
    (a) calcaneus
    (b) interosseous
    (c) clacaneus
    (d) intreosseous

34. Spindle shaped; structure that is tapered at both ends:
    (a) fusiform
    (b) fusform
    (c) pisiform
    (d) pesiform

35. Surgical removal of a meniscus:
    (a) menisectomy
    (b) mellelus
    (c) melleolus
    (d) meniscectomy

36. Symptoms of a specific disease:
    (a) asympmatic
    (b) symptomatology
    (c) symptomology
    (d) asymptomatic

37. To bend the joint toward the posterior aspect of the body:
    (a) dorsiflexion
    (b) flixion
    (c) abduction
    (d) dorsflexion

38. Uncontrolled twitching of a group of muscle fibers:
    (a) acromon
    (b) faciculations
    (c) acromion
    (d) fasciculations

39. Without symptoms:
    (a) asympmatic
    (b) symptomatology
    (c) symptomology
    (d) asymptomatic

PART I / CHECK YOUR PROGRESS *continued*

40. The muscles of the back of the neck and shoulder:
    (a) metatarsus
    (b) trapezius
    (c) trapezsus
    (d) metatarus

41. The disease of the lymph nodes:
    (a) lymphadenopathy
    (b) lymphenopathy
    (c) lymphedema
    (d) lymphodema

42. Crescent-shaped fibrocartilage in the knee joint:
    (a) meniscus
    (b) malelus
    (c) menscus
    (d) malleolus

43. The long, medial bone of the forearm:
    (a) radius
    (b) radious
    (c) ulna
    (d) unla

44. Any of the five long bones of the foot between the ankle and toes:
    (a) metatarsus
    (b) trapezius
    (c) trapezsus
    (d) metatarus

45. Either of the two rounded projections on either side of the ankle joint:
    (a) meniscus
    (b) malelus
    (c) menscus
    (d) malleolus

46. The heel bone or os calcis:
    (a) colcaneus
    (b) calcaneus
    (c) ulna
    (d) unla

47. Inflammation involving the folds of tissue surrounding the nail:
    (a) synovia
    (b) synomvia
    (c) parychia
    (d) paronychia

48. Trade name for a beta-adrenergic blocker:
    (a) Lopressor
    (b) Percocet
    (c) Lopresor
    (d) Percoset

49. Generic name for an antibiotic:
    (a) tetrasysline
    (b) spironolactone
    (c) spironlactone
    (d) tetracycline

50. Trade name for an opioid analgesic:
    (a) Lopressor
    (b) Percocet
    (c) Lopresor
    (d) Percoset

51. Trade name for an antihyperlipidemic:
    (a) Linoxin
    (b) Lipitor
    (c) Lanoxin
    (d) Lippitor

52. Trade name for an antiarrhythmic cardiotonic:
    (a) Linoxin
    (b) Lipitor
    (c) Lanoxin
    (d) Lippitor

PART I / CHECK YOUR PROGRESS *continued*

53. Generic name for a corticosteroid:
    (a) codeine
    (b) cortisone
    (c) codenine
    (d) cortisome

54. Generic name for an opioid analgesic:
    (a) codeine
    (b) cortisone
    (c) codenine
    (d) cortisome

55. Trade name for an antiarrhythmic; local anesthetic:
    (a) Xylocaine
    (b) Biaxin
    (c) Baixin
    (d) Xylacane

56. Generic name for a diuretic:
    (a) tetrasysline
    (b) spironolactone
    (c) spironlactone
    (d) tetracycline

57. Trade name for an antibiotic:
    (a) Xylocaine
    (b) Biaxin
    (c) Baixin
    (d) Xylacane

58. Trade name for a narcotic analgesic:
    (a) Keflex
    (b) Keplex
    (c) Vicoprofen
    (d) Vicoprophen

59. Trade name for an antibiotic:
    (a) Keflex
    (b) Keplex
    (c) Vicoprofen
    (d) Vicoprophen

60. Trade name for an anti-inflammatory:
    (a) Dolibid
    (b) Dolobid
    (c) Vicodin
    (d) Vicidin

61. Trade name for a narcotic analgesic:
    (a) Dolibid
    (b) Dolobid
    (c) Vicodin
    (d) Vicidin

62. Generic name for any of a large group of antibacterial antibiotics derived from the strains of fungi:
    (a) pencilin
    (b) pennicilin
    (c) penicilin
    (d) penicillin

Part II/Pretest (6T-2)

Textbook Users

Launch your word processing package.

Insert the appropriate audiocassette in your transcribing machine and find dictation *6T-2*.

On the open screen, transcribe and proofread dictation *6T-2*.

Identify and correct all errors.

Save your work on your student disk.

After completing the transcription, refer to the answer key.

Manually complete the error analysis chart.

If you score below 90%, continue on to *Activities 4 and 5: Proofreading Worksheet Exercises*.

If you score 90% or above, congratulations. If you wish, you can immediately move on to Part III.

Software Users

Click on *Chapter 6, Part II, Pretest (6T-2)*.

Insert the appropriate audiocassette tape in your transcribing machine and find dictation *6T-2*.

Click on *Start Watch*, then transcribe and proofread dictation *6T-2*. Identify and correct all errors.

When you are finished, click on *Done*, then *Save Document* to display your production for pay.

Click on *Display Error Analysis* to reveal your score.

Save your work (with errors showing) on your student disk by clicking on *File*, then *Save As*.

If you score below 90%, continue on to *Activities 4 and 5: Proofreading Worksheet Exercises*.

If you score 90% or above, congratulations. If you wish, you can immediately move on to Part III.

Activities 4–5

Proofreading Worksheet Exercises

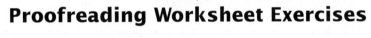

Textbook Users

Proofread and correct errors in the medical documents shown in *Activities 4–5*. Identify and correct all errors.

After completing the exercises, refer to the answer key.

Manually complete the error analysis chart for each document.

Software Users

Click on *Chapter 6, Part II, Activity 4*. Proofread and correct errors found in the medical document.

Click *File*, then *Done* and a pop-up window will appear.

Click on *Score Document* to reveal your score and on *View Errors* to see your errors.

Save your work (with errors showing) on your student disk by clicking on *File*, then *Save As*.

Click on *File*, then *Exit*, to proceed. Follow the same process to complete *Activity 5*.

PART II / ACTIVITY 4
PROOFREADING WORKSHEET EXERCISE

Directions: Proofread this medical document that contains multiple errors using full block, open punctuation, and all other formatting guidelines established in this textbook.

HITORY AND PHYSICAL EXAMINATION REPORT
Winster, Penny
File Number: 41390
Date of birth: March 17, 19xx
Examination Date: *current date*
James P. Osseous, MD
HISTORY:
HISTORY OF PRESENT ILLNESS: I had the pleasure of seeing Penny in the office today. This is a 43 year old right hand dominant woman who saw Dr.Zart for left rotator cuff tendinitis. She has impingment. A MRI shown acromial spur, no sign of a rotator cuff tear. He has an early syst formation. She has undergone two injections. The first did not help. The second seemed to help her for a few days. She has had physical therapy for three months.
PAST MEDICAL HISTORY: Significant for cardiac arhythmia.
MEDICATIONS: She is intermittently on Lopresor. She hasn't always been real compliant with that if she is not having any problems. Codine.
REVIEW OF SYMPTOMS: She denies liver or kidney disease. She has had an ulcer in the remote past. She has not had any problems with it recently.
FAMILY HISTORY: 1/2 pack per day smoker for fifteen years.
PHYSICAL EXAMINATION: On examination, this is a welldeveloped woman in no a cute distress. She has full pain less range of motion of her neck. Has has pain in the Neer and Hawkins impingments tests. Active adduction is 135 degrees. Forward flexion is 125 degrees. Passively, I could take her the rest of the way. Her strength is mildly diminished in external rotation, good in internal and abduction. She has a negative lift-off test. She is missing about two levels internal rotation up her back. She has pain with cross chest adduction. There is no pain at the SC or AC joint. No clavicular tenderness is noted. Neurovascularly, she is intact.

DIAGNOSTIC TESTS: I reviewed the MRI as above. We got an AP and outlet x-ray which shows a type III acronion.

PLAN: Penny has chronic impingment. We discussed the options. We are going to procede with arthoscopic subacromial decompresion. We discussed the surgery and the risks involved which she understands. All questions were answered and an instruction booklet given. We will schedule this in a timely fashion after appropriate postoperative testing.

_____

James P. Osseous, MD/xx D: 6/28/xx

PART II / ACTIVITY 5
PROOFREADING WORKSHEET EXERCISE

Directions: Proofread this medical document that contains multiple errors using full block, open punctuation, and all other formatting guidelines established in this textbook.

CHART NOTE
Lucy Smith
DOB: February 28, 19xx
Examination Date: *current date*

SUBJECTIVE: Lucy is an 84 year old female who falled directly onto her right hand yesterday.

OBJECTIVE: She suffered a wrist fracture. She is right hand dominant. He can move his fingers okay and has good perpheral circulation and sensation. There is considerable echymosis and a little bit of deformity of the wrist. X rays show a reversed Coles or Smith fracture.

ASSESSMENT: Reversed Coles fracture, left wrist.

PLAN: I have proceeded with reduction of the fracture with 1% Xylocane local anesthesia and have placed her in a sugar tong splint. Post reduction x-rays shows essentially an anatomic reduction. I am going to plan to keep her immobilized for six weeks. I will have her return to the office in one wk for an x-ray throught the cast.

_____

James P. Osseous, M.D

Part II / Activities 6–7
Proofreading Transcription Exercises (*6T-3, 6T-4*)

Now you are ready to make the transition from simply proofreading printed material to both transcribing and proofreading dictated material. This is the time to concentrate on building your medical vocabulary, which ultimately will improve your speed and accuracy. There are two activities in this section.

This learning activity is a two-step process for **Activity 6 (document 6T-3) only.**

Textbook Users

Step 1: Launch your word processing packages. Insert the appropriate audiocassette in your transcribing machine and find dictation *6T-3.* Listen to the entire dictation to gain an understanding of the medical concepts and terms involved in the report. Rewind the tape to the beginning of the dictation and transcribe what you hear. Do not worry about formatting, style, or speed. Simply type what you hear being dictated, using correct punctuation, capitalization, and spelling. Stop as needed to look up words you do not understand or cannot spell. Adjust the speed control of the transcriber to a comfortable level, starting slowly to assure no dictated words are missed, and then increase the speed as your accuracy improves.

Step 2: Rewind the tapes again, and using your created template, transcribe document *6T-3* again, including correct spacing and formatting. Proofread the report. Identify and correct all errors. Save your work on your student disk. Refer to the answer key and manually complete the error analysis and production for pay charts. Repeat the same process for dictation *6T-4.*

Software Users

Click on *Chapter 6, Activity 6, Proofreading Transcription Exercise.*
Insert the appropriate audiocassette in your transcribing machine and find dictation *6T-3.*

Step 1: Listen to the entire dictation to gain an understanding of the medical concepts and terms involved. Rewind the tape to the beginning of the dictation, click *Start Watch,* and transcribe what you hear. Do not worry about formatting, style, or speed. Simply type what you hear being dictated, using correct punctuation, capitalization, and spelling. Stop as needed to look up words you do not understand or cannot spell. Adjust the speed control of the transcriber to a comfortable level, starting slowly to assure no dictated words are missed, and then increase the speed as your accuracy improves. When you are finished, click on *Done,* then choose *Return to Main Menu.*

Step 2: Click on *Chapter 6, Activity 6* again. Rewind the tapes again, click on *Start Watch,* and transcribe dictation *6T-3* again, including correct spacing and formatting. Proofread the report. Identify and correct all errors. When you are finished, click on *Done,* then on *Score Document* to display your production for pay. Click on *Display Error Analysis* to reveal your score and *View Errors* to see your errors. Save your work (with errors showing) on your student disk by clicking on *File,* then *Save As.* Follow the same process for dictation *6T-4.*

Part II/Check Your Progress (6T-2)

Let's pause a minute and see how well you are doing. This section will allow you to evaluate your success at transcribing and proofreading orthopaedic reports.

Textbook Users

Launch your word processing package.

Insert the appropriate audiotape in your transcribing machine and find dictation *6T-2.*

On the open screen, transcribe and proofread dictation *6T-2.*

Use formatting guidelines established in Chapter 2. Save your work on your student disk.

Identify and correct all errors.

After completing the transcription, refer to the answer key.

Manually complete the error analysis and production for pay charts.

If you score below 90%, you are recommended to redo the Part II activities.

If you score 90% or above, congratulations. You can immediately move on to Part III.

Software Users

Click on *Chapter 6, Part II, Check Your Progress (6T-2).*

Insert the appropriate audiocassette in your transcribing machine and find dictation *6T-2.*

Click on *Start Watch,* then transcribe and proofread dictation *6T-2.*

Identify and correct all errors.

When you are finished, click on *Done,* then on *Score Document* to display your production for pay.

Click on *Display Error Analysis* to reveal your score.

Click on View Errors to see your errors.

Save your work (with errors showing) on your student disk by clicking on *File,* then *Save As.*

If you score below 90%, you are recommended to redo the Part II activities.

If you score 90% or above, congratulations. You can immediately move on to Part III.

Pretest (6T-5, 6T-6)

Professional transcriptionists can transcribe and proofread their own work. Can you? Scoring 90% or better proves it!

Textbook Users

Launch your word processing package.

Insert the appropriate audiocassette in your transcribing machine and find dictation *6T-5*.

On the open screen, transcribe and proofread dictation *6T-5*.

Identify and correct all errors.

Use formatting guidelines established in Chapter 2.

Save your work on your student disk.

Follow the same process for dictation *6T-6*.

After completing the transcription, refer to the answer key.

Manually complete the error analysis chart for each document.

Manually complete the production for pay summary chart for each document.

If you score below 90%, continue with *Orthopaedic Transcription at FedDes Wellness Center*.

If you score 90% or above, congratulations. If you wish, you can immediately move on to the next chapter.

Software Users

Click on *Chapter 6, Part III, Pretest (6T-5 and 6T-6)*.

Insert the appropriate audiocassette in your transcribing machine and find dictation *6T-5*.

Click on *Start Watch*, then transcribe and proofread dictation *6T-5*.

Identify and correct all errors.

When you are finished, click on *Done*, then on *Score Document:* a pop-up window will display your production for pay.

Click on *Display Error Analysis* to reveal your score.

Click on *View Errors* to see your errors.

Save your work (with errors showing) on your student disk by clicking on *File*, then *Save As*.

Follow the same process for dictation *6T-6*.

If you score below 90%, complete *Orthopaedic Transcription at FedDes Wellness Center*.

If you score 90% or above, congratulations. If you wish, you can immediately move on to the next chapter.

ORTHOPAEDIC TRANSCRIPTION AT FEDDES WELLNESS CENTER

You finally made it! You have been hired as a transcriptionist at FedDes Wellness Center in the orthopaedic division. Your supervisor has asked you to transcribe today's dictation.

Textbook Users

Launch your word processing package.

Insert the appropriate audiocassette in your transcribing machine and find dictation *6T-7.*

Create or use an existing template for the six types of reports: chart note, chart note using history and physical format, history and physical examination report, x-ray report, procedure report, and consultation letter.

On the open screen, transcribe and proofread dictation *6T-7.*

Identify and correct all errors.

Use formatting guidelines established in Chapter 2.

Save your work on your student disk.

Follow the same process for dictations *6T-8* through *6T-19.*

After completing the transcriptions, refer to the answer key.

Manually complete the error analysis chart for each document.

Manually complete the production for pay summary chart for each document.

Software Users

Click on *Chapter 6, Part III, Orthopaedic Transcription at FedDes Wellness Center (6T-7).*

Insert the appropriate audiocassette in your transcribing machine and find dictation *6T-7.*

Click on *Start Watch,* then transcribe and proofread dictation *6T-7.*

Identify and correct all errors.

When you are finished, click on *Done,* then on *Score Document:* a pop-up window will display your production for pay.

Click on *Display Error Analysis* to reveal your score.

Click on *View Errors* to see your errors.

Save your work (with errors showing) on your student disk by clicking on *File,* then *Save As.*

Follow the same process for dictations *6T-8* and *6T-9.*

NOTE: Continue with medical dictations *6T-10* through *6T-19* using your word processing package and manually complete the error analysis chart and production for pay summary sheet.

Index of Dictations and Associated Transcription Tips

Please remember to follow the guidelines pertaining to capitalization, numbers, punctuation, abbreviations, measurements, symbols, and use of templates to create medical reports at FedDes Wellness Center. Review of this material is found in Unit 1.

6T-7
X-ray Report
Patient's Name: Mary Ann Dubroy
Ordering Physician: Izzy Sertoli, MD
Physician: Harry A. Medulla, MD

● **TRANSCRIPTION TIP**
- A hyphen is used between numbers and *year old*.
  You will hear the dictator say: twenty one old female.
  You should transcribe as: 21-year-old female.

- Ordinal numbers first through ninth are spelled out: fifth metacarpal.

6T-8
Chart Note Using History and Physical Format
Patient's Name: Peter Hammer
Physician: James P. Osseous, MD

● **TRANSCRIPTION TIP**
- A hyphen is used when two or more words are viewed as a single word.
  You will hear the dictator say: Steri strips were removed.
  You should transcribe as: Steri-strips were removed.

- A hyphen is used to join two or more words when used as an adjective that proceeds a noun. The word pair is not hyphenated because the term is not used as an adjective: follow up.

- A hyphen is used between two "like" vowels: re-evaluation.

- Numbers one through ten are spelled out when they do not refer to technical items and the sentence does not contain numbers over ten.

You hear the dictator say: He started weightbearing approximately nine days ago and felt his cast was very loose.
You should transcribe this sentence as: He started weightbearing approximately nine days ago and felt his cast was very loose.

6T-9
X-ray Report
Patient's Name: Rachel Winterman
Ordering Physician: Charles P. Davis, MD
Physician: David Treppe, MD

6T-10
X-ray Report
Patient's Name: Lance Newhouse
Ordering Physician: P. H. Waters, MD
Physician: Harry A. Medulla, MD

● **TRANSCRIPTION TIP**
- The following abbreviation is dictated in this report:
  PIP joint: proximal interphalangeal joint, articulation between proximal and middle phalanx.

- Words beginning with *pre, re, post,* and *non* are generally not hyphenated: nondisplaced.

6T-11
Chart Note Using History and Physical Format
Patient's Name: Tommy Butger
Physician: David Treppe, MD

● **TRANSCRIPTION TIP**
- Words beginning with *pre, re, post,* and *non* are generally not hyphenated: nontender.

- The following term is transcribed as one word: weightbearing (supporting one's own weight).

6T-12
Chart Note Using History and Physical Format
Patient's Name: James Harris
Physician: David Treppe, MD

- A hyphen is used to join two or more words when it is used within an adjective clause that proceeds a noun. The following word pair is dictated in this report: eight-week.

- Figures are used for measurements and Latin terms.

- Figures are used in ranges and ratios.

- A hyphen is used to take the place of the word *to* or *through* to identify ranges.

- Remember that the figure and the word *degree* must remain on the same line of the chart note.
  You hear the dictator say: Dorsiflexion is ten to fifteen degrees with plantar flexion to twenty-five degrees.
  You should transcribe it as: Dorsiflexion is 10-15 degrees with plantar flexion to 25 degrees.

6T-13
Chart Note Using History and Physical Format
Patient's Name: Patricia Willis
Physician: James P. Osseous, MD

TRANSCRIPTION TIPS

- A hyphen is used with words beginning with *ex* and *self*: self-referred.

- The following new term is dictated in this report:
  Lipomatous (li-po-mah-tus): affected with or of the nature of lipoma

- The following acronym is dictated in this report. Remember that acronyms are typed in all capital letters.
  MRI: magnetic resonance imaging

6T-14
History and Physical Examination in Letter Format
Patient's Name: Juan Rodriquez
Physician: Harry A. Medulla, MD
Inside Address: John Mastersetti, MD, Pleasantville Family Health, 792 West Walnut Street, Westerville, OH 78910

TRANSCRIPTION TIP

- The following abbreviations are dictated in this report and are keyed in all capital letters:
  I&D: incision and drainage
  ER: emergency room
  DIP joint: distal interphalangeal joint, articulation between middle and distal phalanx

- A hyphen is used to join two or more words it is when used within an adjective clause that proceeds a noun. The following word pair is dictated in this report: right-hand.

- Latin abbreviations are expressed in lowercase letters with periods: p.o. (per os, by mouth).

- Capitalize the name of specific departments or sections in a hospital or institution.
  You will hear the dictator say: He was seen in the county hospital emergency room.
  You should transcribe this sentence as: He was seen in the County Hospital Emergency Room.

6T-15
Chart Note Using History and Physical Format
Patient's Name: William Grant
Physician: Harry A. Medulla, MD

TRANSCRIPTION TIP

- The following term is transcribed as two words: a lot.

- The following is a troublesome spelling term: posteromedial.

- The term *status post* means *after the condition* and may be abbreviated as *S/P.*

- The following abbreviation is dictated in this report:
  MCL: medial collateral ligament

- A hyphen is used between two "like" vowels: re-evaluation.

6T-16
Chart Note Using History and Physical Format
Patient's Name: John Phillips
Physician: Harry A. Medulla, MD

● **TRANSCRIPTION TIP**
- The following medication is dictated in this report:
  Vicodin: the brand name for the drug classification opioid analgesic

- The following acronym is dictated in this report. Remember that acronyms are typed in all capital letters.
  MRI: magnetic resonance imaging

- The following abbreviation is dictated in this report:
  AP: directional term for anterior to posterior

- A hyphen is used between two "like" vowels: re-evaluation.

6T-17
History and Physical Examination Report
Patient's Name: Sam Evertson
Physician: Harry A. Medulla, MD

● **TRANSCRIPTION TIP**
- The following are new terms:
  Radiation (ra-de-a-shun) is the process by which energy travels through space or matter. In clinical medicine, it often refers to the divergence of pain from the site of injury to other areas of the body.
  Impingement is an abnormal contact or pressure between two structures.

- Figures are used for age, weight, height, blood pressure, pulse, and respiration.
  You hear the dictator say: Blood pressure one hundred twelve over seventy-four pulse sixty-four and regular respirations sixteen per minute.
  You should transcribe it as: BP 112/74, pulse 64 and regular, respirations 16/min.

- The following abbreviation is dictated in this report.
  AC joint: acromioclavicular joint, articulation between acromion and clavicle

- A hyphen is used to join two or more words when used as an adjective that proceeds a noun. The following word pair is dictated in this report: three-month.

- The following drug is dictated in this report:
  Pencillin: the generic name for any of the large group of natural or semisynthetic antibacterial antibiotics

6T-18
History and Physical Examination Report
Patient's Name: Jerry Madison
Physicians: James P. Osseous, MD; Enrique Hernandez, MD

● **TRANSCRIPTION TIPS**
- A hyphen is used to join two or more words when used as an adjective that proceeds a noun. The following word pairs are dictated in this report: light-duty, two-week, follow-up.

- Capitalize eponyms. Eponyms are surnames teamed with a disease, instrument, or surgical procedure. The following eponym is dictated in this report: Achilles reflexes.

- An apostrophe is used to form the possessive of singular and plural nouns.
  You will hear the dictator say: I reviewed the patients x rays.
  You should transcribe it as: I reviewed the patient's x-rays.

- The following drugs are dictated in this report:
  Vicoprofen: the brand name for the drug classification opioid analgesic
  Dolobid: the brand name for a drug classified as an NSAID, a nonsteroidal anti-inflammatory drug

- Latin abbreviations are expressed in lowercase letters with periods: b.i.d. (bis in die, twice a day).

- Figures are used for measurements and Latin terms. No period follows metric abbreviations unless the abbreviation ends a sentence.

You hear the dictator say: I have changed his prescription to Dolobid five hundred milligrams to be taken on a b I d basis. You should transcribe it as: I have changed his prescription to Dolobid 500 mg to be taken on a b.i.d. basis.

- The following procedure is dictated in this report:
  Valsalva's maneuver (val-<u>sal</u>-vahz) is an attempt to forcibly exhale with the glottis, nose, and mouth closed.

- Figures are used with the + or − symbols.

- Reflexes are usually graded on a scale from zero to four plus as follows: 4+ is very brisk and may indicate disease; 3+ is brisker than average but not necessarily indicative of disease; 2+ is normal; 1+ is low normal; and 0 is no response and may indicate neuropathy.
  You hear the dictator say: He had two plus and symmetric patella as well as Achilles reflexes. You should transcribe it as: He had 2+ and symmetric patella as well as Archilles reflexes.

- Figures and capital letters are used to refer to the vertebral column and spinal nerves.
  You hear the dictator say: There is evidence of discogenic abnormality at L four through five. You should transcribe it as: There is evidence of discogenic abnormality at L4-5.

- If a sentence contains numbers under and over ten, use figures for all.
  You hear the dictator say: The patient smokes two packs per day and has done so for twenty-four years.
  You should transcribe it as: The patient smokes 2 packs per day and has done so for 24 years.

6T-19

History and Physical Examination Using Letter Format
Patient's Name: Clara B. Jackson
Physician: James P. Osseous, MD
Inside Address: Peter R. Desman, MD, Orange Hill Family Practice, 214 Orchard Road, Brooklyn, NY 11245

● **TRANSCRIPTION TIP**

- Figures are used for measurements and Latin terms. No period follows metric abbreviations unless the abbreviation ends a sentence: p.r.n. (pro re nata, as circumstances may require).

- A hyphen is used to join two or more words when used as an adjective that proceeds a noun. The following word pairs are dictated in this report: follow-up, work-up.

- The following procedure is dictated in this report.
  lupus test: a test to determine lupus vulgaris or lupus erythematosus

Part III / Check Your Progress

Professional transcriptionists can transcribe and proofread their own work with speed and accuracy. Have you mastered the orthopaedic transcription rotation at FedDes Wellness Center?

Textbook Users

Launch your word processing package.

Insert the appropriate audiocassette in your transcribing machine and find dictation *6T-5*.

On the open screen, transcribe and proofread dictation *6T-5*.

Identify and correct all errors.

Use formatting guidelines established in Chapter 2.

Save your work on your student disk.

Follow the same process for dictation *6T-6*.

After completing the transcriptions, refer to the answer key.

Manually complete the error analysis chart for each document.

Manually complete the production for pay summary chart for each document.

If you score below 90%, you are recommended to repeat Part III.

If you score 90% or above, congratulations. You have mastered the material presented in Part III.

Software Users

Click on *Chapter 6, Part III, Check Your Progress (6T-5)*.

Insert the appropriate audiocassette in your transcribing machine and find dictation *6T-5*.

Click on *Start Watch*, then transcribe and proofread dictation *6T-5*.

Identify and correct all errors.

When you are finished, click on *Done*, then *Score Document:* a pop-up window will display your production for pay.

Click on *Display Error Analysis* to reveal your score.

Click on *View Errors* to see your errors.

Save your work (with errors showing) on your student disk by clicking on *File*, then *Save As*.

Follow the same process for dictation *6T-6*.

If you score below 90%, you are recommended to repeat Part III.

If you score 90% or above, congratulations. You have mastered the material presented in Part III.

Chapter 7

Office Medical Transcription from the Urology Practice

OBJECTIVES

At the completion of Chapter 7, you should be able to do the following:

1. Match medical terms associated with the urology specialty with their definitions.

2. Spell medical terms associated with the urology specialty with their definitions.

3. Transcribe medical terms in sentence structure.

4. Proofread, edit, and correct medical documents associated with the urology specialty containing various errors.

5. Transcribe and proofread authentic medical documents associated with the urology specialty.

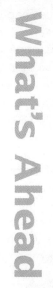

What's Ahead

173

The Urology Rotation

The FedDes Wellness Center has three urologists (specialists in urology) on staff. *Urology* is the study of the urinary tract in both women and men and the genital tract in men. The urologist treats male patients for problems with the urogenital system, which includes the male sexual organs.

In this unit, you assume the role of a medical transcriptionist employed at FedDes Wellness Center. **Please remember to follow the guidelines pertaining to capitalization, numbers, punctuation, abbreviations, measurements, symbols, and use of templates to create medical reports at FedDes Wellness Center.** Review of this material can be found in Unit 1. A list of the patient's name and the type of report as well as associated transcription tips are included in this chapter.

You will work with the textbook, CD-ROM, and accompanying audiocassettes. Your mastery of urology transcription is assessed through worksheets, timed transcription exercises, the error analysis chart, and the production for pay summary.

All answer keys are found in the textbook and CD-ROM, providing immediate feedback. After transcribing a report, you will proofread your work and correct any errors. Then you will compare your proofread work against a master transcript, categorize all errors, and tabulate the errors on the error analysis chart. The production for pay summary correlates your production to the FedDes Wellness Center pay scale, which is based on industry compensation standards. The scale is also linked to your grade. This system allows you to assess your mastery of transcription skills in a real-world scenario.

PART I ▪ GETTING CLOSE TO THE REAL THING

Pretest

Let's find out if you can define and spell selected terminology and drugs of the urology specialty that are included in this chapter by scoring 90% or better.

Textbook Users
Select the correctly spelled term that matches its definition.
Refer to the answer key for immediate feedback.
If you score below 90%, continue on to *Activities 1 through 3.*
If you score 90% or above, congratulations. You have mastered the material covered in Part I. If you wish, you can immediately move on to Part II.

Software Users
Click on *Chapter 7, Part I, Pretest.*
Key the correctly spelled term that matches its definition.
When you are finished, click on *End Test.*
A pop-up screen will reveal your score.
If you score below 90%, continue on to *Activities 1 through 3.*
If you score 90% or above, congratulations. You have mastered the material covered in Part I. If you wish, you can immediately move on to Part II.

PART I / PRETEST

Directions: Select the correctly spelled term that matches its definition.

1. Generic name for a bactericidal antibiotic:
   (a) bacitracin
   (b) bactracine
   (c) meclizine
   (d) mecizine

2. A colorless blood corpuscle:
   (a) occlude
   (b) oclude
   (c) leukocyte
   (d) leuocyte

3. A cystoscope that gives a wide-angle view of the bladder:
   (a) syncope
   (b) synscope
   (c) pandoscope
   (d) panendoscope

4. A discharge or escape of fluid from a vessel into the tissues:
   (a) extravasation
   (b) extrevasation
   (c) fulguration
   (d) fulgeration

5. Generic name for a diuretic, antihypertensive agent:
   (a) hydrochlorozide
   (b) hydrochlorothiazide
   (c) hydrocele
   (d) hydrosele

6. A diagnostic x-ray study of kidneys, ureter, and bladder:
   (a) nephrogram
   (b) nepherogram
   (c) urogram
   (d) urologram

7. A herniation of part of the rectum into the vagina:
   (a) cystocele
   (b) cystosele
   (c) rectosele
   (d) rectocele

8. A hollow or depressed area:
   (a) fossa
   (b) fosa
   (c) meatus
   (d) metus

9. A normal alkaline constituent of urine and blood:
   (a) creatinine
   (b) creatine
   (c) incontinence
   (d) incontinance

10. An accumulation of fluid in a sac-like cavity:
    (a) hydrosele
    (b) hydrocele
    (c) urethrosele
    (d) urethrocele

11. A radiograph of an artery:
    (a) arterogram
    (b) arterigram
    (c) arteriogram
    (d) arteiogram

12. A sac or pouch in the walls of a canal or organ:
    (a) verumontanum
    (b) verumonum
    (c) diverticulum
    (d) diverticum

PART I / PRETEST continued

13. A seam or ridge noting the line of junction of halves of a part:
    (a) coapte
    (b) coapt
    (c) rafe
    (d) raphe

14. A skin discoloration caused by a hemorrhage:
    (a) hydronephrosis
    (b) hydronphrosis
    (c) ecchymosis
    (d) echymosis

15. A small beam or supporting structure:
    (a) trabeculation
    (b) traculation
    (c) concomitant
    (d) concommitant

16. A triangular area:
    (a) staghorn
    (b) staghorne
    (c) trigon
    (d) trigone

17. Above the pubis:
    (a) periumbilical
    (b) supraumbilical
    (c) suprapubic
    (d) peripubic

18. An abnormal concretion, stone:
    (a) calculus
    (b) calcus
    (c) coudé
    (d) coudus'

19. Generic name for an angiotensin-converting enzyme inhibitor:
    (a) captopril
    (b) amoxicillin
    (c) catopril
    (d) amoxcillin

20. Generic name for an antibiotic:
    (a) captopril
    (b) amoxicillin
    (c) catopril
    (d) amoxcillin

21. Generic name for an antiemetic, antihistamine, motion sickness relief:
    (a) bacitracin
    (b) bactracine
    (c) meclizine
    (d) mecizine

22. An endoscope especially designed for passing through the urethra into the bladder:
    (a) cystoscope
    (b) cystourethroscope
    (c) cystscope
    (d) cystourescope

23. An incision of a duct or organ for the removal of calculi:
    (a) laminectomy
    (b) laminotomy
    (c) lithotomy
    (d) lithectomy

24. An instrument for examining the posterior urethra and bladder:
    (a) cystoscope
    (b) cystourethroscope
    (c) cystscope
    (d) cystourescope

25. An instrument placed in the vagina to support the uterus or rectum:
    (a) pessary
    (b) pesary
    (c) pissary
    (d) pisary

PART I / PRETEST *continued*

26. An opening:
    (a) fossa
    (b) fosa
    (c) meatus
    (d) metus

27. Around the umbilicus:
    (a) periumbilical
    (b) supraumbilical
    (c) suprapubic
    (d) peripubic

28. Bent or elbowed:
    (a) calculus
    (b) calcus
    (c) coude'
    (d) coudus'

29. Labored or difficult breathing:
    (a) dispneic
    (b) dyspneic
    (c) diuresis
    (d) dyuresis

30. Pertains to an atrium and the ventricle of the heart:
    (a) vas deferens
    (b) atriventricular
    (c) vas defens
    (d) atrioventricular

31. Pertains to the genitalia and urinary organs:
    (a) genitorinary
    (b) genitourinary
    (c) pyruia
    (d) pyuria

32. Pus in the urine:
    (a) genitorinary
    (b) genitourinary
    (c) pyruia
    (d) pyuria

33. Takes place at the same time:
    (a) trabeculation
    (b) traculation
    (c) concomitant
    (d) concommitant

34. A calculus of the renal pelvis usually extending into multiple calices:
    (a) staghorn
    (b) staghorne
    (c) trigon
    (d) trigone

35. The removal of the gallbladder:
    (a) cholecystectomy
    (b) cystometrography
    (c) chocystectomy
    (d) cystorography

36. The destruction of living tissue by electric sparks generated by a high-frequency current:
    (a) extravasation
    (b) extrevasation
    (c) fulguration
    (d) fulgeration

37. The discharge of blood in the urine:
    (a) heme
    (b) hematuria
    (c) heman
    (d) hemeturia

38. The distention of the renal pelvis and calices with urine:
    (a) hydronephrosis
    (b) hydronphrosis
    (c) ecchymosis
    (d) echymosis

PART I / PRETEST *continued*

39. The elevation on the floor of the prostatic portion of the urethra where the seminal ducts enter:
    (a) verumontanum
    (b) verumonum
    (c) diverticulum
    (d) diverticum

40. The essential elements of an organ:
    (a) perenchyma
    (b) parenchyma
    (c) bardycardia
    (d) bradycardia

41. To cut a portion of a tissue or organ:
    (a) flank
    (b) flanke
    (c) desect
    (d) resect

42. The excision of one or both ovaries:
    (a) oophorectomy
    (b) colporrhaphy
    (c) ophorectomy
    (d) colporhaphy

43. The excretory duct of the testis:
    (a) vas deferens
    (b) atriventricular
    (c) vas defens
    (d) atrioventricular

44. The x-ray study of the renal pelvis and uterus:
    (a) pyleogram
    (b) pylegram
    (c) cystorograph
    (d) cystumetrogram

45. The graphic record of the pressure in the bladder at varying stages of filling:
    (a) cholecystectomy
    (b) cystometrography
    (c) chocystectomy
    (d) urogram

46. The herniation of the urinary bladder into the vagina:
    (a) cystocele
    (b) cystosele
    (c) rectosele
    (d) rectocele

47. The inability to control excretory functions:
    (a) creatinine
    (b) creatine
    (c) incontinence
    (d) incontinance

48. An increased excretion of urine:
    (a) dispneic
    (b) dyspneic
    (c) diuresis
    (d) dyuresis

49. The inflammation of the gallbladder:
    (a) cystitis
    (b) cystisis
    (c) cholcystitis
    (d) cholecystitis

50. The inflammation of the kidney and renal pelvis:
    (a) urethrogonitis
    (b) urethrotrigonitis
    (c) pyelonephritis
    (d) pyelonphritis

51. The inflammation of the urethra and trigone of the bladder:
    (a) urethrogonitis
    (b) urethrotrigonitis
    (c) pyelonephritis
    (d) pyelonphritis

52. The inflammation of the urinary bladder:
    (a) cystitis
    (b) cystisis
    (c) cholcystitis
    (d) cholecystitis

PART I / PRETEST *continued*

53. The nonprotein, insoluble, iron constituent of hemoglobin:
    (a) heme
    (b) hematuria
    (c) heman
    (d) hemeturia

54. The penis:
    (a) fallus
    (b) fallis
    (c) phalus
    (d) phallus

55. The poisoning from retained and absorbed urinary substances:
    (a) urosepsis
    (b) urethrocele
    (c) urethepsis
    (d) urothcele

56. The prolapse of the female urethra through the urinary meatus:
    (a) urosepsis
    (b) urethrocele
    (c) urethepsis
    (d) urothcele

57. The side of the body between the ribs and ilium:
    (a) flank
    (b) flanke
    (c) desect
    (d) resect

58. The slowness of the heart beat:
    (a) perenchyma
    (b) parenchyma
    (c) bardycardia
    (d) bradycardia

59. The supply of vessels to a specific region:
    (a) vasculature
    (b) vaculature
    (c) nephrectomy
    (d) neprectomy

60. The surgical excision of the lamina:
    (a) laminectomy
    (b) laminotomy
    (c) lithotomy
    (d) lithectomy

61. The surgical removal of the kidney:
    (a) vasculature
    (b) vaculature
    (c) nephrectomy
    (d) neprectomy

62. The suture of the vagina:
    (a) oophorectomy
    (b) colporrhaphy
    (c) ophorectomy
    (d) colporhaphy

63. The temporary suspension of consciousness; fainting:
    (a) syncope
    (b) synscope
    (c) pandoscope
    (d) panendoscope

64. To bring together, as suturing a laceration:
    (a) coapte
    (b) coapt
    (c) rafe
    (d) raphe

65. To close tight:
    (a) occlude
    (b) oclude
    (c) leukocyte
    (d) leuocyte

PART I / PRETEST *continued*

66. Trade name for a diuretic:
    (a) Calen
    (b) Calan
    (c) Aldatone
    (d) Aldactone

67. Trade name for a diuretic, antiglaucoma agent:
    (a) Neptazane
    (b) Netazane
    (c) Noroxin
    (d) Norxin

68. Trade name for an antibacterial, urinary tract anti-infective:
    (a) Neptazane
    (b) Netazane
    (c) Noroxin
    (d) Norxin

69. Trade name for an antibacterial, antibiotic:
    (a) Maxquine
    (b) Maxaquin
    (c) Lopressor
    (d) Lopresor

70. Trade name for an antibacterial, antibiotic:
    (a) Ciprro
    (b) Cipro
    (c) Cardura
    (d) Carduro

71. Trade name for an antiarrhythmic, anesthetic:
    (a) Xylocine
    (b) Perpine
    (c) Propine
    (d) Xylocaine

72. Trade name for a nonsteroidal anti-inflammatory drug; analgesic for acute, moderately severe pain:
    (a) Toradol
    (b) Torodol
    (c) Tolinase
    (d) Tolenase

73. Trade name for a topical antiglaucoma agent:
    (a) Timoptic
    (b) Timptic
    (c) Trimpix
    (d) Trimpex

74. Trade name for an antianginal, antiarrhythmic, antihypertensive:
    (a) Calen
    (b) Calan
    (c) Aldatone
    (d) Aldactone

75. Trade name for an antianginal, antihypertensive:
    (a) Maxquine
    (b) Maxaquin
    (c) Lopressor
    (d) Lopresor

76. Trade name for an antidiarrheal:
    (a) Imadium
    (b) Imodium
    (c) Emadium
    (d) Emodium

77. Trade name for an antiglaucoma agent, eyedrops:
    (a) Xylocine
    (b) Perpine
    (c) Propine
    (d) Xylocaine

78. Trade name for an antihypertensive, antiadrenergic:
    (a) Ciprro
    (b) Cipro
    (c) Cardura
    (d) Carduro

PART I / PRETEST *continued*

79. Trade name for an antibacterial, antibiotic:
    (a) Timoptic
    (b) Timptic
    (c) Trimpix
    (d) Trimpex

80. Trade name for an antibiotic:
    (a) Bactrim
    (b) Betadine
    (c) Backrim
    (d) Betdine

81. Trade name for a topical antibacterial, antiseptic:
    (a) Bactrim
    (b) Betadine
    (c) Backrim
    (d) Betdine

82. Trade name for an antidiabetic agent:
    (a) Toradol
    (b) Torodol
    (c) Tolinase
    (d) Tolenase

Part I / Activity 1
Keyboarding Medical Terms and Definitions

Let's learn to spell and define selected terminology and drugs of the urology specialty that are included in this chapter. Keyboarding these terms is an innovative and fun way to improve your skills.

Textbook Users
Launch your word processing package.
On the open screen, read and type each word and its definition as shown below.
Save your work on your student disk.

1. Amoxicillin (ah-moks-I-<u>sil</u>-in) is a generic name for an antibiotic.
2. Arteriogram (ar-<u>te</u>-re-o-gram) is a radiograph of an artery.
3. Atrioventricular (a-tre-o-ven-<u>trik</u>-I-lar) pertains to the atrium and the ventricle of the heart.
4. Bacitracin (bas-I-<u>tra</u>-sin) is a generic name for an antibacterial.
5. Bradycardia (brad-e-<u>kar</u>-de-ah) is the slowness of the heart beat.
6. Calculus (<u>kal</u>-ku-lus) is an abnormal concretion, stone.

7. Captopril (<u>kap</u>-to-pril) is a generic name for an angiotensin-converting enzyme inhibitor.
8. Cholecystectomy (ko-le-sis-<u>tos</u>-to-me) is the removal of the gallbladder.
9. Cholecystitis (ko-le-sis-<u>ti</u>-tis) is the inflammation of the gallbladder.
10. Coapt (ko-<u>apt</u>) is to bring together, as suturing a laceration.
11. Colporrhaphy (kol-<u>por</u>-ah-fe) is the suture of the vagina.
12. Concomitant (kon-<u>kom</u>-I-tant) takes place at the same time.

13. Coudé (koo-dae) is bent or elbowed.
14. Creatinine (kre-at-I-nin) is a normal alkaline constituent of urine and blood.
15. Cystitis (sis-ti-tis) is the inflammation of the urinary bladder.
16. Cystocele (sis-to-sel) is the herniation of the urinary bladder into the vagina.
17. Cystometrography (sis-to-me-trog-ra-fe) is the graphic record of the pressure in the bladder at varying stages of filling.
18. Cystoscope (sis-to-skop) is an endoscope especially designed to permit visual inspection of the interior of the bladder.
19. Cystourethroscope (sis-to-u-re-thro-skop) is an instrument for examining the posterior urethra and bladder.
20. Diuresis (di-u-re-sis) is an increased excretion of urine.
21. Diverticulum (di-ver-tik-u-lum) is a sac or pouch in the walls of a canal or organ.
22. Dyspneic (disp-ne-ah) is labored or difficult breathing.
23. Ecchymosis (ek-I-mo-sis) is a skin discoloration caused by a hemorrhage.
24. Extravasation (eks-trav-ah-za-shun) is a discharge or escape of fluid from a vessel into the tissues.
25. Flank (flangk) is the side of the body between the ribs and ilium.
26. Fossa (fos-ah) is a hollow or depressed area.
27. Fulguration (ful-gu-ra-shun) is the destruction of living tissue by electric sparks generated by a high-frequency current.
28. Genitourinary (jen-I-to-u-ri-ner-e) pertains to the genitalia and urinary organs.
29. Hematuria (hem-ah-tu-re-ah) is the discharge of blood in the urine.
30. Heme (hem) is the nonprotein, insoluble, iron constituent of hemoglobin.
31. Hydrocele (hi-dro-sel) is the accumulation of fluid in a sac-like cavity.
32. Hydrochlorothiazide (hi-dro-klor-o-thi-ah-zid) is a generic name for a diuretic, antihypertensive agent.
33. Hydronephrosis (hi-dro-ne-fro-sis) is the distention of the renal pelvis and calices with urine.
34. Incontinence (in-kon-ti-nens) is the inability to control excretory functions.
35. Laminectomy (lam-I-nek-to-me) is the surgical excision of the lamina.
36. Leukocytes (loo-ko-sit) is a colorless blood corpuscle.
37. Lithotomy (li-thot-o-me) is an incision of a duct or organ for the removal of calculi.
38. Meatus (me-a-tus) is an opening.
39. Meclizine (mek-li-zen) is a generic name for an antiemetic, antihistamine, motion sickness relief.
40. Nephrectomy (ne-frek-to-me) is the surgical removal of the kidney.
41. Occlude (o-klood) is to close tight.
42. Oophorectomy (o-of-o-rek-to-me) is the excision of one or both ovaries.
43. Panendoscope (pan-en-do-skop) is a cystoscope that gives a wide-angle view of the bladder.
44. Parenchyma (pah-reng-ki-mah) are the essential elements of an organ.
45. Periumbilical (per-e-um-bil-I-kal) is around the umbilicus.
46. Pessary (pes-ah-re) is an instrument placed in the vagina to support the uterus or rectum.
47. Phallus (fal-us) is the penis.
48. Pyelogram (pi-e-lo-gram) is a x-ray study of the renal pelvis and uterus.
49. Pyelonephritis (pi-e-lo-ne-fri-tis) is the inflammation of the kidney and renal pelvis.
50. Pyuria (pi-u-re-ah) is pus in the urine.
51. Raphe (ra-fe) is a seam or ridge noting the line of junction of halves of a part.
52. Rectocele (rek-to-sel) is a hernia protrusion of part of the rectum into the vagina.
53. Resect (re-sekt) is to cut off or cut out a portion of a tissue or organ.
54. Staghorn (stag-horn) is the calculus of the renal pelvis usually extending into multiple calices.
55. Suprapubic (soo-prah-pu-bik) is above the pubis.
56. Syncope (sing-ko-pe) is the temporary suspension of consciousness; fainting.
57. Trabeculation (trah-bek-u-lah) is a small beam or supporting structure.
58. Trigone (tri-gon) is a triangular area.
59. Urethrocele (u-re-thro-sel) is the prolapse of the female urethra through the urinary meatus.

60. Urethrotrigonitis (u-re-thro-tri-go-<u>ni</u>-tis) is the inflammation of the urethra and trigone of the bladder.
61. Urogram (<u>u</u>-ro-gram) is a diagnostic x-ray study of the kidneys, ureter, and bladder.
62. Urosepsis (u-ro-<u>sep</u>-sis) is the poisoning from retained and absorbed urinary substances.
63. Vas deferens (vas <u>def</u>-er-ens) is the excretory duct of the testis.
64. Vasculature (<u>vas</u>-ku-lah-tur) is the supply of vessels to a specific region.
65. Verumontanum (ver-oo-mon-<u>ta</u>-num) is the elevation on the floor of the prostatic portion of the urethra where the seminal ducts enter.
66. Aldactone (al <u>dak</u>-ton) is the trade name for a diuretic.
67. Bactrim (bak-trim) is the trade name for an antibiotic.
68. Betadine (<u>bat</u>-ah-den) is the trade name for a topical antibacterial, antiseptic.
69. Calan (<u>kal</u>-an) is the trade name for an antianginal, antiarrhythmic, antihypertensive.
70. Cardura (<u>kar</u>-du-rah) is the trade name for an antihypertensive, antiadrenergic.
71. Cipro (<u>si</u>-pro) is the trade name for a fluoroquinolone antibiotic, antibacterial drug.
72. Imodium (I-mo-<u>de</u>-um) is the trade name for an antidiarrheal.
73. Lopressor (lo-<u>pres</u>-or) is the trade name for an antianginal, antihypertensive.
74. Maxaquin (mak-<u>sa</u>-kwin) is the trade name for a fluoroquinolone antibiotic, antibacterial.
75. Neptazane (nep-<u>ta</u>-zan) is the trade name for a diuretic, antiglaucoma agent.
76. Noroxin (<u>nor</u>-o-sin) is the trade name for an antibacterial, urinary tract anti-infective.
77. Propine (<u>pro</u>-pine) is the trade name for an antiglaucoma agent, eyedrops.
78. Timoptic (tim-<u>op</u>-tik) is the trade name for a topical antiglaucoma agent.
79. Tolinase (<u>tol</u>-I-nas) is the trade name for an antidiabetic agent.
80. Toradol (<u>tor</u>-a-dol) is the trade name for a nonsteroidal anti-inflammatory drug; analgesic for acute, moderately severe pain.
81. Trimpex (tri-<u>mip</u>-eks) is the trade name for an antibacterial, antibiotic.
82. Xylocaine (zi-<u>lo</u>-kan) is the trade name for an anesthetic, antiarrhythmic.

Part I / Activity 2
Spelling Medical Terms

Do you remember back in school when you had to write each spelling word ten times? Because you had to physically write each word, your mind and body were focused on the assignment and the method worked! Let's follow this successful method by reinforcing the spelling of selected terms and drugs found in the urology specialty through keyboarding drills.

Textbook and Software Users
Launch your word processing package.
On the open screen, read, mentally spell, and type each word in its sequence.
Save your work on your student disk.

1. amoxicillin arteriogram atrioventricular amoxicillin arteriogram atrioventricular
2. bacitracin bradycardia calculus bacitracin bradycardia calculus bacitracin bradycardia
3. captopril cholecystectomy cholecystitis captopril cholecystectomy cholecystitis
4. coapt colporrhaphy concomitant coapt colporrhaphy concomitant coapt colporrhaphy
5. coude creatinine cystitis coude creatinine cystitis coude creatinine cystitis coude
6. cystocele cystometrography cystoscope cystocele cystometrography cystoscope
7. cystourethroscope diuresis diverticulum cystourethroscope diuresis diverticulum
8. dyspneic ecchymosis extravasation dyspneic ecchymosis extravasation dyspneic
9. flank fossa fulguration flank fossa fulguration flank fossa fulguration flank fossa
10. genitourinary hematuria heme genitourinary hematuria heme genitourinary hematuria
11. hydrocele hydrochlorothiazide hydronephrosis hydrocele hydrochlorothiazide
12. incontinence laminectomy leukocytes incontinence laminectomy leukocytes
13. lithotomy meatus meclizine lithotomy meatus meclizine lithotomy meatus meclizine
14. nephrectomy occlude oophorectomy nephrectomy occlude oophorectomy occlude

15. panendoscope parenchyma periumbilical panendoscope parenchyma periumbilical
16. pessary phallus pyelogram pessary phallus pyelogram pessary phallus pyelogram
17. pyelonephritis pyuria raphe pyelonephritis pyuria raphe pyelonephritis pyuria raphe
18. rectocele resect staghorn rectocele resect staghorn rectocele resect staghorn rectocele
19. suprapubic syncope trabeculation suprapubic syncope trabeculation suprapubic
20. trigone urethrocele urethrotrigonitis trigone urethrocele urethrotrigonitis trigone
21. urogram urosepsis vas deferens urogram urosepsis vas deferens urogram urosepsis
22. vasculature verumontanum vasculature verumontanum vasculature verumontanum
23. Aldactone Bactrim Betadine Aldactone Bactrim Betadine Aldactone Bactrim
24. Calan Cardura Cipro Calan Cardura Cipro Calan Cardura Cipro Calan Cardura Cipro
25. Imodium Lopressor Maxaquin Imodium Lopressor Maxaquin Imodium Lopressor
26. Neptazane Noroxin Propine Neptazane Noroxin Propine Neptazane Noroxin Propine
27. Timoptic Tolinase Toradol Timoptic Tolinase Toradol Timoptic Tolinase Toradol
28. Trimpex Xylocaine Trimpex Xylocaine Trimpex Xylocaine Trimpex Xylocaine

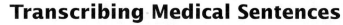

Part I / Activity 3
Transcribing Medical Sentences

Now you are ready to make the transition from keyboarding medical terms, which is a visual process, to transcribing medical terms, an aural process. You are going to use audiocassette tapes rather than printed material.

Textbook Users
Insert the appropriate audiocassette in your transcribing machine and find dictation *7T-1*.
You will be transcribing spelling words in sentence structure.
Launch your word processing software.
Listen carefully to each sentence on the audiocassette before transcribing.
Rewind and type (transcribe) the sentences.
Save your work on your student disk.
Refer to the answer key.

Part I / Check Your Progress

Let's pause a minute and see how well you are doing. This section will allow you to evaluate your mastery of keyboarding and spelling selected terms and drugs found in the urology specialty.

Textbook Users
Select the correctly spelled term that matches its definition.
Refer to the answer key for immediate feedback.
If you score below 90%, you are recommended to redo the Part I Activities.
If you score 90% or above, congratulations. You have mastered the material covered in Part I. You can immediately move on to Part II.

Software Users
Click on *Chapter 7, Part I, Check Your Progress*.
Key the correctly spelled term that matches its definition.
When you are finished, click on *End Test*.
A pop-up screen will reveal your score.
If you score below 90%, you are recommended to redo the Part I Activities.
If you score 90% or above, congratulations. You have mastered the material covered in Part I. You can immediately move on to Part II.

PART I / CHECK YOUR PROGRESS

Directions: Select the correctly spelled term that matches its definition.

1. Generic name for a bactericidal antibiotic:
   (a) bacitracin
   (b) bactracine
   (c) meclizine
   (d) mecizine

2. A colorless blood corpuscle:
   (a) occlude
   (b) oclude
   (c) leukocyte
   (d) leuocyte

3. A cystoscope that gives a wide-angle view of the bladder:
   (a) syncope
   (b) synscope
   (c) pandoscope
   (d) panendoscope

4. A discharge or escape of fluid from a vessel into the tissues:
   (a) extravasation
   (b) extrevasation
   (c) fulguration
   (d) fulgeration

5. Generic name for a diuretic, antihypertensive agent:
   (a) hydrochlorozide
   (b) hydrochlorothiazide
   (c) hydrocele
   (d) hydrosele

6. A diagnostic x-ray study of kidneys, ureter, and bladder:
   (a) nephrogram
   (b) nepherogram
   (c) urogram
   (d) urologram

7. A hernia protrusion of part of the rectum into the vagina:
   (a) cystocele
   (b) cystosele
   (c) rectosele
   (d) rectocele

8. A hollow or depressed area:
   (a) fossa
   (b) fosa
   (c) meatus
   (d) metus

9. A normal alkaline constituent of urine and blood:
   (a) creatinine
   (b) creatine
   (c) incontinence
   (d) incontinance

10. An accumulation of fluid in a sac-like cavity:
    (a) hydrosele
    (b) hydrocele
    (c) urethrosele
    (d) urethrocele

11. A radiograph of an artery:
    (a) arterogram
    (b) arterigram
    (c) arteriogram
    (d) arteiogram

12. A sac or pouch in the walls of a canal or organ:
    (a) verumontanum
    (b) verumonum
    (c) diverticulum
    (d) diverticum

PART I / CHECK YOUR PROGRESS *continued*

13. A seam or ridge noting the line of junction of halves of a part:
    (a) coapte
    (b) coapt
    (c) rafe
    (d) raphe

14. A skin discoloration caused by a hemorrhage:
    (a) hydronephrosis
    (b) hydronphrosis
    (c) ecchymosis
    (d) echymosis

15. A small beam or supporting structure:
    (a) trabeculation
    (b) traculation
    (c) concomitant
    (d) concommitant

16. A triangular area:
    (a) staghorn
    (b) staghorne
    (c) trigon
    (d) trigone

17. Above the pubis:
    (a) periumbilical
    (b) supraumbilical
    (c) suprapubic
    (d) peripubic

18. An abnormal concretion, stone:
    (a) calculus
    (b) calcus
    (c) coudé
    (d) coudus'

19. Generic name for an angiotensin-converting enzyme inhibitor:
    (a) captopril
    (b) amoxicillin
    (c) catopril
    (d) amoxcillin

20. Generic name for an antibiotic:
    (a) captopril
    (b) amoxicillin
    (c) catopril
    (d) amoxcillin

21. Generic name for an antiemetic, antihistamine, motion sickness relief:
    (a) bacitracin
    (b) bactracine
    (c) meclizine
    (d) mecizine

22. An endoscope especially designed for passing through the urethra into the bladder:
    (a) cystoscope
    (b) cystourethroscope
    (c) cystscope
    (d) cystourescope

23. An incision of a duct or organ for the removal of calculi:
    (a) laminectomy
    (b) laminotomy
    (c) lithotomy
    (d) lithectomy

24. An instrument for examining the posterior urethra and bladder:
    (a) cystoscope
    (b) cystourethroscope
    (c) cystscope
    (d) cystourescope

25. An instrument placed in the vagina to support the uterus or rectum:
    (a) pessary
    (b) pesary
    (c) pissary
    (d) pisary

PART I / CHECK YOUR PROGRESS *continued*

26. An opening:
    (a) fossa
    (b) fosa
    (c) meatus
    (d) metus

27. Around the umbilicus:
    (a) periumbilical
    (b) supraumbilical
    (c) suprapubic
    (d) peripubic

28. Bent or elbowed:
    (a) calculus
    (b) calcus
    (c) coudé
    (d) coudus'

29. Labored or difficult breathing:
    (a) dispneic
    (b) dyspneic
    (c) diuresis
    (d) dyuresis

30. Pertains to an atrium and the ventricle of the heart:
    (a) vas deferens
    (b) atriventricular
    (c) vas defens
    (d) atrioventricular

31. Pertains to the genitalia and urinary organs:
    (a) genitorinary
    (b) genitourinary
    (c) pyruia
    (d) pyuria

32. Pus in the urine:
    (a) genitorinary
    (b) genitourinary
    (c) pyruia
    (d) pyuria

33. Takes place at the same time.
    (a) trabeculation
    (b) traculation
    (c) concomitant
    (d) concommitant

34. A calculus of the renal pelvis usually extending into multiple calices:
    (a) staghorn
    (b) staghorne
    (c) trigon
    (d) trigone

35. The removal of the gallbladder:
    (a) cholecystectomy
    (b) cystometrography
    (c) chocystectomy
    (d) cystorography

36. The destruction of living tissue by electric sparks generated by a high-frequency current:
    (a) extravasation
    (b) extrevasation
    (c) fulguration
    (d) fulgeration

37. The discharge of blood in the urine:
    (a) heme
    (b) hematuria
    (c) heman
    (d) hemeturia

38. The distention of the renal pelvis and calices with urine:
    (a) hydronephrosis
    (b) hydronphrosis
    (c) ecchymosis
    (d) echymosis

PART I / CHECK YOUR PROGRESS *continued*

39. The elevation on the floor of the prostatic portion of the urethra where the seminal ducts enter.
    (a) verumontanum
    (b) verumonum
    (c) diverticulum
    (d) diverticum

40. The essential elements of an organ:
    (a) perenchyma
    (b) parenchyma
    (c) bardycardia
    (d) bradycardia

41. To cut a portion of a tissue or organ:
    (a) flank
    (b) flanke
    (c) desect
    (d) resect

42. The excision of one or both ovaries:
    (a) oophorectomy
    (b) colporrhaphy
    (c) ophorectomy
    (d) colporhaphy

43. The excretory duct of the testis:
    (a) vas deferens
    (b) atriventricular
    (c) vas defens
    (d) atrioventricular

44. X-ray study of the renal pelvis and ureter:
    (a) pyelogram
    (b) pyleogram
    (c) urogram
    (d) urologram

45. The graphic record of the pressure in the bladder at varying stages of filling:
    (a) cholecystectomy
    (b) cystometrography
    (c) chocystectomy
    (d) cystorography

46. The herniation of the urinary bladder into the vagina:
    (a) cystocele
    (b) cystosele
    (c) rectosele
    (d) rectocele

47. The inability to control excretory functions:
    (a) creatinine
    (b) creatine
    (c) incontinence
    (d) incontinance

48. An increased excretion of urine:
    (a) dispneic
    (b) dyspneic
    (c) diuresis
    (d) dyuresis

49. The inflammation of the gallbladder:
    (a) cystitis
    (b) cystisis
    (c) cholcystitis
    (d) cholecystitis

50. The inflammation of the kidney and renal pelvis:
    (a) urethrogonitis
    (b) urethrotrigonitis
    (c) pyelonephritis
    (d) pyelonphritis

51. The inflammation of the urethra and trigone of the bladder:
    (a) urethrogonitis
    (b) urethrotrigonitis
    (c) pyelonephritis
    (d) pyelonphritis

52. The inflammation of the urinary bladder:
    (a) cystitis
    (b) cystisis
    (c) cholcystitis
    (d) cholecystitis

PART I / CHECK YOUR PROGRESS *continued*

53. The nonprotein, insoluble, iron constituent of hemoglobin:
    (a) heme
    (b) hematuria
    (c) heman
    (d) hemeturia

54. The penis:
    (a) fallus
    (b) fallis
    (c) phalus
    (d) phallus

55. The poisoning from retained and absorbed urinary substances:
    (a) urosepsis
    (b) urethrocele
    (c) urethepsis
    (d) urothcele

56. The prolapse of the female urethra through the urinary meatus:
    (a) urosepsis
    (b) urethrocele
    (c) urethepsis
    (d) urothcele

57. The area between the ribs and ilium:
    (a) flank
    (b) flanke
    (c) desect
    (d) resect

58. The slowness of the heart beat:
    (a) perenchyma
    (b) parenchyma
    (c) bardycardia
    (d) bradycardia

59. The supply of vessels to a specific region:
    (a) vasculature
    (b) vaculature
    (c) nephrectomy
    (d) neprectomy

60. The surgical excision of the lamina:
    (a) laminectomy
    (b) laminotomy
    (c) lithotomy
    (d) lithectomy

61. The surgical removal of the kidney:
    (a) vasculature
    (b) vaculature
    (c) nephrectomy
    (d) neprectomy

62. The suture of the vagina:
    (a) oophorectomy
    (b) colporrhaphy
    (c) ophorectomy
    (d) colporhaphy

63. The temporary suspension of consciousness; fainting:
    (a) syncope
    (b) synscope
    (c) pandoscope
    (d) panendoscope

64. To bring together, as suturing a laceration:
    (a) coapte
    (b) coapt
    (c) rafe
    (d) raphe

65. To close tight:
    (a) occlude
    (b) oclude
    (c) leukocyte
    (d) leuocyte

66. Trade name for a diuretic:
    (a) Calen
    (b) Calan
    (c) Aldatone
    (d) Aldactone

PART I / CHECK YOUR PROGRESS *continued*

67. Trade name for a diuretic, antiglaucoma agent:
    (a) Neptazane
    (b) Netazane
    (c) Noroxin
    (d) Norxin

68. Trade name for an antibacterial, urinary tract anti-infective:
    (a) Neptazane
    (b) Netazane
    (c) Noroxin
    (d) Norxin

69. Trade name for a fluoroquinolone antibiotic, antibacterial:
    (a) Maxquine
    (b) Maxaquin
    (c) Lopressor
    (d) Lopresor

70. Trade name for a fluoroquinolone antibiotic, antibacterial drug:
    (a) Ciprro
    (b) Cipro
    (c) Cardura
    (d) Carduro

71. Trade name for an anesthetic, antiarrhythmic:
    (a) Xylocine
    (b) Perpine
    (c) Propine
    (d) Xylocaine

72. Trade name for a nonsteroidal anti-inflammatory drug; analgesic for acute, moderately severe pain:
    (a) Toradol
    (b) Torodol
    (c) Tolinase
    (d) Tolenase

73. Trade name for a topical antiglaucoma agent:
    (a) Timoptic
    (b) Timptic
    (c) Trimpix
    (d) Trimpex

74. Trade name for an antianginal, antiarrhythmic, antihypertensive:
    (a) Calen
    (b) Calan
    (c) Aldatone
    (d) Aldactone

75. Trade name for an antianginal, antihypertensive:
    (a) Maxquine
    (b) Maxaquin
    (c) Lopressor
    (d) Lopresor

76. Trade name for an antidiarrheal:
    (a) Imadium
    (b) Imodium
    (c) Emadium
    (d) Emodium

77. Trade name for an antiglaucoma agent, eyedrops:
    (a) Xylocine
    (b) Perpine
    (c) Propine
    (d) Xylocaine

78. Trade name for an antihypertensive, antiadrenergic:
    (a) Ciprro
    (b) Cipro
    (c) Cardura
    (d) Carduro

PART I / CHECK YOUR PROGRESS *continued*

79. Trade name for an antibacterial, antibiotic:
    (a) Timoptic
    (b) Timptic
    (c) Trimpix
    (d) Trimpex

80. Trade name for an antibiotic:
    (a) Bactrim
    (b) Betadine
    (c) Backrim
    (d) Betdine

81. Trade name for a topical antibacterial, antiseptic:
    (a) Bactrim
    (b) Betadine
    (c) Backrim
    (d) Betdine

82. Trade name for an antidiabetic agent:
    (a) Toradol
    (b) Torodol
    (c) Tolinase
    (d) Tolenase

Pretest (7T-2)

Professional transcriptionists proofread their own work. Can you? Scoring 90% or better proves it!

Textbook Users

Launch your word processing package.

Insert the appropriate audiocassette in your transcribing machine and find dictation *7T-2.*

On the open screen, transcribe and proofread dictation *7T-2.*

Identify and correct all errors.

Use formatting guidelines established in Chapter 2.

Save your work on your student disk.

After completing the transcription, refer to the answer key.

Manually complete the error analysis chart.

Manually complete the production for pay summary chart.

If you score below 90%, continue on to *Activities 4 through 5: Proofreading Worksheet Exercises* as well as *Activities 6 through 7: Proofreading Transcription Exercises.*

If you score 90% or above, congratulations. You have mastered the material covered in Part II. If you wish, you can immediately move on to Part III.

Software Users

Click on *Chapter 7, Part II, Pretest (7T-2).*

Insert the appropriate audiocassette in your transcribing machine and find dictation *7T-2.*

Click on *Start Watch,* then transcribe and proofread dictation *7T-2.*

Identify and correct all errors.

When you are finished, click on *Done,* then on *Score Document;* a pop-up window will display your production for pay.

Click on *Display Error Analysis* to reveal your score.

Click on *View Errors* to see your errors.

Save your work (with errors showing) on your student disk by clicking on *File,* then *Save As.*

If you score below 90%, continue on to *Activities 4 through 5: Proofreading Worksheet Exercises* as well as *Activities 6 through 7: Proofreading Transcription Exercises.*

If you score 90% or above, congratulations. You have mastered the material covered in Part II. If you wish, you can immediately move on to Part III.

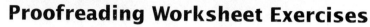

Part II / Activities 4–5
Proofreading Worksheet Exercises

Finding your own errors and correcting them is not easy, but it is an essential skill for your success as a medical transcriptionist. The worksheets in this activity will help you develop your proofreading skills.

Textbook Users

Proofread and correct errors in the medical documents shown in *Activities 4 through 5*.
After completing the exercises, refer to the answer key.
Manually complete the error analysis chart for each document.

Software Users

Click on *Chapter 7, Part II, Activity 4.*
Proofread and correct errors found in the medical document.
Click on *File*, the *Done*, and a pop-up window will appear.
Click on *Score Document* to reveal your score.
Click on *View Errors* to see your errors.
Save your work (with errors showing) on your student disk by clicking on *File*, then *Save As*.
Click on *File*, then *Exit*, to proceed.
Follow the same process to complete *Activity 5*.

PART II / ACTIVITY 4
PROOFREADING WORKSHEET EXERCISE

Directions: Proofread this medical document that contains multiple errors using full block, open punctuation, and all other formatting guidelines established in this textbook.

CONSULTATION REPORT

Patient Name: Barnes, Franklyn

File Number: 003416

Date of Birth: February 13, 19xx

Examination Date: *current date*

Requesting Physician: Izzy Sertoli, MD

HISTORY OF PRESENT ILLNESS: This 22 year old gentleman fell approximately twenty seven ft off a scaffold. He landed on a stack of concete blocks, and sustained a abrasion of his right flank. The patient informs me that he did not have much pain immediately after the fall and therefore did not come to see you for evaluation until later in the day. A urine analyses performed in your office showed 20-50 rbc's. Due to your concern about fight flank trauma I was asked to evaluate the patient.

The patient is alerted and oriented. There is no tenderness over the abdomen. There is a left flank abrasion measuring about 4 c.m. No hemotoma or echymosis are noted. The left flank area is smooth and un-remarkable. There is no tenderness in the lower abdomen. The testicles are normal. The prostrate is 1+, smooth and nontender. His hemogloben is fourteen.
An IVP was performed that showed a large gass pattern over the entire adbomen. The left kidney functions promply and is smooth. The right kidney shows good function in both the upper and lower poles. There is some decreased filing of the renal penvis but there is good excetion of contast. The renal pelvis does not really fill out will in the entire mid-line area which I think is consistent with a renal contrusion. Thre is no sign of any exvasation.
A renal sonagram also shows the kidney to be totally entact. No deformity to the parencyma or fluid loss is noted. It is essentially a normal appearing kidney.
IMPRESSION: Right renal contusion. No signs of any exvasation.
PLAN: The patient will be admitted to university hospital and placed on bedrest, with observation. I will order a urine culture, and sensitivity test. He will be started on IV antibiotics and I will follow along with you in his care. Thank you for refering this patient to us.

_____

Benjamin Keytone, MD/xx

PART II / ACTIVITY 5
PROOFREADING WORKSHEET EXERCISE

Directions: Proofread this medical document that contains multiple errors using full block, open punctuation, and all other formatting guidelines established in this textbook.

OPERATIVE REPORT

Patient Name: Cruise, Jason

File Number: 0045612

Date of Birth: March 16, 19XX

Examination Date: *current date*

Operation: FLEXIBLE CYSTOSCOPY

PREOPERATIVE DIAGNOSIS: Carcinoma of the prostrate.
POSTOPERATIVE DIAGNOSIS: Carcinoma of the prostrate.

PROCEDURE: Flexible cystioscopy
The patient was identified by me prepped and drapped in the usual fashion. The panindoscopy was performed with a number sixteen french flexible panendoscope. The anterior urethra was unremarkable. The membranous urethra is entact. There is no evidence of any structure.
The prostratic fosa demonstrates grade 2/IV obstruction as viewed from the verue. This probably represents fifteen to twenty grams of resectable adenoma. Thre is no evidence of tumor within the prostratic fosa. The bladder neck anatomy is unremarkable. The bladder mucosa is healthy thruout. There were no stones, tumors, or diverticula identified.

Right and left ureteral orifices were in normal position and normal configuration. Clear refflux is seen bilaterally. The bladder neck anatomy isunremarkable as noted from a retroflex postion. There is no evidence of any tumor envasion into the bladder base.

The scope was withdrawn. The patent tolerated the procedure well.
PLAN:Trimpex 100 mgs. bid
Schedule a followup appointment in 2 weeks to discuss treatment options for carcinoma of the prostrate.

_____

Theodore Trigone, MD/xx

Part II / Activities 6–7
Proofreading Transcription Exercises *(7T-3, 7T-4)*

Now you are ready to make the transition from simply proofreading printed material to both transcribing and proofreading dictated material. This is the time to concentrate on building your medical vocabulary, which ultimately will improve your speed and accuracy. There are two activities in this section.

Textbook Users

Step 1: Launch your word processing package. Insert the appropriate audiocassette in your transcribing machine and find dictation *7T-3.* Listen to the entire dictation to gain an understanding of the medical concepts and terms involved. Rewind the tape to the beginning of the dictation and transcribe what you hear. Do not worry about formatting, style, or speed. Simply type what you hear being dictated, using correct punctuation, capitalization, and spelling. Stop as needed to look up words you do not understand or cannot spell correctly. Adjust the speed control of the transcriber to a comfortable level, starting slowly to assure no dictated words are missed, and then increase the speed as your accuracy improves.

Step 2: Rewind the tape again, and using your created template, transcribe dictation *7T-3* again including correct spacing and formatting. Proofread the report. Identify and correct all errors. Save your work on your student disk. Refer to the answer key and manually complete the error analysis and production for pay charts.

Repeat the same process for dictation *7T-4.*

Activity 7 (audio/transcription document *7T-4*)

Software Users

Click on *Chapter 7, Activity 6, Proofreading Transcription Exercise.*

Insert the appropriate audiocassette in your transcribing machine and find dictation *7T-3.*

Step 1: Listen to the entire dictation to gain an understanding of the medical concepts and terms involved. Rewind the tape to the beginning of the dictation, click Start Watch, and transcribe what you hear. Do not worry about formatting, style, or speed. Simply type what you hear being dictated, using correct punctuation, capitalization, and spelling. Stop as needed to look up words you do not understand or cannot spell. Adjust the speed control of the transcriber to a comfortable level, starting slowly to assure no dictated words are missed, and then increase the speed as your accuracy improves. When you are finished, click on *Done,* then choose *Return to Main Menu.*

Step 2: Click on *Chapter 7, Activity 6* again. Rewind the tapes again, click on *Start Watch,* and transcribe dictation *7T-3* again, including correct spacing and formatting. Proofread the report. Identify and correct all errors. When you are finished, click on *Done,* then *Score Document* to display your production for pay. Click on *Display Error Analysis* to reveal your score and *View Errors* to see the errors you made. Save your work (with errors showing) on your student disk by clicking on *File,* then *Save As.*

Follow the same process for dictation *7T-4.*

Part II / Check Your Progress *(7T-2)*

Let's pause a minute and see how well you are doing. This section will allow you to evaluate your success at transcribing and proofreading urology reports.

Textbook Users

Launch your word processing package.

Insert the appropriate audiotape in your transcribing machine and find dictation *7T-2.*

On the open screen, transcribe and proofread dictation *7T-2.*

Identify and correct all errors.

After completing the transcription, refer to the answer key.

Manually complete the error analysis chart.

Manually complete the production for pay chart.

If you score below 90%, you are recommended to redo the Part II activities.

If you score 90% or above, congratulations. You have mastered the material covered in Part II. You can immediately move on to Part III.

Software Users

Click on *Chapter 7, Part II, Check Your Progress (7T-2).*

Insert the appropriate audiocassette in your transcribing machine and find dictation *7T-2.*

Click on *Start Watch,* then transcribe and proofread dictation *7T-2.*

Identify and correct all errors.

When you are finished, click on *Done,* then *Score Document:* a pop-up window will display your production for pay.

Click on *Display Error Analysis* to reveal your score.

Click on *View Errors* to see your errors.

Save your work (with errors showing) on your student disk by clicking on *File,* then *Save As.*

If you score below 90%, you are recommended to redo the Part II activities.

If you score 90% or above, congratulations. You have mastered the material covered in Part II. You can immediately move on to Part III.

Pretest (7T-5, 7T-6)

Professional transcriptionists can transcribe and proofread their own work. Can you? Scoring 90% or better proves it!

Textbook Users

Launch your word processing package.

Insert the appropriate audiocassette in your transcribing machine and find dictation *7T-5*.

On the open screen, transcribe and proofread dictation *7T-5*.

Identify and correct all errors.

Use formatting guidelines established in Chapter 2.

Save your work on your student disk.

Follow the same process for dictation *7T-6*.

After completing the transcriptions, refer to the answer key.

Manually complete the error analysis chart for each document.

Manually complete the production for pay chart for each document.

If you score below 90%, continue with *Urology Transcription at FedDes Wellness Center*.

If you score 90% or above, congratulations. You have mastered the material covered in Part III. If you wish, you can immediately move on to the next chapter.

Software Users

Click on *Chapter 7, Part III, Pretest (7T-5)*.

Insert the appropriate audiocassette in your transcribing machine and find dictation *7T-5*.

Click on *Start Watch*, then transcribe and proofread dictation *7T-5*.

Identify and correct all errors.

When you are finished, click on *Done*, then *Score Document*; a pop-up window will display your production for pay.

Click on *Display Error Analysis* to reveal your score.

Click on *View Errors* to see the errors you made.

Save your work (with errors showing) on your student disk by clicking on *File*, then *Save As*.

Follow the same process for dictation *7T-6*.

If you score below 90%, continue with *Urology Transcription at FedDes Wellness Center*.

If you score 90% or above, congratulations. You have mastered the material covered in Part III. If you wish, you can immediately move on to the next chapter.

Urology Transcription at Fed Des Wellness Center

You finally made it! You have been hired as a transcriptionist at FedDes Wellness Center in the urology division. Your supervisor has asked you to transcribe today's dictation.

Textbook Users

Launch your word processing package.

Insert the appropriate audiocassette in your transcribing machine and find dictation *7T-7*.

Create or use an existing template for the six types of reports.

Transcribe and proofread dictation *7T-7*. Identify and correct all errors.

Save your work on your student disk.

Follow the same process for dictations *7T-8* through *7T-15*.

After completing the transcriptions, refer to the answer key.

Manually complete the error analysis and production for pay charts.

Software Users

Click on *Chapter 7, Part III, Urology Transcription at FedDes Wellness Center (7T-7)*.

Insert the appropriate audiocassette in your transcribing machine and find dictation *7T-7*.

Click on *Start Watch*, then transcribe and proofread dictation *7T-7*.

Identify and correct all errors.

When you are finished, click on *Done*, then *Score Document* to display your production for pay.

Click on *Display Error Analysis* to reveal your score.

Save your work (with errors showing) on your student disk by clicking on *File*, then *Save As*.

Follow the same process for dictations *7T-8* and *7T-9*.

NOTE: Continue with dictations *7T-11* through *7T-15* using your word processing package and manually complete the error analysis and production for pay charts.

Index of Dictations and Associated Transcription Tips

Please remember to follow the guidelines pertaining to capitalization, numbers, punctuation, abbreviations, measurements, symbols, and use of templates. Review of this material can be found in Unit 1.

7T-7

Consultation Report

Patient's Name: Jason Stewartson

Requesting Physician: Charles P. Davis, MD

Physician: Helen Loop, MD

● **TRANSCRIPTION TIPS**

- A hyphen is used between numbers and *year old*.

You will hear the dictator say: twenty four year old mother.

You should transcribe as: 24-year-old mother.

- Generic drugs are not capitalized: amoxicillin.

- Words beginning with *pre, re, post,* and *non* are generally not hyphenated.
  For example: nontender

7T-8

Procedure Report

Patient's Name: Soshia Yonie

Ordering Physician: Charles P. Davis, MD

Physician: Helen Loop, MD

- A hyphen is used to join two or more words when used as an adjective that proceeds a noun. The following word pair is dictated in this report: three-month.

- The following drugs are dictated in this report:
  Betadine: the trade name for a topical antibacterial, antiseptic
  Xylocaine: the trade name for an anesthetic, antiarrhythmic

7T-9
History and Physical Examination Report
Patient's Name: Roal Diaz
Physician: Benjamin Keytone, MD

TRANSCRIPTION TIPS

- The following abbreviations are dictated in this report:
  TURP: transurethral resection of the prostate
  BPH: benign prostatic hypertrophy

- A hyphen is used when two or more words are viewed as a single word: well-developed.

- Figures are used to express the day of the month and the year.
  You will hear the dictator say: The patient underwent prostatic resection and hernia repair in nineteen ninety eight.
  You should transcribe as: The patient underwent prostatic resection and hernia repair in 1998.

- Words beginning with *pre, re, post,* and *non* are generally not hyphenated.
  For example: noncontributory

7T-10
Chart Note using History and Physical Format
Patient's Name: Betty Ann Jackson-Jones
Physician: Helen Loop, MD

TRANSCRIPTION TIPS

- A period is used to separate a decimal fraction from its whole number and is used to take the place of the word *point.*

You will hear the dictator say: Her white blood count is six point eight.
You should transcribe as: Her white blood count is 6.8.

- Figures are used to express vital signs. Commas are used to separate vital signs.
  You will hear the dictator say: Temperature ninety seven point eight pulse seventy nine respirations twenty two per minute blood pressure one hundred fifty seven over eighty six.
  You should transcribe as: Temperature 97.8, pulse 79, respirations 22/min., BP 157/86.

- A hyphen is used to join two or more words when used as an adjective that proceeds a noun. The following word pairs are dictated in this report: follow-up, high-powered.

- The following abbreviation is dictated in this report:
  CVA: costovertebral angle

- The following drug is dictated in this report:
  Noroxin: the trade name for an antibacterial, urinary tract anti-infective

- A hyphen is used to take the place of the words *to* or *through* to identify ranges.
  You will hear the dictator say: Urinalysis reveals three to five white cells.
  You should transcribe as: Urinalysis reveals 3-5 white cells.

- Words beginning with *pre, re, post,* and *non* are generally not hyphenated.
  For example: nonpalpable, rebound

- The following procedure is dictated in this report:
  Marshall-Marchetti-Krantz bladder neck suspension: an examination that is performed to correct a cystocele and urinary incontinence

7T-11
History and Physical Examination Report
Patient's Name: Julie Pierre
Physician: Helen Loop, MD

- The following abbreviations are dictated in this report:
  CT: computerized tomography

- The following diseases are dictated in this report:
  Crohn's disease: inflammation of the terminal portion of the ileum
  diverticulitis: inflammation of the diverticula of the colon

- The following drugs are dictated in this report:
  Lopressor: the trade name for an antianginal, antihypertensive
  Aldactone: the trade name for a diuretic
  Imodium: the trade name for an antidiarrheal

- Words beginning with *pre, re, post,* and *non* are generally not hyphenated:
  noncontributory, nontender, pretibial.

7T-12

History and Physical Examination Report
Patient's Name: Dawson, Thomas
Physician: Theodore Trigone, MD

TRANSCRIPTION TIPS

- The following drugs are dictated in this report:
  Bactrim DS: the trade name for an antibiotic
  Trimpex: the trade name for an antibacterial, antibiotic

- Figures are used with the + or − symbols.
  You will hear the dictator say: Urinalysis shows two plus leukocytes.
  You should transcribe as: Urinalysis shows 2+ leukocytes.
  You will hear the dictator say: three plus heme.
  You should transcribe as: 3+ heme.

- A hyphen is used to join two or more words when used as an adjective that proceeds a noun. The following word pair is dictated in this report: follow-up.

- Figures are used for Latin terms. Latin terms are expressed in lower case letters.

You will hear the dictator say: a follow up appointment in three months or P R N basis.
You should transcribe as: a follow-up appointment in three months or p.r.n. basis.

- The letter *x* is used to abbreviate the word *by* and the word *times* when it precedes a number or another abbreviation. The dosage of medicine is never separated by line spacing.
  You will hear the dictator say: The patient will resume a regimen of Bactrim DS one B I D times ten days.
  You should transcribe as: The patient will resume a regimen of Bactrim DS 1 b.i.d. x 10 days.

- The following disease is dictated in this report:
  Parkinson's disease: a slowly progressive disease characterized by degeneration within the nuclear masses of the extrapyramidal system

- The following abbreviations are dictated in this report:
  CVA: costovertebral angle
  UA: urinalysis
  C&S: culture and sensitivity

7T-13

Consultation Letter
Patient's Name: Ross, Mary
Requesting Physician: J. Thomas Geiger, MD
Physician: Helen Loop, MD

TRANSCRIPTION TIPS

- A hyphen is used in place of *to* or *through* to identify ranges.

- You will hear the dictator say: vague abdominal pain three to four days ago.
  You should transcribe as: vague abdominal pain 3-4 days ago.

- Capitalize the name of specific departments or sections in a hospital or institution.
  You will hear the dictator say: She presented to the university hospital emergency room last night.

You should transcribe as: She presented to the University Hospital Emergency Room last night.

- Quotation marks are used to indicate a direct quote.
  You will hear the dictator say: The urinalysis was described as turbid yellow.
  You should transcribe as: The urinalysis was described as "turbid yellow."

- The following abbreviation is dictated in this report:
  KUB: kidneys, ureters, bladder
  CVA: costovertebral angle

7T-14
History and Physical Examination Report
Patient's Name: Resch, Gladys
Physician: Helen Loop, MD

● TRANSCRIPTION TIPS

- The following procedure is dictated in this report:
  Marshall test: performed to determine stress-related urinary incontinence

- The following device is dictated in this report:
  Gellhorn pessary: an inflexible device made of acrylic resin or plastic in the form of a large collar button. It has a canal through the stem that allows drainage of vaginal sections.

- A hyphen is used when two or more words are viewed as a single word: well-developed, well-nourished.

- The following generic drugs are dictated in this report:
  hydrochlorothiazide: a generic name for a diuretic, antihypertensive agent
  meclizine: a generic name for an antiemetic, antihistamine, motion sickness relief

7T-15
Consultation Report
Patient's Name: Sever, Jed
Requesting Physician: Izzy Sertoli, MD
Physician: Benjamin Keytone, MD

● TRANSCRIPTION TIPS

- The following drugs are dictated in this report:
  Maxaquin: the trade name for a fluoroquinolone antibiotic, antibacterial

- A hyphen is used to join two or more words when used as an adjective that proceeds a noun. The following word pairs are dictated in this report: worm-like, moderate-sized, seven-day, blood-tinged.

- The number or pound sign (#) is used to abbreviate the word *number* followed by medical instrument or apparatus.
  You will hear the dictator say: He had a number eighteen french foley catheter.
  You should transcribe as: He had a #18 French Foley catheter.

- Words beginning with *pre, re, post,* and *non* are generally not hyphenated: nondraining

Part III / Check Your Progress (7T-5, 7T-6)

Professional transcriptionists can transcribe and proofread their own work with speed and accuracy. Have you mastered the urology transcription rotation at FedDes Wellness Center?

Textbook Users

Launch your word processing package.

Insert the appropriate audiocassette in your transcribing machine and find dictation *7T-5*.

On the open screen, transcribe and proofread dictation *7T-5*.

Identify and correct all errors.

Use formatting guidelines established in Chapter 2.

Save your work on your student disk.

Follow the same process for dictation *7T-6*.

After completing the transcriptions, refer to the answer key.

Manually complete the error analysis chart for each document.

Manually complete the production for pay chart for each document.

If you score below 90%, you are recommended to repeat Part III.

If you score 90% or above, congratulations. You have mastered the material presented in Part III.

Software Users

Click on *Chapter 7, Part III, Check Your Progress (7T-5)*.

Insert the appropriate audiocassette in your transcribing machine and find dictation *7T-5*.

Click on *Start Watch*, then transcribe and proofread dictation *7T-5*.

Identify and correct all errors.

When you are finished, click on *Done*, then *Score Document:* a pop-up window will display your production for pay.

Click on *Display Error Analysis* to reveal your score.

Click on *View Errors* to see the errors you made.

Save your work (with errors showing) on your student disk by clicking on *File*, then *Save As.*

Follow the same process for dictation *7T-6*.

If you score below 90%, you are recommended to repeat Part III.

If you score 90% or above, congratulations. You have mastered the material presented in Part III.

Chapter 8

Office Medical Transcription from the Pulmonary Medicine Practice

OBJECTIVES

At the completion of Chapter 8, you should be able to do the following:

1. Match medical terms associated with the pulmonary medicine specialty with their definitions.

2. Spell medical terms associated with the pulmonary medicine specialty with their definitions.

3. Transcribe medical terms in sentence structure.

4. Proofread, edit, and correct medical documents associated with the pulmonary medicine specialty containing various errors.

5. Transcribe and proofread authentic medical documents associated with the pulmonary medicine specialty.

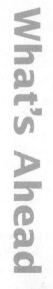

What's Ahead

205

The Pulmonary Medicine Rotation

The FedDes Wellness Center has three pulmonologists, or specialists in pulmonary medicine, on staff. Pulmonary medicine is the study of the respiratory system and its organs, including the nose, mouth, pharynx, epiglottis, esophagus, trachea, lungs, bronchi, bronchioles, and alveoli.

The pulmonologist assesses abnormalities that decrease the amount of air entry, cause restrictive breathing, and affect lung parenchyma. The physicians in FedDes Pulmonary medicine division perform laboratory tests and procedures including pulmonary function tests, bronchoscopy, metabolic cart study, indirect calorimetry, thoracentesis, and pleural biopsy.

In this unit, you assume the role of a medical transcriptionist employed at FedDes Wellness Center. **Please remember to follow the guidelines pertaining to capitalization, numbers, punctuation, abbreviations, measurements, symbols, and use of templates to create medical reports at FedDes Wellness Center. Review of this material can be found in Unit 1.** A list of the patient's name and the type of report as well as associated transcription tips is included in this chapter.

You will work with the textbook, CD-ROM, and accompanying audiocassettes. Your mastery of pulmonary medicine transcription is assessed through worksheets, timed transcription exercises, the error analysis chart, and the production for pay summary.

All the answer keys are found in the textbook and CD-ROM, providing immediate feedback. After transcribing a report, you will proofread your work and correct any errors. Then you will compare your proofread work against a master transcript, categorize all errors, and tabulate the errors on the error analysis chart. The production for pay summary correlates your production to the FedDes Wellness Center pay scale, which is based on industry compensation standards. The scale is also linked to your grade. This system allows you to assess your mastery of transcription skills in a real-world scenario.

PART I ▪ GETTING CLOSE TO THE REAL THING

Pretest

Let's find out if you can define and spell selected terminology and drugs of the pulmonary medicine specialty that are included in this chapter by scoring 90% or better.

Textbook Users
Select the correctly spelled term that matches its definition.
Refer to the answer key for immediate feedback.
If you score below 90%, continue on to *Activities 1–3*.
If you score 90% or above, congratulations. You have mastered of the material covered in Part I. If you wish, you can immediately move on to Part II.

Software Users
Click on *Chapter 8, Part I, Pretest*.
Key the correctly spelled term that matches its definition. When you are finished, click on *End Test*.
A pop-up screen will reveal your score.
If you score below 90%, continue on to *Activities 1–3*.
If you score 90% or above, congratulations on your mastery of the material covered in Part I! If you wish, you can immediately move on to Part II.

PART I / PRETEST

Directions: Select the correctly spelled term that matches its definition.

1. Ability to control urination and defecation urges:
   (a) continent
   (b) contenint
   (c) empiric
   (d) impiric

2. Abnormal crackle sound heard on chest auscultation:
   (a) rale
   (b) rub
   (c) ralle
   (d) rube

3. Abnormal heart condition characterized by the increased size of the right ventricle:
   (a) cor pulmonale
   (b) cor pulmonary
   (c) pulmonary toilet
   (d) pulmon toilet

4. Abnormal heart rhythm:
   (a) sequela
   (b) gallop
   (c) sequelia
   (d) galop

5. Abnormal slowing or stopping of fluid flowing through a vessel:
   (a) atelectasis
   (b) stasis
   (c) atellectasis
   (d) stacis

6. Abnormal sound heard on chest auscultation due to an obstructed airway:
   (a) hemotysis
   (b) hemoptysis
   (c) rhonchus
   (d) ronchus

7. Abnormally fast heartbeat:
   (a) tachycardia
   (b) dyrhythmia
   (c) tachcardia
   (d) dysrhythmia

8. Accumulation of excess fluid in the tissues of the body:
   (a) sputum
   (b) edena
   (c) spitum
   (d) edema

9. Accumulation of fluid in the peritoneal cavity:
   (a) caries
   (b) ascites
   (c) caires
   (d) acites

10. Act of closure or state of being closed:
    (a) oclusion
    (b) auscultation
    (c) auscutation
    (d) occlusion

11. Act of fainting:
    (a) somnolence
    (b) somolence
    (c) syncope
    (d) synscope

12. Act of listening for sounds produced within the body with an unaided ear or with a stethoscope:
    (a) oclusion
    (b) auscultation
    (c) auscutation
    (d) occlusion

PART I / PRETEST *continued*

13. Affecting both sides:
    (a) afebrile
    (b) bilateral
    (c) afevrile
    (d) bilaral

14. Any abnormal condition that follows and is the result of a disease, treatment, or injury:
    (a) erythema
    (b) sequea
    (c) erytema
    (d) sequela

15. Any drug that has the capacity of increasing the capacity of the pulmonary air passages and improving ventilation to the lungs:
    (a) efflusion
    (b) bronchidilator
    (c) bronchodilator
    (d) effusion

16. Aspiration of fluid from the chest cavity:
    (a) metastasis
    (b) thoracentesis
    (c) metasis
    (d) thorasis

17. Bluish-purple discoloration of the skin due to lack of oxygenated blood:
    (a) cyanesis
    (b) cyanosis
    (c) emesis
    (d) enesis

18. Calf pain with dorsiflexion of foot:
    (a) Homan's sign
    (b) theophylline
    (c) Homans' sign
    (d) theophyline

19. Cleansing of the trachea and bronchial tree:
    (a) cor pulmonale
    (b) cor pulmonary
    (c) pulmonary toilet
    (d) pulmon toilet

20. Collapse of a portion of the lung:
    (a) atelectasis
    (b) stasis
    (c) atellectasis
    (d) stacis

21. Compound containing water molecules:
    (a) hydrate
    (b) hidrate
    (c) infiltrate
    (d) enfiltrate

22. Condition of decay and destruction of a tooth:
    (a) caries
    (b) ascites
    (c) caires
    (d) acites

23. Containing pus:
    (a) pedol
    (b) purlent
    (c) purulent
    (d) pedal

24. Coughing or spitting up blood from the respiratory tract:
    (a) hemotysis
    (b) hemoptysis
    (c) rhonchus
    (d) ronchus

25. Cramping pains of the calves caused by poor circulation to the leg muscles:
    (a) dention
    (b) claudication
    (c) caudication
    (d) dentition

PART I / PRETEST *continued*

26. Decreased supply of oxygenated blood to a body part:
    (a) ischemia
    (b) ischema
    (c) dyspneia
    (d) dyspnea

27. Diagnostic procedure using ultrasound to study heart structure and motion:
    (a) echocardiogram
    (b) echiocardogram
    (c) arteriogram
    (d) arterogram

28. Disordered rhythm:
    (a) rhonchus
    (b) dyrhythmia
    (c) ronchis
    (d) dysrhythmia

29. Drowsiness:
    (a) somnolence
    (b) somolence
    (c) syncope
    (d) synscope

30. Enlargement of the glands, especially the lymph nodes:
    (a) thyromegaly
    (b) adenogaly
    (c) adenopathy
    (d) thyropathy

31. Enlargement of the thyroid gland:
    (a) thyromegaly
    (b) adenogaly
    (c) adenopathy
    (d) thyropathy

32. Escape of fluid into a body cavity:
    (a) efflusion
    (b) bronchidilator
    (c) bronchodilator
    (d) effusion

33. Fluid, cells, or other substances pass into tissue spaces:
    (a) hydrate
    (b) hidrate
    (c) infiltrate
    (d) enfiltrate

34. Generic antianxiety drug:
    (a) lorazepam
    (b) lorasepam
    (c) isorbide
    (d) isosorbide

35. Generic calcium channel blocker drug:
    (a) haperin
    (b) heparin
    (c) nifedipin
    (d) nifedipine

36. Generic corticosteroid drug:
    (a) prednisone
    (b) prenisone
    (c) cephalosporin
    (d) cephalsporin

37. Generic name for a broad-spectrum antibiotic:
    (a) nitroglyserin
    (b) erythromycin
    (c) nitroglycerin
    (d) erythromysin

38. Generic name for a bronchodilator:
    (a) Homan's sign
    (b) theophylline
    (c) Homans' sign
    (d) theophyline

39. Generic name for a coronary vasodilator, antianginal:
    (a) nitroglyserin
    (b) erythromycin
    (c) nitroglycerin
    (d) erythromysin

PART I / PRETEST *continued*

40. Generic name for a nitrate-based antianginal agent:
    (a) lorazepam
    (b) lorasepam
    (c) isorbide
    (d) isosorbide

41. Generic name for an aminopenicillin antibiotic:
    (a) amoxicillin
    (b) amoxicilin
    (c) doxepin
    (d) dozepin

42. Generic name for an anticoagulant:
    (a) haperin
    (b) heparin
    (c) nifedipin
    (d) nifedipine

43. Generic name for an antidepressant:
    (a) amoxicillin
    (b) amoxicilin
    (c) doxepin
    (d) dozepin

44. Generic name for any of the large group of broad-spectrum antibiotics:
    (a) prednisone
    (b) prenisone
    (c) cephalosporin
    (d) cephalsporin

45. Increased excretion of urine:
    (a) duiresis
    (b) diuresis
    (c) duiretic
    (d) diuretic

46. Involuntary, rapid, rhythmic movement of the eyeball:
    (a) nystagus
    (b) nystagmus
    (c) adencarcinoma
    (d) adenocarcinoma

47. Labored or difficult breathing:
    (a) ischemia
    (b) ischema
    (c) dyspneia
    (d) dyspnea

48. Localized dilitation of the wall of a blood vessel:
    (a) aneurysm
    (b) embolus
    (c) aneruysm
    (d) emblous

49. Malignant tumor of the glands:
    (a) nystagus
    (b) nystagmus
    (c) adencarcinoma
    (d) adenocarcinoma

50. Mass that is brought by the blood from another vessel that obstructs blood circulation:
    (a) aneurysm
    (b) embolus
    (c) aneruysm
    (d) emblous

51. Material coughed up from the lungs and ejected through the mouth:
    (a) sputum
    (b) edena
    (c) spitum
    (d) edema

PART I / PRETEST *continued*

52. Normally occurring microrganisms living within the body that provide natural immunity against certain organisms:
    (a) fora
    (b) saphenous
    (c) flora
    (d) sapenous

53. Occuring at night:
    (a) intrauterine
    (b) nocturnal
    (c) interuterine
    (d) noctural

54. Pertains to the two main superficial veins of the lower leg:
    (a) fora
    (b) saphenous
    (c) flora
    (d) sapenous

55. Position and condition of the teeth:
    (a) dention
    (b) claudication
    (c) caudication
    (d) dentition

56. Presence of air or gas in the pleural cavity:
    (a) pneumontomy
    (b) pneumonectomy
    (c) pneumotorax
    (d) pneumothorax

57. Radiographic visualization of an artery after injection of a contrast medium:
    (a) echocardiogram
    (b) echiocardogram
    (c) arteriogram
    (d) arterogram

58. Redness of the skin:
    (a) erythema
    (b) sequea
    (c) erytema
    (d) sequela

59. Relating to the foot:
    (a) pedol
    (b) purlent
    (c) purulent
    (d) pedal

60. Situated or occurring above the ventricles:
    (a) superventricular
    (b) supraventricular
    (c) suberventricular
    (d) suparventricular

61. Sound caused by the rubbing together of two surfaces:
    (a) rale
    (b) rub
    (c) ralle
    (d) rube

62. Sound or murmur heard on auscultation:
    (a) bruit
    (b) gallop
    (c) briut
    (d) galop

63. Substance that promotes the excretion of urine:
    (a) duiresis
    (b) diuresis
    (c) duiretic
    (d) diuretic

64. Surgical removal of all or a segment of the lung:
    (a) pneumontomy
    (b) pneumonectomy
    (c) pneumotorax
    (d) pneumothorax

PART I / PRETEST *continued*

65. To vomit:
    (a) cyanesis
    (b) cyanosis
    (c) emesis
    (d) enesis

66. Transfer of disease from one organ or part to another not directly connected with it:
    (a) metastasis
    (b) thoracentesis
    (c) metasis
    (d) thorasis

67. Treating a disease based upon observation and experience rather than reasoning alone:
    (a) continent
    (b) contenint
    (c) empiric
    (d) impiric

68. Treatment by a spray:
    (a) nebulization
    (b) nebullization
    (c) fibrillation
    (d) fibrilation

69. Uncoordinated twitching of muscle fibers:
    (a) nebulization
    (b) nebullization
    (c) fibrillation
    (d) fibrilation

70. Within the uterus:
    (a) intrauterine
    (b) nocturnal
    (c) interuterine
    (d) noctural

71. Without fever:
    (a) afebrile
    (b) bilateral
    (c) afevrile
    (d) bilaral

72. Trade name for a bronchodilator, metered dose inhaler:
    (a) Proventil MDI
    (b) Provintel MDI
    (c) Vanceril
    (d) Vanseril

73. Trade name for a bronchodilator:
    (a) Ventlin
    (b) Ventolin
    (c) Paxil
    (d) Pasil

74. Trade name for a bronchodilator:
    (a) Theo-Dur
    (b) Xanaz
    (c) Xanax
    (d) Theo-Dure

75. Trade name for a bulk-forming laxative:
    (a) Dilantin
    (b) Dylantin
    (c) FiberCon
    (d) Fiberkon

76. Trade name for a calcium channel blocker for atrial fibrillation:
    (a) Cardizem
    (b) Cardisem
    (c) Colase
    (d) Colace

77. Trade name for a coronary vasodilator:
    (a) Procardia
    (b) Serevent
    (c) Procariodia
    (d) Servent

78. Trade name for a corticosteroid for the prevention or treatment of bronchial asthma:
    (a) Azamcort
    (b) Bumex
    (c) Azmacort
    (d) Bumez

PART I / PRETEST *continued*

79. Trade name for a corticosteroid:
    (a) Proventil MDI
    (b) Provintel MDI
    (c) Vanceril
    (d) Vanseril

80. Trade name for a loop diuretic:
    (a) Azamcort
    (b) Bumex
    (c) Azmacort
    (d) Bumez

81. Trade name for a narcotic analgesic:
    (a) Compazine
    (b) Darvon
    (c) Compasine
    (d) Darvin

82. Trade name for a nasal spray, bronchodilator:
    (a) Ascriptin
    (b) Asriptin
    (c) Atrovent
    (d) Atovent

83. Trade name for a preparation of aspirin with Maalox, an analgesic and anti-inflammatory:
    (a) Ascriptin
    (b) Asriptin
    (c) Atrovent
    (d) Atovent

84. Trade name for a sedative-hypnotic:
    (a) Pepsid
    (b) Restoril
    (c) Pepcid
    (d) Restoral

85. Trade name for a stool softener:
    (a) Cardizem
    (b) Cardisem
    (c) Colase
    (d) Colace

86. Trade name for a tranquilizer and antiemetic:
    (a) Compazine
    (b) Darvon
    (c) Compasine
    (d) Darvin

87. Trade name for an acid controller for heartburn and acid indigestion:
    (a) Pepsid
    (b) Restoril
    (c) Pepcid
    (d) Restoral

88. Trade name for an acid controller for heartburn and acid indigestion:
    (a) Zantac
    (b) Vasotec
    (c) Zantak
    (d) Vasotek

89. Trade name for an aerosol bronchodilator:
    (a) Procardia
    (b) Serevent
    (c) Procariodia
    (d) Servent

90. Trade name for an antianxiety agent:
    (a) Theo-Dur
    (b) Xanaz
    (c) Xanax
    (d) Theo-Dure

91. Trade name for an anticonvulsant used in the treatment of epilepsy:
    (a) Dilantin
    (b) Dylantin
    (c) Fibercon
    (d) Fiberkon

92. Trade name for an antidepressant:
    (a) Ventlin
    (b) Ventolin
    (c) Paxil
    (d) Pasil

PART I / PRETEST *continued*

93. Trade name for an antihyperlipidemic:
    (a) Lopressor
    (b) Metacor
    (c) Lopresor
    (d) Mevacor

94. Trade name for an antihypertensive:
    (a) Lopressor
    (b) Metacor
    (c) Lopresor
    (d) Mevacor

95. Trade name for an antihypertensive:
    (a) Zantac
    (b) Vasotec
    (c) Zantak
    (d) Vasotek

96. Trade name for a cephalosporin antibiotic:
    (a) Ancef IV
    (b) Ansef IV
    (c) NPH
    (d) PNH

97. Trade name for an extended-release bronchodilator:
    (a) Slow-bid
    (b) Slo-bide
    (c) Slow-bide
    (d) Slo-bid

98. Trade name for an insulin that decreases blood sugar:
    (a) Ancef IV
    (b) Ansef IV
    (c) NPH
    (d) PNH

Part I / Activity 1
Keyboarding Medical Terms and Definitions

Let's learn to spell and define selected terminology and drugs of the pulmonary medicine specialty that are included in this chapter. Keyboarding these terms is an innovative and fun way to improve your skills.

Textbook Users
Launch your word processing package.
On the open screen, read and type each word and its definition as shown below.
Save your work on your student disk.

1. Adenocarcinoma (ade-no-kar-si-no-mah) is a malignant tumor of the glands.
2. Adenopathy (ade-nop-ah-the) is the enlargement of the glands, especially the lymph nodes.
3. Afebrile (a-feb-ril) is without fever.
4. Amoxicillin (ah-moks-i-sil-in) is the generic name for an aminopenicillin antibiotic.

5. Aneurysm (an-u-rizm) is a localized dilitation of the wall of a blood vessel.
6. Arteriogram (ar-te-re-o-gram) is the radiographic visualization of an artery after injection of a contrast medium.
7. Ascites (ah-si-tez) is the accumulation of fluid in the peritoneal cavity.

8. Atelectasis (ate-<u>lek</u>-tah-sis) is the collapse of a portion of the lung.

9. Auscultation (aw-skul-<u>ta</u>-shun) is the act of listening for sounds produced within the body with an unaided ear or with a stethoscope.

10. Bilateral (bi-<u>lat</u>-er-al) is affecting both sides.

11. Bronchodilator (brong-ko-di-<u>la</u>-tor) is any drug that has the capacity of increasing the capacity of the pulmonary air passages and improving ventilation to the lungs.

12. Bruit (broot) is a sound or murmur heard on auscultation.

13. Caries (<u>ka</u>-re-ez) is the condition of decay and destruction of a tooth.

14. Cephalosporin (sef-ah-lo-<u>spor</u>-in) is a generic name for any of the large group of broad-spectrum antibiotics.

15. Claudication (klaw-di-<u>ka</u>-shun) is cramping pains of the calves caused by poor circulation to the leg muscles.

16. Continent (<u>kon</u>-ti-ent) is the ability to control urination and defecation urges.

17. Cor pulmonale (kor pul-<u>mona</u>-le) is an abnormal heart condition characterized by the increased size of the right ventricle.

18. Cyanosis (si-ah-<u>no</u>-sis) is the bluish-purple discoloration of the skin due to lack of oxygenated blood.

19. Dentition (den-<u>tish</u>-un) refers to the position and condition of the teeth.

20. Diuresis (di-u-<u>re</u>-sis) is increased urine excretion.

21. Diuretic (di-u-<u>ret</u>-ik) is a substance that promotes the excretion of urine.

22. Doxepin (<u>dok</u>-se-pin) is the generic name for an antidepressant.

23. Dyspnea (disp-<u>ne</u>-ah) is labored or difficult breathing.

24. Dysrhythmia (dis-<u>rith</u>-me-ah) is a disordered rhythm.

25. Echocardiogram (eko-<u>kar</u>-de-o-gram) is a diagnostic procedure using ultrasound to study heart structure and motion.

26. Edema (<u>ede</u>-mah) is the accumulation of excess fluid in the tissues of the body.

27. Effusion (e-<u>fu</u>-zhun) is the escape of fluid into a body cavity.

28. Embolus (<u>em</u>-bo-lus) is a mass that is brought by the blood from another vessel that obstructs blood circulation.

29. Emesis (<u>em</u>-e-sis) is to vomit.

30. Empiric (em-<u>pir</u>-i-kl) is treating a disease based upon observation and experience rather than reasoning alone.

31. Erythema (eri-<u>the</u>-mah) is redness of the skin.

32. Erythromycin (e-rith-ro-<u>mi</u>-sin) is a generic name for a broad-spectrum antibiotic.

33. Fibrillation (fi-bri-<u>la</u>-shun) is the uncoordinated twitching of muscles fibers.

34. Flora (<u>flo</u>-rah) are normally occurring microorganisms living within the body that provide natural immunity against certain organisms.

35. Gallop (<u>gal</u>-op) is an abnormal heart rhythm.

36. Hemoptysis (he-<u>mop</u>-ti-sis) is the coughing or spitting up of blood from the respiratory tract.

37. Heparin (<u>hep</u>-ah-rin) is the generic name for an anticoagulant.

38. Homans' sign (<u>ho</u>-manz sin) is a calf pain with dorsiflexion of foot.

39. Hydrate (<u>hi</u>-drat) is a compound containing water molecules.

40. Infiltrate (in-<u>fil</u>-trat) is when fluid, cells, or other substances pass into tissue spaces.

41. Intrauterine (in-trah-<u>u</u>-ter-in) is within the uterus.

42. Ischemia (is-<u>ke</u>-me-ah) is a decreased supply of oxygenated blood to a body part.

43. Isosorbide (i-so-<u>sor</u>-bid) is the generic name for a nitrate-based antianginal agent.

44. Lorazepam (lor-a-<u>zep</u>-am) is a generic antianxiety drug.

45. Metastasis (me-<u>tas</u>-tah-sis) is the transfer of disease from one organ or part to another not directly connected with it.

46. Nebulization (neb-u-li-<u>za</u>-shun) is a treatment by a spray.

47. Nifedipine (ni-<u>fed</u>-i-pen) is a generic calcium channel blocker drug.

48. Nitroglycerin (ni-tro-<u>glis</u>-er-in) is a generic name for a coronary vasodilator, antianginal.

49. Nocturnal (nok-<u>tur</u>-nal) is something that occurs at night.

50. Nystagmus (nis-<u>tag</u>-mus) is the involuntary, rapid, rhythmic movement of the eyeball.

51. Occlusion (o-<u>kloo</u>-zhun) is the act of closure or state of being closed.

52. Pedal (<u>ped</u>-al) is a term relating to the foot.

53. Pneumonectomy (nu-mo-<u>nek</u>-to-me) is the surgical removal of all or a segment of the lung.

54. Pneumothorax (nu-mo-<u>tho</u>-raks) is the presence of air or gas in the pleural cavity.
55. Prednisone (<u>pred</u>-ni-son) is a generic corticosteroid drug.
56. Pulmonary toilet (<u>pul</u>-mo-ner-e <u>toi</u>-let) is the cleansing of the trachea and bronchial tree.
57. Purulent (<u>pu</u>-roo-lent) is containing pus.
58. Rale (rahl) is an abnormal crackle sound heard on chest auscultation.
59. Rhonchus (<u>rong</u>-kus) is an abnormal sound heard on chest auscultation due to an obstructed airway.
60. Rub (rub) is a sound caused by the rubbing together of two surfaces.
61. Saphenous (sah-<u>fe</u>-nus) pertains to the two main superficial veins of the lower leg.
62. Sequela (se-<u>kwel</u>-lah) is any abnormal condition that follows and is the result of a disease, treatment or injury.
63. Somnolence (<u>som</u>-no-lens) is drowsiness.
64. Sputum (<u>spu</u>-tum) is the material coughed up from the lungs and ejected through the mouth.
65. Stasis (<u>sta</u>-sis) is an abnormal slowing or stopping of fluid flowing through a vessel.
66. Supraventricular (soo-prah-ven-<u>trik</u>-u-lar) is situated or occurring above the ventricles.
67. Syncope (<u>sing</u>-ko-pe) is the act of fainting.
68. Tachycardia (take-<u>kar</u>-de-ah) is an abnormally fast heartbeat.
69. Theophylline (the-o-<u>fil</u>-in) is a generic name for a bronchodilator.
70. Thoracentesis (tho-rah-sen-<u>te</u>-sis) is the aspiration of fluid from the chest cavity.
71. Thyromegaly (thi-ro-<u>meg</u>-ah-le) is the enlargement of the thyroid gland.
72. Ancef IV (an-<u>sef</u>) is the trade name for an cephalosporin antibiotic.
73. Ascriptin (ah-<u>skrip</u>-tin) is the trade name for a preparation of aspirin with Maalox, an analgesic and anti-inflammatory.
74. Atrovent (at-ro-<u>vent</u>) is the trade name for a nasal spray, bronchodilator.
75. Azmacort (<u>az</u>-ma-kort) is the trade name for a corticosteroid for the prevention or treatment of bronchial asthma.
76. Bumex (bu-<u>meks</u>) is the trade name for a loop diuretic.
77. Cardizem (kar-<u>di</u>-zem) is the trade name for a calcium channel blocker for atrial fibrillation.
78. Colace (ko-<u>las</u>) is the trade name for a stool softener.
79. Compazine (<u>kom</u>-pah-zen) is the trade name for a tranquilizer and antiemetic.
80. Darvon (<u>dar</u>-von) is the trade name for a narcotic analgesic.
81. Dilantin (di-<u>lan</u>-tin) is the trade name for an anticonvulsant used in the treatment of epilepsy.
82. Fibercon (<u>fi</u>-ber-kon) is the trade name for a bulk-forming laxative.
83. Lopressor (lo-<u>pres</u>-or) is the trade name for an antihypertensive.
84. Mevacor (me-<u>va</u>-kor) is the trade name for an antihyperlipidemic.
85. NPH (neutral protamine Hagedorn) insulin is trade name for an insulin that decreases blood sugar.
86. Paxil (pa-<u>ksil</u>) is the trade name for an antidepressant.
87. Pepcid (<u>pep</u>-sid) is the trade name for an acid controller for heartburn and acid indigestion.
88. Procardia (pro-<u>kar</u>-de-ah) is the trade name for a coronary vasodilator.
89. Proventil MDI (pro-<u>ven</u>-til) is a trade name for a bronchodilator, metered dose inhaler.
90. Restoril (<u>res</u>-to-ril) is the trade name for a sedative-hypnotic.
91. Serevent (<u>ser</u>-e-vent) is the trade name for an aerosol bronchodilator.
92. Slo-bid (<u>slo</u>-bid) is the trade name for an extended-release bronchodilator.
93. Theo-Dur (<u>the</u>-o-dur) is the trade name for a bronchodilator.
94. Vanceril (<u>van</u>-ser-il) is the trade name for a corticosteroid.
95. Vasotec (<u>vah</u>-so-tek) is the trade name for an antihypertensive.
96. Ventolin (<u>ven</u>-to-lin) is the trade name for a bronchodilator.
97. Xanax (<u>zan</u>-aks) is the trade name for an antianxiety agent.
98. Zantac (<u>zan</u>-tak) is the trade name for an acid controller for heartburn and acid indigestion.

Do you remember back in school when you had to write each spelling word ten times? Because you had to physically write each word, your mind and body were focused on the assignment, and the method worked! Let's follow this successful method by reinforcing the spelling of selected terms and drugs found in the pulmonary medicine specialty through keyboarding drills.

Textbook Users
Launch your word processing package.
On the open screen, read, mentally spell, and type each word in its sequence.
Save your work on your student disk.

1. adenocarcinoma adenopathy afebrile adenocarcinoma adenopathy afebrile adenocarcinoma
2. amoxicillin aneurysm arteriogram amoxicillin aneurysm arteriogram amoxicillin aneurysm
3. ascites atelectasis auscultation ascites atelectasis auscultation ascites atelectasis auscultation
4. bilateral bronchodilator bruit bilateral bronchodilator bruit bilateral bronchodilator bruit
5. caries cephalosporin claudication caries cephalosporin claudication caries cephalosporin
6. continent cor pulmonale cyanosis continent cor pulmonale cyanosis continent cor pulmonale
7. dentition diuresis diuretic dentition diuresis diuretic dentition diuresis diuretic dentition
8. doxepin dyspnea dysrhythmia doxepin dyspnea dysrhythmia doxepin dyspnea dysrhythmia
9. echocardiogram edema effusion echocardiogram edema effusion echocardiogram edema
10. embolus emesis empiric embolus emesis empiric embolus emesis empiric embolus emesis
11. erythema erythromycin fibrillation erythema erythromycin fibrillation erythema fibrillation
12. flora gallop hemoptysis flora gallop hemoptysis flora gallop hemoptysis flora gallop flora
13. heparin Homans' sign hydrate heparin Homans' sign hydrate heparin Homans' sign hydrate
14. infiltrate intrauterine ischemia infiltrate intrauterine ischemia infiltrate intrauterine ischemia
15. isosorbide lorazepam metastasis isosorbide lorazepam metastasis isosorbide lorazepam
16. nebulization nifedipine nitroglycerin nebulization nifedipine nitroglycerin nebulization
17. nocturnal nystagmus occlusion nocturnal nystagmus occlusion nocturnal nystagmus
18. pedal pneumonectomy pneumothorax pedal pneumonectomy pneumothorax pneumonectomy
19. prednisone pulmonary toilet purulent prednisone pulmonary toilet purulent prednisone
20. rale rhonchus rub rale rhonchus rub rale rhonchus rub rale rhonchus rub rale rhonchus rub
21. saphenous sequela somnolence saphenous sequela somnolence saphenous sequela
22. sputum stasis supraventricular sputum stasis supraventribular sputum stasis supraventricular
23. syncope tachycardia theophylline syncope tachycardia theophylline syncope tachycardia
24. thoracentesis thyromegaly thoracentesis thyromegaly thoracentesis thyromegaly
25. Ancef IV Ascriptin Atrovent Ancef IV Ascriptin Atrovent Ancef IV Ascriptin Atrovent
26. Azmacort Bumex Cardizem Azmacort Bumex Cardizem Azmacort Bumex Cardizem
27. Colace Compazine Darvon Colace Compazine Darvon Colace Compazine Darvon Colace
28. Dilantin Fibercon Lopressor Dilantin Fibercon Lopressor Dilantin Fibercon Lopressor
29. Mevacor Paxil Pepcid Mevacor Paxil Pepcid Mevacor Paxil Pepcid Mevacor Paxil Pepcid
30. Procardia Proventil MDI Restoril Procardia Proventil MDI Restoril Procardia Proventil MDI
31. Serevent Slo-bid Theo-Dur Serevent Slo-bid Theo-Dur Serevent Slo-bid Theo-Dur Serevent
32. Vanceril Vasotec Ventolin Vanceril Vasotec Ventolin Vanceril Vasotec Ventolin Vanceril
33. Xanax Zantac Xanax Zantac Xanax Zantac Xanax Zantac Xanax Zantac Xanax Zantac

Part I / Activity 3
Transcribing Medical Sentences

Now you are ready to make the transition from keyboarding medical terms, which is a visual process, to transcribing medical terms, an aural process. You are going to use audiocassette tapes rather than printed material.

Textbook Users
Launch your word processing package.
Insert the appropriate audiocassette in your transcribing machine and find dictation *87-1*.
You will be transcribing spelling words in sentence structure.
Listen carefully to each sentence on the audiocassette before transcribing.
Rewind and type (transcribe) the sentences.
Save your work on your student disk.
Refer to the answer key.

Part I / Check Your Progress

Let's pause a minute and see how well you are doing. This section will allow you to evaluate your mastery of keyboarding and spelling selected terms and drugs found in the pulmonary medicine specialty.

Textbook Users
Select the correctly spelled term that matches its definition.
Refer to the answer key for immediate feedback.
If you score below 90%, you are recommended to redo the Part I activities.
If you score 90% or above, congratulations. You have mastered the material covered in Part I. If you wish, you can immediately move on to Part II.

Software Users
Click on *Chapter 8, Part I, Check Your Progress.*
Key the correctly spelled term that matches its definition.
When you are finished, click on *End Test.*
A pop-up screen will reveal your score.
If you score below 90%, you are recommended to redo the Part I activities.
If you score 90% or above, congratulations. You have mastered the material covered in Part I. If you wish, you can immediately move on to Part II.

PART I / CHECK YOUR PROGRESS

Directions: Select the correctly spelled term that matches its definition.

1. Increased excretion of urine:
   (a) duiresis
   (b) diuresis
   (c) duiretic
   (d) diuretic

2. Involuntary, rapid, rhythmic movement of the eyeball:
   (a) nystagus
   (b) nystagmus
   (c) adencarcinoma
   (d) adenocarcinoma

3. Labored or difficult breathing:
   (a) ischemia
   (b) ischema
   (c) dyspneia
   (d) dyspnea

4. Localized dilitation of the wall of a blood vessel:
   (a) aneurysm
   (b) embolus
   (c) aneruysm
   (d) emblous

5. Malignant tumor of the glands:
   (a) nystagus
   (b) nystagmus
   (c) adencarcinoma
   (d) adenocarcinoma

6. Containing pus:
   (a) pedol
   (b) purlent
   (c) purulent
   (d) pedal

7. Coughing or spitting up blood from the respiratory tract:
   (a) hemotysis
   (b) hemoptysis
   (c) rhonchus
   (d) ronchus

8. Cramping pains of the calves caused by poor circulation to the leg muscles:
   (a) dention
   (b) claudication
   (c) caudication
   (d) dentition

9. Any drug that has the capacity of increasing the capacity of the pulmonary air passages and improving ventilation to the lungs:
   (a) efflusion
   (b) bronchidilator
   (c) bronchodilator
   (d) effusion

10. Aspiration of fluid from the chest cavity:
    (a) metastasis
    (b) thoracentesis
    (c) metasis
    (d) thorasis

11. Bluish-purple discoloration of the skin due to lack of oxygenated blood:
    (a) cyanesis
    (b) cyanosis
    (c) emesis
    (d) enesis

12. Calf pain with dorsiflexion of foot:
    (a) Homan's sign
    (b) theophylline
    (c) Homans' sign
    (d) theophyline

PART I / CHECK YOUR PROGRESS *continued*

13. Accumulation of fluid in the peritoneal cavity:
    (a) caries
    (b) ascites
    (c) caires
    (d) acites

14. Act of closure or state of being closed:
    (a) oclusion
    (b) auscultation
    (c) auscutation
    (d) occlusion

15. Act of fainting:
    (a) somnolence
    (b) somolence
    (c) syncope
    (d) synscope

16. Abnormal heart condition characterized by the increased size of the right ventricle:
    (a) cor pulmonale
    (b) cor pulmonary
    (c) pulmonary toilet
    (d) pulmon toilet

17. Abnormal heart rhythm:
    (a) sequela
    (b) gallop
    (c) sequelia
    (d) galop

18. Abnormal slowing or stopping of fluid flowing through a vessel:
    (a) atelectasis
    (b) stasis
    (c) atellectasis
    (d) stacis

19. Ability to control urination and defecation urges:
    (a) continent
    (b) contenint
    (c) empiric
    (d) impiric

20. Abnormal crackle sound heard on chest auscultation:
    (a) rale
    (b) rub
    (c) ralle
    (d) rube

21. Abnormal sound heard on chest auscultation due to an obstructed airway:
    (a) hemotysis
    (b) hemoptysis
    (c) rhonchus
    (d) ronchus

22. Abnormally fast heartbeat:
    (a) tachycardia
    (b) dyrhythmia
    (c) tachcardia
    (d) dysrhythmia

23. Accumulation of excess fluid in the tissues of the body:
    (a) sputum
    (b) edena
    (c) spitum
    (d) edema

24. Act of listening for sounds produced within the body with an unaided ear or with a stethoscope:
    (a) oclusion
    (b) auscultation
    (c) auscutation
    (d) occlusion

25. Drowsiness:
    (a) somnolence
    (b) somolence
    (c) syncope
    (d) synscope

PART I / CHECK YOUR PROGRESS *continued*

26. Enlargement of the glands, especially the lymph nodes:
    (a) thyromegaly
    (b) adenogaly
    (c) adenopathy
    (d) thyropathy

27. Enlargement of the thyroid gland:
    (a) thyromegaly
    (b) adenogaly
    (c) adenopathy
    (d) thyropathy

28. Escape of fluid into a body cavity:
    (a) efflusion
    (b) bronchidilator
    (c) bronchodilator
    (d) effusion

29. Affecting both sides:
    (a) afebrile
    (b) bilateral
    (c) afevrile
    (d) bilaral

30. Any abnormal condition that follows and is the result of a disease, treatment, or injury:
    (a) erythema
    (b) sequea
    (c) erytema
    (d) sequela

31. Cleansing of the trachea and bronchial tree:
    (a) cor pulmonale
    (b) cor pulmonary
    (c) pulmonary toilet
    (d) pulmon toilet

32. Collapse of a portion of the lung:
    (a) atelectasis
    (b) stasis
    (c) atellectasis
    (d) stacis

33. Decreased supply of oxygenated blood to a body part:
    (a) ischemia
    (b) ischema
    (c) dyspneia
    (d) dyspnea

34. Mass that is brought by the blood from another vessel that obstructs blood circulation:
    (a) aneurysm
    (b) embolus
    (c) aneruysm
    (d) emblous

35. Material coughed up from the lungs and ejected through the mouth:
    (a) sputum
    (b) edena
    (c) spitum
    (d) edema

36. Normally occurring microrganisms living within the body that provide natural immunity against certain organisms:
    (a) fora
    (b) saphenous
    (c) flora
    (d) sapenous

37. Occuring at night:
    (a) intrauterine
    (b) nocturnal
    (c) interuterine
    (d) noctural

38. Pertains to the two main superficial veins of the lower leg:
    (a) fora
    (b) saphenous
    (c) flora
    (d) sapenous

PART I / CHECK YOUR PROGRESS continued

39. Diagnostic procedure using ultrasound to study heart structure and motion:
    (a) echocardiogram
    (b) echiocardogram
    (c) arteriogram
    (d) arterogram

40. Disordered rhythm:
    (a) rhonchus
    (b) dyrhythmia
    (c) ronchis
    (d) dysrhythmia

41. Treatment by a spray:
    (a) nebulization
    (b) nebullization
    (c) fibrillation
    (d) fibrilation

42. Uncoordinated twitching of muscle fibers:
    (a) nebulization
    (b) nebullization
    (c) fibrillation
    (d) fibrilation

43. Within the uterus:
    (a) intrauterine
    (b) nocturnal
    (c) interuterine
    (d) noctural

44. Without fever:
    (a) afebrile
    (b) bilateral
    (c) afevrile
    (d) bilaral

45. Compound containing water molecules:
    (a) hydrate
    (b) hidrate
    (c) infiltrate
    (d) enfiltrate

46. Condition of decay and destruction of a tooth:
    (a) caries
    (b) ascites
    (c) caires
    (d) acites

47. Generic antianxiety drug:
    (a) lorazepam
    (b) lorasepam
    (c) isorbide
    (d) isosorbide

48. Generic name for a nitrate-based antianginal agent:
    (a) lorazepam
    (b) lorasepam
    (c) isorbide
    (d) isosorbide

49. Generic name for an aminopenicillin antibiotic:
    (a) amoxicillin
    (b) amoxicilin
    (c) doxepin
    (d) dozepin

50. Generic name for an anticoagulant:
    (a) haperin
    (b) heparin
    (c) nifedipin
    (d) nifedipine

51. Generic name for an antidepressant:
    (a) amoxicillin
    (b) amoxicilin
    (c) doxepin
    (d) dozepin

52. Position and condition of the teeth:
    (a) dention
    (b) claudication
    (c) caudication
    (d) dentition

PART I / CHECK YOUR PROGRESS *continued*

53. Situated or occurring above the ventricles:
    (a) superventricular
    (b) supraventricular
    (c) suberventricular
    (d) suparventricular

54. Sound caused by the rubbing together of two surfaces:
    (a) rale
    (b) rub
    (c) ralle
    (d) rube

55. Sound or murmur heard on auscultation:
    (a) bruit
    (b) gallop
    (c) briut
    (d) galop

56. Substance that promotes the excretion of urine:
    (a) duiresis
    (b) diuresis
    (c) duiretic
    (d) diuretic

57. Surgical removal of all or part of the lung:
    (a) pneumontomy
    (b) pneumonectomy
    (c) pneumotorax
    (d) pneumothorax

58. To vomit:
    (a) cyanesis
    (b) cyanosis
    (c) emesis
    (d) enesis

59. Transfer of disease from one organ or part to another not directly connected with it:
    (a) metastasis
    (b) thoracentesis
    (c) metasis
    (d) thorasis

60. Treating a disease based upon observation and experience rather than reasoning alone:
    (a) continent
    (b) contenint
    (c) empiric
    (d) impiric

61. Presence of air or gas in the pleural cavity:
    (a) pneumontomy
    (b) pneumonectomy
    (c) pneumotorax
    (d) pneumothorax

62. Radiographic visualization of an artery after injection of a contrast medium:
    (a) echocardiogram
    (b) echiocardogram
    (c) arteriogram
    (d) arterogram

63. Redness of the skin:
    (a) erythema
    (b) sequea
    (c) erytema
    (d) sequela

64. Relating to the foot:
    (a) pedol
    (b) purlent
    (c) purulent
    (d) pedal

65. Generic name for any of the large group of broad-spectrum antibiotics:
    (a) prednisone
    (b) prenisone
    (c) cephalosporin
    (d) cephalsporin

66. Generic calcium channel blocker drug:
    (a) haperin
    (b) heparin
    (c) nifedipin
    (d) nifedipine

PART I / CHECK YOUR PROGRESS *continued*

67. Generic corticosteroid drug:
    (a) prednisone
    (b) prenisone
    (c) cephalosporin
    (d) cephalsporin

68. Generic name for a broad-spectrum antibiotic:
    (a) nitroglyserin
    (b) erythromycin
    (c) nitroglycerin
    (d) erythromysin

69. Generic name for a bronchodilator:
    (a) Homan's sign
    (b) theophylline
    (c) Homans' sign
    (d) theophyline

70. Generic name for a coronary vasodilator, antianginal:
    (a) nitroglyserin
    (b) erythromycin
    (c) nitroglycerin
    (d) erythromysin

71. Trade name for a bronchodilator, metered dose inhaler:
    (a) Proventil MDI
    (b) Provintel MDI
    (c) Vanceril
    (d) Vanseril

72. Trade name for a bronchodilator:
    (a) Ventlin
    (b) Ventolin
    (c) Paxil
    (d) Pasil

73. Trade name for a bronchodilator:
    (a) Theo-Dur
    (b) Xanaz
    (c) Xanax
    (d) Theo-Dure

74. Trade name for a bulk-forming laxative:
    (a) Dilantin
    (b) Dylantin
    (c) Fibercon
    (d) Fiberkon

75. Trade name for a calcium channel blocker for atrial fibrillation:
    (a) Cardizem
    (b) Cardisem
    (c) Colase
    (d) Colace

76. Trade name for a coronary vasodilator:
    (a) Procardia
    (b) Serevent
    (c) Procariodia
    (d) Servent

77. Trade name for a corticosteroid for the prevention or treatment of bronchial asthma:
    (a) Azamcort
    (b) Bumex
    (c) Azmacort
    (d) Bumez

78. Trade name for a corticosteroid:
    (a) Proventil MDI
    (b) Provintel MDI
    (c) Vanceril
    (d) Vanseril

79. Trade name for a loop diuretic:
    (a) Azamcort
    (b) Bumex
    (c) Azmacort
    (d) Bumez

80. Trade name for a narcotic analgesic:
    (a) Compazine
    (b) Darvon
    (c) Compasine
    (d) Darvin

PART I / CHECK YOUR PROGRESS *continued*

81. Trade name for a nasal spray, bronchodilator:
    (a) Ascriptin
    (b) Asriptin
    (c) Atrovent
    (d) Atovent

82. Trade name for a preparation of aspirin with Maalox, an analgesic and anti-inflammatory:
    (a) Ascriptin
    (b) Asriptin
    (c) Atrovent
    (d) Atovent

83. Trade name for a sedative-hypnotic:
    (a) Pepsid
    (b) Restoril
    (c) Pepcid
    (d) Restoral

84. Trade name for a stool softener:
    (a) Cardizem
    (b) Cardisem
    (c) Colase
    (d) Colace

85. Trade name for a tranquilizer and antiemetic:
    (a) Compazine
    (b) Darvon
    (c) Compasine
    (d) Darvin

86. Trade name for an acid controller for heartburn and acid indigestion:
    (a) Pepsid
    (b) Restoril
    (c) Pepcid
    (d) Restoral

87. Trade name for an acid controller for heartburn and acid indigestion:
    (a) Zantac
    (b) Vasotec
    (c) Zantak
    (d) Vasotek

88. Trade name for an aerosol bronchodilator:
    (a) Procardia
    (b) Serevent
    (c) Procariodia
    (d) Servent

89. Trade name for an antianxiety agent:
    (a) Theo-Dur
    (b) Xanaz
    (c) Xanax
    (d) Theo-Dure

90. Trade name for an anticonvulsant used in the treatment of epilepsy:
    (a) Dilantin
    (b) Dylantin
    (c) Fibercon
    (d) Fiberkon

91. Trade name for an antidepressant:
    (a) Ventlin
    (b) Ventolin
    (c) Paxil
    (d) Pasil

92. Trade name for an antihyperlipidemic:
    (a) Lopressor
    (b) Metacor
    (c) Lopresor
    (d) Mevacor

93. Trade name for an antihypertensive:
    (a) Lopressor
    (b) Metacor
    (c) Lopresor
    (d) Mevacor

94. Trade name for an antihypertensive:
    (a) Zantac
    (b) Vasotec
    (c) Zantak
    (d) Vasotek

PART I / CHECK YOUR PROGRESS *continued*

95. Trade name for a cephalosporin antibiotic:
    (a) Ancef IV
    (b) Ansef IV
    (c) NPH
    (d) PNH

96. Trade name for an extended-release bronchodilator:
    (a) Slow-bid
    (b) Slo-bide
    (c) Slow-bide
    (d) Slo-bid

97. Trade name for an insulin that decreases blood sugar:
    (a) Ancef IV
    (b) Ansef IV
    (c) NPH
    (d) PNH

98. An abnormal heart rhythm:
    (a) galop
    (b) rale
    (c) gallop
    (d) ralle

Pretest (8T-2)

Textbook Users

Launch your word processing package.

Insert the appropriate audiocassette in your transcribing machine and find dictation *8T-2*.

On the open screen, transcribe and proofread dictation *8T-2*. Identify and correct all errors.

Save your work on your student disk.

After completing the transcription, refer to the answer key.

Manually complete the error analysis and production for pay charts.

If you scored below 90%, continue on to *Activities 4–7*.

If you scored 90% or above, congratulations. If you wish, you can immediately move on to Part III.

Software Users

Click on *Chapter 8, Part II, Pretest (8T-2)*.

Insert the appropriate audiocassette in your transcribing machine and find dictation *8T-2*.

Click on *Start Watch*, then transcribe and proofread dictation *8T-2*. Identify and correct all errors.

When you are finished, click on *Done*, then *Score Document* to display your production for pay.

Click on *Display Error Analysis* to reveal your score.

Click on *View Errors* to see your errors.

Save your work (with errors showing) on your student disk by clicking on *File*, then *Save As*.

If you score below 90%, continue on to *Activities 4–7*.

If you score 90% or above, congratulations. If you wish, you can immediately move on to Part III.

Activities 4–5
Proofreading Worksheet Exercises

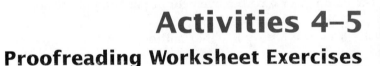

Textbook Users

Proofread and correct errors in the medical documents *Activities 4–5*.

After completing the exercises, refer to the answer key.

Manually complete the error analysis chart for each report.

Software Users

Click on *Chapter 8, Part II, Activities 4–5*.

Proofread and correct errors found in the medical documents.

Click on *File*, then *Done*.

Click on *Score Document* to see the errors you made.

Save your work (with errors showing) on your student disk by clicking on *File*, then *Save As*.

Click on *File*, then *Exit*, to proceed.

PART II / ACTIVITY 4
PROOFREADING WORKSHEET EXERCISE

Directions: Proofread this medical document using all formatting guidelines established in this textbook.

CONSULTATION REPORT

Patient Name: Calabretta, Gregory

File Number: 09451

Date of Birth: January 15, 19xx

Examination Date: *current date*

Requesting Physician: Izzy Sertoli, MD

HISTORY OF PRESENT ILLNESS: The patient is a 42 year old white male who presented to the Hospital with some vague chest pain as well as a history of shortness of breathe. The patient states to me that he has had shortness of breathe for approximately a year and 1/2. The dispnea is worse on excursion especially when climbing stairs and doing his job as a janitor. He has had a dry cough which on occasion was productive of clear sputume but has not been productive of blood or puss. Her complains of vague substernal left sided chest pain. The pain is worse with movement or papation of the area.

PAST HISTORY: Her past history is significant for asthma. He had a bilateral hernia repair 3 yrs ago.

REVIEW OF SYSTEMS: Neg.

PHYSICAL EXAMINATION

GENERAL: His blood pressure is 120 over 70 pulse seventy respirations 12 per minute.

HEENT: Negative. Neck veins are not extended. Trachea is mid line. There are no knodes in the superclavicular or cervical chain.

CHEST: Breath sounds reveal some krackles at the basis but are otherwise negative.

HEART: Heart sounds are normal but distant.

EXTREMITIES: No clubing cyanosis or edema noted.

LABORATORY DATA: Room air abg shows a po2 of fifty nine without co2 retention. Chest x-ray reveals a diffuse inter-stitial process with no hilar knodes.

Continued

PART II / ACTIVITY 4 *continued*

CONSULTATION REPORT
Patient Name: Calabretta, Gregory
File Number: 09451
Date of Birth: January 15, 19xx
Examination Date: *current date*
Requesting Physician: Izzy Sertoli, MD

IMPRESSION: I suspect that we are dealing with an inflammatory precess in his lungs. A illness such as sarciod is a extinct possibility as we discussed on the phone last night. Additionally this could be chf although clinically it does not look like it. We will have an answer if the next chest x ray results show improvement with dyuresis. If it does not than a more intensive work up shall take place. Clinically I doubt an infection. I suspect we end up doing a bronchscopy with a biopsy.

PLAN: If there is no improvement on tomorrows x-ray we will proceed with a more agressive workup. The patient states she has no previous chest x-rays for comparison.

_____

Allan Bolus MD

PART II / ACTIVITY 5
PROOFREADING WORKSHEET EXERCISE

Directions: Proofread this medical document using all formatting guidelines established in this textbook.

FedDes Wellness Center
Pulmonary medicine Division, Suite 451
Wellness Way Drive
New York, NY 10036

Current date

Charles P. Davis, MD
FedDes Wellness Center
Family Practice Division, Suite 300
Wellness Way Drive
New York, NY 10036

Re: Lawrence a. Rabia
Date of Birth: Janaury 20, 19xx

Dear Dr. Davis

Mr. Rabai is a 62 year old white male with a past history of smoking. He is 6 weeks status post aortic aneurysm repair. Postoperatively she did well and was discharged. At home, she has been fairly home bound but not bedridden. He was in his usual state of health without an upper respiratory illness cough congestion or aches when he developed the a cute on set of left sided pleuritic chest pain. The pleurtic component of the pain has entensified and is actually positional at this time. He denied any hemotysis. He has some mild shortness of breathe and mild dispnea or exertion. He has no history of ankle edema or deep vein thrombsis all though he has had coronary artery by pass grafting and a safenous vein harvest on the left side.

On physical examination the patients temperature was ninety nine. His other vital signs were stable. HENT was benign. Neck showed no mass or adenpathy. Lungs showed diminished breathe sounds bilaterally with scratchie rublike sounds on the left side. Cardiovascular exam shows SI SII within normal limits and grade 1 over 6 systolic injection murmur at the lower left sternal border. There was no cardiac rub. Adbomen was soft. Extremities showed no edema. Calfs were benign and non-tender.

Chest x ray showed no evidence of neumothorax with some hyper inflation and chronic obstructive pulmonary disease changes. Her ventilation prefusion scan showed an abnormal perfusion study with 3 matched defects.

IMPRESSION: Pleuritic left sided chest pain 6 weeks post operative and an abnormal perfusion scan. Given the indeterminate scan I suspect there is a substantial chance this may yet be a pulmonary imbolus. I would empirically haperinize at this time and procede with pulmonary angoigraphy. I have discussed this with the patient and he understands and agrees.

Thank-you for this referral.

PART II / ACTIVITY 5 *continued*

Charles P. Davis, MD
Current date
Page 3

Sincerely

Allan Bolus MD

xx

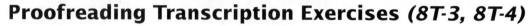

Part II / Activities 6–7
Proofreading Transcription Exercises (8T-3, 8T-4)

Now you are ready to make the transition from simply proofreading printed material to both transcribing and proofreading dictated material. There are two activities in this section.

Textbook Users

Launch your word processing package. Insert the appropriate audiocassette in your transcribing machine and find dictation *8T-3*.

Step 1: Listen to the entire dictation to gain an understanding of the medical concepts and terms involved. Rewind the tape to the beginning of the dictation and transcribe what you hear. Do not worry about formatting, style, or speed. Simply type what you hear being dictated, using correct punctuation, capitalization, and spelling. Stop as needed to look up words you do not understand or cannot spell. Adjust the speed control of the transcriber to a comfortable level, starting slowly to assure no dictated words are missed, and then increase the speed as your accuracy improves.

Step 2: Rewind the tape again, and using your created template, transcribe dictation *8T-3* again. Proofread the report and correct all errors. Save your work on your student disk. Refer to the answer key and manually complete the error analysis and production for pay charts.

Repeat the same process for dictation *8T-4*.

Software Users

Click on *Chapter 8, Activity 6: Proofreading Transcription Exercise.*

Insert the appropriate audiocassette in your transcribing machine and find dictation *8T-3*.

Step 1: Listen to the entire dictation to gain an understanding of the medical concepts and terms involved. Rewind the tape to the beginning of the dictation, click *Start Watch,* and transcribe what you hear. Do not worry about formatting, style, or speed. Simply type what you hear being dictated, using correct punctuation, capitalization, and spelling. Stop as needed to look up words you do not understand or cannot spell. Adjust the speed control of the transcriber to a comfortable level, starting slowly to assure no dictated words are missed, and then increase the speed as your accuracy improves. When you are finished, click on *Done,* then choose *Return to Main Menu.*

Step 2: Click on *Chapter 8, Activity 6* again. Rewind the tapes again, click on *Start Watch,* and transcribe dictation *8T-3* again. Proofread the report and correct all errors. When you are finished, click on *Done,* then *Score Document* to display your production for pay. Click on *Display Error Analysis* to reveal your score and then *View Errors* to see the errors you made. Save your work (with errors showing) on your student disk by clicking *File,* then *Save As.*

Follow the same process for dictation *8T-4*.

Part II / Check Your Progress (8T-2)

Let's pause a minute and see how well you are doing. This section will allow you to evaluate your success at transcribing and proofreading pulmonary medicine reports.

Textbook Users

Launch your word processing package.

Insert the appropriate audiocassette in your transcribing machine and find dictation *8T-2*.

On the open screen, transcribe and proofread dictation *8T-2*.

Identify and correct all errors.

Use formatting guidelines established in Chapter 2.

Save your work on your student disk.

After completing the transcription, refer to the answer key.

Manually complete the error analysis chart.

Manually complete the production for Pay summary chart.

If you score below 90%, you are recommended to redo the Part II Activities.

If you score 90% or above, congratulations. You have mastered the material covered in Part II. If you wish, you can immediately move on to Part III.

Software Users

Click on *Chapter 8, Part II, Check Your Progress (8T-2)*.

Insert the appropriate audiocassette in your transcribing machine and find dictation *8T-2*.

Click on *Start Watch*, then transcribe and proofread dictation *8T-2*.

Identify and correct all errors.

When you are finished, click on *Done*, then *Score Document*: a pop-up window will display your production for pay.

Click on *Display Error Analysis* to reveal your score.

Click on *View Errors* to see the errors you made.

Save your work (with errors showing) on your student disk by clicking on *File*, then *Save As*.

If you score below 90%, you are recommended to redo the Part II Activities.

If you score 90% or above, congratulations. You have mastered the material covered in Part II. If you wish, you can immediately move on to Part III.

Pretest (8T-5, 8T-6)

Professional transcriptionists can transcribe and proofread their own work. Can you? Scoring 90% or better proves it!

Textbook Users
Launch your word processing package.
Insert the appropriate audiocassette in your transcribing machine and find dication *8T-5.*
On the open screen, transcribe and proofread dictation *8T-5.*
Identify and correct all errors.
Use formatting guidelines established in Chapter 2.
Save your work on your student disk.
Follow the same process for dictation *8T-6.*
After completing the transcriptions, refer to the answer key.
Manually complete the error analysis chart for each document.
Manually complete the production for pay chart for each document.
If you score below 90%, continue with *Pulmonary Medicine Transcription at FedDes Wellness Center.*
If you score 90% or above, congratulations. You have mastered the material covered in Part III. If you wish, you can immediately move on to the next chapter.

Software Users
Click on *Chapter 8, Part III, Pretest (8T-5).*
Insert the appropriate audiocassette in your transcribing machine and find dictation *8T-5.*
Click on *Start Watch,* then transcribe and proofread dictation *8T-5.*
Identify and correct all errors.
When you are finished, click on *Done,* then *Score Document:* a pop-up window will display your production for pay.
Click on *Display Error Analysis* to reveal your score.
Click on *View Errors* to see the errors you made.
Save your work (with errors showing) on your student disk by clicking on *File,* then *Save As.*
Follow the same process for dictation *8T-6.*
If you score below 90%, continue with *Pulmonary Medicine Transcription at FedDes Wellness Center.*
If you score 90% or above, congratulations. You have mastered the material covered in Part III. If you wish, you can immediately move on to the next chapter.

Pulmonary Medicine Transcription at FedDes Wellness Center

You finally made it! You have been hired as a transcriptionist at FedDes Wellness Center in the Pulmonary Medicine Division. Your supervisor has asked you to transcribe today's dictation.

Textbook Users
Launch your word processing package.
Insert the appropriate audiocassette in your transcribing machine and find dictation *8T-7*.
Create or use an existing template for the six types of reports.
On the open screen, transcribe and proofread dictation *8T-7*.
Identify and correct all errors.
Save your work on your student disk.
Follow the same process for dictations *8T-8 through 8T-12*.
After completing the transcription, refer to the answer key.
Manually complete the error analysis chart and production for pay charts for each document.

Software Users
Click on *Chapter 8, Part III, Pulmonary Medicine Transcription at FedDes Wellness Center (8T-7)*.
Insert the appropriate audiocassette in your transcribing machine and find dictation *8T-7*.
Click on *Start Watch,* then transcribe and proofread dictation *8T-7*.
Identify and correct all errors.
When you are finished, click on *Done,* then *Score Document:* to display your production for pay.
Click on *Display Error Analysis* to reveal your score and on *View Errors* to see the errors you made.
Save your work (with errors showing) on your student disk by clicking on *File,* then *Save As.*
Follow the same process for dictations *8T-8 and 8T-9*.
NOTE: Continue with medical documents *8T-10* through *8T-12* using your word processing package and manually complete the Error Analysis and Production for Pay sheets.

Index of Dictations and Associated Transcription Tips

Please remember to follow the guidelines pertaining to capitalization, numbers, punctuation, abbreviations, measurements, symbols, and use of templates to create medical reports at FedDes Wellness Center. Review of this material can be found in Unit 1.

8T-7
History and Physical Examination
Patient's Name: Francine Banks
Physician: Allan Bolus, MD

TRANSCRIPTION TIPS
- A hyphen is used between numbers and *year old.*
  You will hear the dictator say: This is a twenty eight year old white female.
  You will transcribe as: This is a 28-year-old white female.

- A hyphen is used to take the place of the words *to* or *through* to identify ranges.
  You will hear the dictator say: respiratory

infection of seven to ten days duration. You will transcribe as: respiratory infection of 7-10 days duration.

- A hyphen is used to join two or more words when used as an adjective that proceeds a noun.
  The following word pairs are dictated in this report: blood-tinged, follow-up.

- The following drugs are dictated in this report:
  Erythromycin: a generic name for a broad-spectrum antibiotic
  Proventil inhaler: trade name for a bronchodilator, metered dose inhaler

- Words beginning with *pre, re, post,* and *non* are generally not hyphenated.
  For example: noncontributory

- A period is used to take the place of the word *point.*
  You will hear the dictator say: Temperature was one hundred point four.
  You will transcribe as: Temperature was 100.4.

- Figures are used for age, weight, height, blood pressure, pulse, and respiration. The diagonal (/) is used to indicate the word *per* in laboratory values and respirations or the word *over* in blood pressure.
  You will hear the dictator say: b p one hundred over sixty. Respiratory rate twenty to twenty four per minute.
  You will transcribe as: BP 110/60. Respiratory rate 20-24/min.

- The following abbreviations are dictated in this report. The plural is formed by adding the letter *s* only (no added commas).
  TMs: tympanic membranes
  WBC: white blood cell (count)

- Figures and capital letters are used to refer to the vertebral column and spinal nerves. You will hear the dictator say: sinus tachycardia without murmur or s three.
  You should transcribe this sentence as follows: Sinus tachycardia without murmur or S3.

 8T-8
Consultation Report
Patient's Name: Heather Williams
Requesting Physician: Charles P. Davis, MD
Physician: Douglas Sputum, MD

● TRANSCRIPTION TIPS

- A hyphen is used to join two or more words when used as an adjective that proceeds a noun.
  The following word pair is dictated in this report: innocent-sounding.

- Roman numerals are used to express class, cranial leads (EKG), cranial nerves, limb leads (ECG), factor (blood clotting), grade, phase, pregnancy and delivery, stage, and type.
  You will hear the dictator say: There is a short grade two over six innocent-sounding aortic ejection murmur.
  You should transcribe as: There is a short grade II/VI innocent-sounding aortic ejection murmur.

- Figures are used with the + or − symbols.
  You will hear the dictator say: There is one plus dependent edema.
  You should transcribe as: There is 1+ dependent edema.

- The following procedure is dictated in this report.
  dobutamine MUGA scan: multiple gated acquisition, nuclear medicine imaging

 8T-9
History and Physical Examination
Patient's Name: Quinetta Nelson
Physician: Neal Alveoli, MD

● TRANSCRIPTION TIPS

- The following abbreviations are dictated in this report. The plural is formed by adding the letter *s* only.
  DJD: degenerative joint disease
  TIAs: transient ischemic attacks
  AV: atrioventricular
  TMs: tympanic membranes
  JVD: jugular venous distention
  COPD: chronic obstructive pulmonary disease

- Words beginning with *pre, re, post,* and *non* are generally not hyphenated: postabdominal

- The following drugs are dictated in this report:
  Proventil: trade name for a bronchodilator, metered dose inhaler
  Vanceril: trade name for a corticosteroid
  Atrovent: the trade name for a nasal spray, bronchodilator
  nitroglycerin spray: a generic name for a coronary vasodilator, antianginal
  Darvon: the trade name for a narcotic analgesic
  Slo-bid: the trade name for an extended-release bronchodilator
  Lorazepam: a generic antianxiety drug

- A hyphen is used when two or more words are viewed as a single word. The following word pair is dictated in this report: three-quarters.

- Capital letters are used for electrocardiographic leads, waves, and segments. Waves include P, Q, R, S, T, and U and their combinations.
  You will hear the dictator say: increased p two with a midsystolic murmur
  You should transcribe as: Increased P2 with a midsystolic murmur.

- Words beginning with *pre, re, post,* and *non* are generally not hyphenated: nontender.

- The following disease is dictated in this report:
  cor pulmonale: a serious cardiac condition in which there is a right ventricular heart failure

8T-10
Consultation Report
Patient's Name: Marty Waye
Requesting Physician: Izzy Sertoli, MD
Physician: Allan Bolus, MD

● **TRANSCRIPTION TIPS**
- A hyphen joins two or more words as an adjective that proceeds a noun.
  The following word pair is dictated in this report: left-sided.

- The following abbreviations are dictated in this report:
  CT: computerized tomography
  ENT: ear, nose, throat
  MI: myocardial infarction
  JVD: jugular venous distention
  HEENT: head, eyes, ear, nose, throat
  PT: prothrombin time

- The following procedure is dictated in this report:
  thoracentesis: surgical puncture and drainage of the thoracic cavity

- The following drug is dictated in this report:
  cephalosporin: a generic name for any of the large group of broad-spectrum antibiotics

8T-11
Consultation Report
Patient's Name: John Washington
Requesting Physician: Adam Valence, MD
Physician: Douglas Sputum, MD

● **TRANSCRIPTION TIPS**
- Words beginning with *pre, re, post,* and *non* are generally not hyphenated:
  preoperatively

- The percent sign (%) is used with words and figures.
  You will hear the dictator say: found to have a seventy percent distal left main occlusion
  You should transcribe as: found to have a 70% distal left main occlusion.

- The following drugs are dictated in this report.
  nitroglycerin: generic name for coronary vasodilator, antianginal
  heparin: is the generic name for an anticoagulant.

- The following abbreviations are dictated in this report:
  TB: tuberculosis
  AP: anteroposterior
  FEV1: forced expiratory volume. Pulmonary function test that measures the volume of air expired at 1 second (FEV1).

These tests evaluate pulmonary function. The patient is instructed to inhale slowly and deeply as possible and then to exhale as quickly and completely as possible into the mouthpiece of the spirometer. The procedure is repeated three times and the largest volume is recorded. FEV2 is the volume of air expired in 2 seconds; and FEV3 is the volume of air expired in 3 seconds

BUN: blood urea nitrogen

- Words beginning with *pre, re, post,* and *non* are generally not hyphenated: noncontributory, nontender

- Figures and capital letters are used to refer to the vertebral column and spinal nerves.
  You will hear the dictation say: Cardiac exam reveals soft s four gallop.
  You should transcribe as: Cardiac exam reveals soft S4 gallop.

- A period is used to take the place of the word *point.*
  You will hear the dictator say: hemoglobin of eleven point two
  You should transcribe as: hemoglobin of 11.2

- A comma is used to punctuate large numbers with five or more digits in units of three.
  You will hear the dictator say: white count ten thousand eight hundred
  You should transcribe as: white count 10,800

- An apostrophe is used to form the possessive of singular and plural nouns.
  You will hear the dictator say: The patients pulmonary function tests
  You should transcribe as: The patient's pulmonary function tests

 8T-12
Consultation Report
Patient's Name: Brenda McMurray
Requesting Physician: Charles P. Davis, MD
Physician: Neal Alveoli, MD

TRANSCRIPTION TIPS
- The following abbreviations are dictated in this report:
  TB: tuberculosis
  URI: upper respiratory infection
  MUGA scan: multiple gated acquisition scan

- Ordinal numbers first through ninth are spelled out.
  You will hear the dictator say: normal first and second sounds
  You should transcribe as: normal first and second sounds

- Figures are used with the + or − symbols.
  You will hear the dictator say: There is three plus edema
  You should transcribe as: There is 3+ edema

Part III / Check Your Progress (8T-5, 8T-6)

Professional transcriptionists can transcribe and proofread their own work with speed and accuracy. Have you mastered the pulmonary medicine transcription rotation at FedDes Wellness Center?

Textbook Users

Launch your word processing package.

Insert the appropriate audiocassette in your transcribing machine and find dictation *8T-5*.

On the open screen, transcribe and proofread dictation *8T-5*.

Identify and correct all errors.

Use formatting guidelines established in Chapter 2.

Save your work on your student disk.

Follow the same process for dictation *8T-6*.

After completing the transcriptions, refer to the answer key.

Manually complete the error analysis chart for each document.

Manually complete the production for pay chart for each document.

If you score below 90%, you are recommended to repeat Part III.

If you score 90% or above, congratulations. You have mastered the material covered in this chapter.

Software Users

Click on *Chapter 8, Part III, Check Your Progress (8T-5)*.

Insert the appropriate audiocassette in your transcribing machine and find dictation *8T-5*.

Click on *Start Watch*, then transcribe and proofread dictation *8T-5*.

Identify and correct all errors.

When you are finished, click on *Done*, then *Score Document:* a pop-up window will display your production for pay.

Click on *Display Error Analysis* to reveal your score.

Click on *View Errors* to see the errors you made.

Save your work (with errors showing) on your student disk by clicking on *File*, then *Save As*.

Follow the same process for dictation *8T-6*.

If you score below 90%, you are recommended to repeat Part III.

If you score 90% or above, congratulations. You have mastered the material covered in this chapter.

Chapter 9

Office Medical Transcription from the Gastroenterology Practice

OBJECTIVES

At the completion of Chapter 9, you should be able to do the following:

1. Match medical terms associated with the gastroenterology specialty with their definitions.

2. Spell medical terms associated with the gastroenterology specialty with their definitions.

3. Transcribe medical terms in sentence structure.

4. Proofread, edit, and correct medical documents associated with the gastroenterology specialty containing various errors.

5. Transcribe and proofread authentic medical documents associated with the gastroenterology specialty.

What's Ahead

240

The Gastroenterology Rotation

The FedDes Wellness Center has three gastroenterologists, or specialists in gastroenterology, on staff. Gastroenterology is the study of the digestive tract, liver, and pancreas. The gastroenterologist assesses the function of these organs by performing invasive and noninvasive testing.

Assessment of gastrointestinal problems begin with the patient's complete history from the mouth and teeth to bowel habits. The gastrointestinal tract examination encompasses many organs, including the mouth and pharynx, esophagus, stomach, duodenum, liver, gallbladder, pancreas, small intestine, colon, and rectum.

The physicians in FedDes gastroenterology division perform laboratory tests and procedures using an endoscope, including gastroscopy, exploratory laparoscopy, colonoscopy, and flexible sigmoidoscopy. Other diagnostic tests include an upper GI (gastrointestinal) series and a lower GI series (barium enema). Both of these common x-ray studies use barium sulfate to image the alimentary tract.

In this unit, you assume the role of a medical transcriptionist employed at FedDes Wellness Center. **Please follow the guidelines pertaining to capitalization, numbers, punctuation, abbreviations, measurements, symbols, and use of templates to create medical reports at FedDes Wellness Center. Review of this material can be found in Unit 1.** A list of the patient's name and the type of report as well as associated transcription tips are included in this chapter.

You will work with the textbook, CD-ROM, and accompanying audiocassettes. Your mastery of gastroenterology transcription is assessed through worksheets, timed transcription exercises, the Error analysis chart, and the Production for Pay Summary.

All the answer keys are found in the textbook and CD-ROM, providing immediate feedback. After transcribing a report, you will proofread your work and correct any errors. Then you will compare your proofread work against a master transcript, categorize all errors, and tabulate the errors on the Error analysis chart. The Production for Pay Summary correlates your production to the FedDes Wellness Center pay scale, which is based on industry compensation standards. The scale is also linked to your grade. This system allows you to assess your mastery of transcription skills in a real-world scenario.

Pretest

Let's find out if you can define and spell selected terminology and drugs of the gastroenterology specialty that are included in this chapter by scoring 90% or better.

Textbook Users

Select the correctly spelled term that matches its definition.

Refer to the answer key for immediate feedback.

If you score below 90%, continue on to *Activities 1–3*.

If you score 90% or above, congratulations. You have mastered the material covered in Part I. If you wish, you can immediately move on to Part II.

Software Users

Click on *Chapter 9, Part I, Pretest*.

Key the correctly spelled term that matches its definition.

When you are finished, click on *End Test*.

A pop-up screen will reveal your score.

If you score below 90%, continue on to *Activities 1–3*.

If you score 90% or above, congratulations. You have mastered the material covered in Part I. If you wish, you can immediately move on to Part II.

PART I / PRETEST

Directions: Select the correctly spelled term that matches its definition.

1. A 37% aqueous solution of formaldehyde:
   (a) forlate
   (b) formalen
   (c) formalin
   (d) forlaten

2. A backward or return flow:
   (a) stent
   (b) reflux
   (c) stant
   (d) refluxe

3. A normal component of urine:
   (a) keytone
   (b) ketone
   (c) creatine
   (d) creatinine

4. Generic name for a corticosteroid:
   (a) meclizane
   (b) meclazane
   (c) hydrocortsone
   (d) hydrocortisone

5. A gland in the male that surrounds the neck of the bladder and urethra:
   (a) prostate
   (b) tirate
   (c) postate
   (d) titrate

6. Enlargement of the thyroid gland:
   (a) hepatasplenmegaly
   (b) thyromegaly
   (c) hepatosplenomegaly
   (d) thyomegaly

7. A mold for keeping a skin graft in place:
   (a) stent
   (b) reflux
   (c) stant
   (d) refluxe

8. A radiographic record of an artery after injection of a contrast medium into it:
   (a) pinna
   (b) arterogram
   (c) pina
   (d) arteriogram

9. Ability to move spontaneously:
   (a) bilary
   (b) biliary
   (c) motility
   (d) molity

10. After a meal:
    (a) postprandial
    (b) prophylatic
    (c) posprandial
    (d) prophyacic

11. An agent that tends to ward off disease:
    (a) postprandial
    (b) prophylatic
    (c) posprandial
    (d) prophyacic

12. Generic name for an anticoagulant:
    (a) heparin
    (b) lidocaine
    (c) heparen
    (d) lidacaine

PART I / PRETEST *continued*

13. Generic name for an anti-inflammatory and antiallergic agent:
    (a) prenisone
    (b) prednisone
    (c) lidocaine
    (d) lidocain

14. Generic name for an antinauseant:
    (a) meclizine
    (b) mecizine
    (c) nitroglycerin
    (d) nitoglycerin

15. An elongated endoscope, usually fiberoptic:
    (a) fiberscope
    (b) fiveroscope
    (c) colonoscope
    (d) colonscope

16. An endoscope for use in sigmoidoscopy:
    (a) sigmoidoscope
    (b) sigmiodoscope
    (c) colonoscope
    (d) colonscope

17. An increase in the severity of a disease or symptoms:
    (a) retroflexion
    (b) retroflesion
    (c) exacerbation
    (d) exacerbasion

18. An opening created by surgery, disease, or trauma between two or more organs or structures:
    (a) anastomosis
    (b) anastamosis
    (c) stenosis
    (d) stenasis

19. Any compound containing carbon oxide:
    (a) keytone
    (b) ketone
    (c) creatine
    (d) creatinine

20. Any growth or mass protruding from a mucous membrane:
    (a) polyp
    (b) polpa
    (c) scera
    (d) sclera

21. Any solution compound that conducts electricity:
    (a) lumen
    (b) lumin
    (c) electrilyte
    (d) electrolyte

22. Cavity or channel within a tube:
    (a) lumen
    (b) lumin
    (c) electrilyte
    (d) electrolyte

23. Darkening of the feces by blood pigments:
    (a) malena
    (b) erythema
    (c) melena
    (d) erthema

24. Difficulty in swallowing:
    (a) hematochezia
    (b) dysphagia
    (c) hemotachesia
    (d) dysphogia

25. Disease of the lymph nodes:
    (a) laminectomy
    (b) lymphadenopathy
    (c) lamenectomy
    (d) lympanopathy

PART I / PRETEST *continued*

26. Enlargement of the liver and spleen:
    (a) hepatasplenmegaly
    (b) thyromegaly
    (c) hepatosplenomegaly
    (d) thyomegaly

27. Establishment of a new opening into the stomach:
    (a) gastriparesis
    (b) gastroparesis
    (c) gastristomy
    (d) gastrostomy

28. Feeling of uneasiness:
    (a) targor
    (b) turgor
    (c) malaise
    (d) malise

29. Folic acid:
    (a) folate
    (b) formalen
    (c) formalin
    (d) forlaten

30. Hernia of the bladder usually into the vagina and introitus:
    (a) rectocele
    (b) recocele
    (c) cystocele
    (d) cestocele

31. Hernial protrusion of part of the rectum into the vagina:
    (a) rectocele
    (b) recocele
    (c) cystocele
    (d) cestocele

32. Inflammation of the colon:
    (a) colitis
    (b) colotis
    (c) proctitis
    (d) protitis

33. Inflammation of the otitis interna:
    (a) labrinithitis
    (b) gasritis
    (c) gastritis
    (d) labyrinthitis

34. Inflammation of the rectum:
    (a) colitis
    (b) colotis
    (c) proctitis
    (d) protitis

35. Inflammation of the stomach, especially the mucosal:
    (a) labrinithitis
    (b) gasritis
    (c) gastritis
    (d) labyrinthitis

36. Involuntary, rapid, rhythmic movement of the eyeball:
    (a) adenomatous
    (b) adenamatous
    (c) nistagmus
    (d) nystagmus

37. Jaundice:
    (a) decubitus
    (b) decubetus
    (c) icterus
    (d) ictreus

38. Generic name for a local anesthetic; used as a cardiac antiarrhythmic:
    (a) heparin
    (b) lidocaine
    (c) heparen
    (d) lidacaine

39. Muscular pain:
    (a) myalgia
    (b) odynophagia
    (c) myelgia
    (d) oynophagia

PART I / PRETEST *continued*

40. One of the forms of vitamin B$_6$:
    (a) occult
    (b) ocult
    (c) pyridxine
    (d) pyridoxine

41. Burning, squeezing pain while swallowing:
    (a) myalgia
    (b) odynophagia
    (c) myelgia
    (d) oynophagia

42. Projecting part of the ear lying outside the head:
    (a) pinna
    (b) arterogram
    (c) pina
    (d) arteriogram

43. Redness of the skin due to capillary dilatation:
    (a) malena
    (b) erythema
    (c) melena
    (d) erthema

44. Relates to bile or the biliary tract:
    (a) bilary
    (b) biliary
    (c) motility
    (d) molity

45. Relates to the stomach and esophagus:
    (a) gastroesophageal
    (b) gasointestinal
    (c) gasoesophageal
    (d) gastrointestinal

46. Relates to some types of glandular hyperplasia:
    (a) adenomatous
    (b) adenamatous
    (c) nistagmus
    (d) nystagmus

47. Relates to the stomach and the intestines:
    (a) gastroesophageal
    (b) gasointestinal
    (c) gasoesophageal
    (d) gastrointestinal

48. Removal of the right or left side of the colon:
    (a) hemicolectomy
    (b) hemacolectomy
    (c) cholecystectomy
    (d) colecystectomy

49. Slight degree of gastroparalysis:
    (a) gastriparesis
    (b) gastroparesis
    (c) gastristomy
    (d) gastrostomy

50. Specimen hidden from view:
    (a) occult
    (b) ocult
    (c) pyridxine
    (d) pyridoxine

51. Surgical excision of the lamina:
    (a) laminectomy
    (b) lymphadenopathy
    (c) lamenectomy
    (d) lympanopathy

52. The bending of an organ so that its top is thrust backward:
    (a) retroflexion
    (b) retroflesion
    (c) exacerbation
    (d) exacerbasion

53. The condition of fullness; the expected resiliency of the skin:
    (a) targor
    (b) turgor
    (c) malaise
    (d) malise

PART I / PRETEST *continued*

54. The cul-de-sac, about 6 cm in depth, lying below the terminal ileum forming the first part of the large intestine:
    (a) heme
    (b) cecum
    (c) hema
    (d) cecam

55. The direct examination of the interior of the sigmoid colon:
    (a) endoscopy
    (b) sigmiodoscopy
    (c) endioscopy
    (d) sigmoidoscopy

56. The establishment of an artificial opening into the colon:
    (a) colonscopy
    (b) colonoscopy
    (c) colostomy
    (d) colonstomy

57. The examination of the interior of a canal or hollow viscus by means of endoscope:
    (a) endoscopy
    (b) viscosopy
    (c) endioscopy
    (d) viscuscopy

58. The narrowing of a body passage or opening:
    (a) anastomosis
    (b) anastamosis
    (c) stenosis
    (d) stenasis

59. The oxygen-carrying, color-furnishing group of hemoglobin:
    (a) heme
    (b) cecum
    (c) hema
    (d) cecam

60. The passage of bloody stools:
    (a) hematochezia
    (b) dysphagia
    (c) hemotachesia
    (d) dysphogia

61. A patient in a recumbant position:
    (a) decubitus
    (b) decubetus
    (c) icterus
    (d) ictreus

62. The surgical removal of the gallbladder:
    (a) hemicolectomy
    (b) hemacolectomy
    (c) cholecystectomy
    (d) colecystectomy

63. The tough white outer coat of the eyeball:
    (a) polyp
    (b) polpa
    (c) scera
    (d) sclera

64. The visual examination of the inner surface of the colon by means of a colonoscope:
    (a) colonscopy
    (b) colonoscopy
    (c) colostomy
    (d) colonstomy

65. To analyze a given solution component by adding a liquid reagent:
    (a) prostate
    (b) tirate
    (c) postate
    (d) titrate

66. Generic name for a vasodilator and is used to relieve certain types of pain:
    (a) meclizine
    (b) mecizine
    (c) nitroglycerin
    (d) nitoglycerin

PART I / PRETEST *continued*

67. Vomit blood indicating upper gastrointestinal bleeding:
    (a) hematemesis
    (b) hemetemesis
    (c) emasis
    (d) emesis

68. Vomit:
    (a) hematemesis
    (b) hemetemesis
    (c) emasis
    (d) emesis

69. Trade name for an antianxiety agent:
    (a) Ativan
    (b) Atevan
    (c) Bumex
    (d) Bumix

70. Trade name for an antagonist for the treatment of gastric and duodenal ulcers:
    (a) Axid
    (b) Cheme-7
    (c) Chem-7
    (d) Axide

71. Trade name for a loop diuretic:
    (a) Ativan
    (b) Atevan
    (c) Bumex
    (d) Bumix

72. Trade name for a profile of seven different chemical laboratory tests:
    (a) Axid
    (b) Cheme-7
    (c) Chem-7
    (d) Axide

73. Trade name for an anticoagulant:
    (a) Demerol
    (b) Coumadin
    (c) Demirol
    (d) Doumaden

74. Trade name for a synthetic narcotic analgesic:
    (a) Demerol
    (b) Coumadin
    (c) Demirol
    (d) Doumaden

75. Trade name for an anticonvulsant used in the treatment of epilepsy:
    (a) Delantin
    (b) Dilantin
    (c) Elavil
    (d) Elevil

76. Trade name for an antidepressant:
    (a) Delantin
    (b) Dilantin
    (c) Elavil
    (d) Elevil

77. Trade name for a guaiac test for occult blood:
    (a) Humilin
    (b) Hemoccult
    (c) Humulin
    (d) Hemocult

78. Trade name for an antidiabetic:
    (a) Humilin
    (b) Hemoccult
    (c) Humulin
    (d) Hemocult

79. Trade name for an antihypertensive, sometimes used in the treatment of benign prostatic hyperplasia:
    (a) Indocin
    (b) Indicin
    (c) Hitrin
    (d) Hytrin

PART I / PRETEST *continued*

80. Trade name for a nonsteroidal anti-inflammatory agent:
    (a) Indocin
    (b) Indicin
    (c) Hitrin
    (d) Hytrin

81. Trade name for a potassium supplement:
    (a) K-Dur
    (b) Lopressor
    (c) K-Dura
    (d) Lopresor

82. Trade name for an antihypertensive:
    (a) K-Dur
    (b) Lopressor
    (c) K-Dura
    (d) Lopresor

83. Trade name for an urinary bacteriostatic:
    (a) Mazide
    (b) Maxzide
    (c) Macroid
    (d) Macrobid

84. Trade name for a diuretic and antihypertensive:
    (a) Mazide
    (b) Maxzide
    (c) Macroid
    (d) Macrobid

85. Trade name for a bulk laxative:
    (a) Metamacil
    (b) Naporsyn
    (c) Metamucil
    (d) Naprosyn

86. Trade name for a nonsteroidal anti-inflammatory agent:
    (a) Metamacil
    (b) Naporsyn
    (c) Metamucil
    (d) Naprosyn

87. Trade name for an antianginal and antihypertensive:
    (a) Paxil
    (b) Pasil
    (c) Norvasc
    (d) Norasc

88. Trade name for an antidepressant:
    (a) Paxil
    (b) Pasil
    (c) Norvasc
    (d) Norasc

89. Trade name for an acid controller for heartburn and acid indigestion:
    (a) Maxzide
    (b) Pepcid
    (c) Maxzide
    (d) Pepid

90. Trade name a gastric acid secretion inhibitor:
    (a) Priosec
    (b) K-Dure
    (c) Prilosec
    (d) K-Dur

91. Trade name for a coronary vasodilator:
    (a) Regan
    (b) Procardia
    (c) Porcardia
    (d) Reglan

92. Trade name for a gastrointestinal stimulant, antiemetic:
    (a) Regan
    (b) Procardia
    (c) Porcardia
    (d) Reglan

PART I / PRETEST *continued*

93. Trade name for a mild central nervous system stimulant and antidepressant:
    (a) Ritalin
    (b) Ritilin
    (c) Synthroid
    (d) Synroid

94. Trade name for a thyroid hormone:
    (a) Ritalin
    (b) Ritilin
    (c) Synthroid
    (d) Synroid

95. Trade name for an antihypertensive:
    (a) Tenormin
    (b) Tenorrmin
    (c) Terramycin
    (d) Teramycin

96. Trade name for an antibiotic:
    (a) Tenormin
    (b) Tenorrmin
    (c) Terramycin
    (d) Teramycin

97. Trade name for an antiemetic:
    (a) Timoptic
    (b) Tiggan
    (c) Timptic
    (d) Tigan

98. Trade name for a beta-blocker, antiglaucoma agent:
    (a) Timoptic
    (b) Tiggan
    (c) Timptic
    (d) Tigan

99. Trade name for an antihypertensive:
    (a) Vastec
    (b) Versed
    (c) Vasotec
    (d) Verse

100. Trade name for a short-acting benzodiazepine general anesthetic adjunct for preoperative sedation:
    (a) Vastec
    (b) Versed
    (c) Vasotec
    (d) Verse

101. Trade name for a reductase inhibitor for hypercholesterolemia and coronary heart disease:
    (a) Zoccor
    (b) Zokur
    (c) Zochor
    (d) Zocor

Part I / Activity 1
Keyboarding Medical Terms and Definitions

Let's learn to spell and define selected terminology and drugs of the gastroenterology specialty that are included in this chapter. Keyboarding these terms is an innovative and fun way to improve your skills.

Textbook Users

Launch your word processing package. On the open screen, read and type each word and its definition as shown below.

Save your work on your student disk.

1. Adenomatous (ad-e-<u>no</u>-ma-tus) relates to some types of glandular hyperplasia.
2. Anastomosis (a-nas-to-<u>mo</u>-sis) is an opening created by surgery, disease, or trauma between two or more organs or structures.
3. Arteriogram (ar-<u>ter</u>-e-o-gram) is a radiographic record of an artery after injection of a contrast medium into it.
4. Biliary (<u>bil</u>-e-ar-e) relates to bile or the biliary tract.
5. Cecum (<u>se</u>-kum) is the cul-de-sac, about 6 cm in depth, lying below the terminal ileum forming the first part of the large intestine.
6. Cholecystectomy (<u>ko</u>-le-sis-<u>tek</u>-to-me) is the surgical removal of the gallbladder.
7. Colitis (ko-<u>li</u>-tis) is the inflammation of the colon.
8. Colonoscope (ko-<u>lon</u>-o-skop) is an elongated endoscope, usually fiberoptic.
9. Colonoscopy (ko-lon-<u>os</u>-ko-pe) is the visual examination of the inner surface of the colon by means of a colonoscope.
10. Colostomy (ko-<u>los</u>-to-me) is the establishment of an artificial opening into the colon.
11. Creatinine (kre-<u>ai</u>-I-nen) is a normal component of urine.
12. Cystocele (<u>sis</u>-to-sel) is a hernia of the bladder usually into the vagina and introitus.
13. Decubitus (de-<u>kyu</u>-bi-tus) is a recumbant or horizontal position.
14. Dysphagia (dis-<u>fa</u>-je-a) is the difficulty in swallowing.
15. Electrolytes (e-<u>lek</u>-tro-lit) is any solution compound that conducts electricity.
16. Emesis (<u>em</u>-e-sis) is to vomit.
17. Endoscopy (en-<u>dos</u>-ko-pe) is the examination of the interior of a canal or hollow viscus by means of endoscope.
18. Erythema (er-I-<u>the</u>-ma) is the redness of the skin due to capillary dilatation.
19. Exacerbation (eg-zas-er-<u>ba</u>-shun) is an increase in the severity of a disease or symptoms.
20. Folate (<u>fo</u>-lat) is folic acid.
21. Formalin (<u>for</u>-ma-lin) is a 37% aqueous solution of formaldehyde.
22. Gastritis (gas-<u>tri</u>-tis) is an inflammation of the stomach, especially the mucosal.
23. Gastroesophageal (<u>gas</u>-tro-e-sof-a-je-al) relates to both the stomach and the esophagus.
24. Gastrointestinal (<u>gas</u>-tro-in-tes-tin-al) relates to the stomach and the intestines.
25. Gastroparesis (gas-tro-pa-<u>re</u>-sis) is a slight degree of gastroparalysis.
26. Gastrostomy (gas-<u>tros</u>-to-me) is the establishment of a new opening into the stomach.
27. Hematemesis (he-ma-<u>tem</u>-e-sis) is to vomit blood indicating upper gastrointestinal bleeding.
28. Hematochezia (<u>he</u>-ma-to-<u>ke</u>-ze-a) is the passage of bloody stools.
29. Heme (hem) is the oxygen-carrying, color-furnishing group of hemoglobin.
30. Hemicolectomy (<u>hem</u>-e-ko-<u>lek</u>-to-me) is the removal of the right or left side of the colon.
31. Heparin (<u>hep</u>-ah-rin) is a generic name for an anticoagulant.
32. Hepatosplenomegaly (hep-ah-to-sple-no-<u>meg</u>-ah-le) is the enlargement of the liver and spleen.
33. Hydrocortisone (hi-dro-<u>kor</u>-ti-son) is a generic name for a corticosteroid.
34. Icterus (<u>ik</u>-ter-us) is jaundice.

35. Ketone (<u>ke</u>-ton) is any compound containing carbon oxide.
36. Labyrinthitis (lab-I-rin-<u>thi</u>-tis) is the inflammation of the otitis interna.
37. Laminectomy (lam-I-<u>nek</u>-to-me) is the surgical excision of the lamina.
38. Lidocaine (<u>li</u>-do-kan) is a generic name for a local anesthetic; used as a cardiac antiarrhythmic.
39. Lumen (<u>lu</u>-men) is the cavity or channel within a tube.
40. Lymphadenopathy (lim-fad-e-<u>nop</u>-ah-the) is the disease of the lymph nodes.
41. Malaise (mal-<u>az</u>) is a feeling of uneasiness.
42. Meclizine (<u>mek</u>-li-zen) is a generic name for an antinauseant.
43. Melena (me-<u>le</u>-nah) is the darkening of the feces by blood pigments.
44. Motility (mo-<u>til</u>-I-te) is the ability to move spontaneously.
45. Myalgia (mi-<u>al</u>-je-ah) is muscular pain.
46. Nitroglycerin (ni-tro-<u>glis</u>-er-in) is a generic name for a vasodilator and is used to relieve certain types of pain.
47. Nystagmus (nis-<u>tag</u>-mus) is the involuntary, rapid, rhythmic movement of the eyeball.
48. Occult (o-<u>kult</u>) is hidden from view.
49. Odynophagia (o-din-o-<u>fa</u>-je-ah) is the burning, squeezing pain while swallowing
50. Pinna (<u>pin</u>-ah) is the projecting part of the ear lying outside the head.
51. Polyp (<u>pol</u>-ip) is any growth or mass protruding from a mucous membrane.
52. Postprandial (post-<u>pran</u>-de-al) is after a meal.
53. Prednisone (<u>pred</u>-ni-son) is a generic name for an anti-inflammatory and antiallergic agent.
54. Proctitis (prok-<u>ti</u>-tis) is the inflammation of the rectum.
55. Prophylatic (pro-fi-<u>lak</u>-tik) is an agent that tends to ward off disease.
56. Prostate (<u>pros</u>-tat) is a gland in the male that surrounds the neck of the bladder and urethra.
57. Pyridoxine (pir-o-<u>dok</u>-sen) is one of the forms of vitamin B_6.
58. Rectocele (<u>rek</u>-to-sel) is the hernial protrusion of part of the rectum into the vagina.
59. Reflux (<u>re</u>-fluks) is a backward or return flow.
60. Retroflexion (ret-ro-<u>flek</u>-shun) is the bending of an organ so that its top is thrust backward.
61. Sclera (<u>skle</u>-rah) is the tough white outer coat of the eyeball.
62. Sigmoidoscope (sig-<u>moi</u>-do-skop) is an endoscope for use in sigmoidoscopy.
63. Sigmoidoscopy (sig-moi-<u>dos</u>-ko-pe) is the direct examination of the interior of the sigmoid colon.
64. Stenosis (ste-<u>no</u>-sis) is the narrowing of a body passage or opening.
65. Stent (stent) is a mold for keeping a skin graft in place.
66. Thyromegaly (thi-ro-<u>meg</u>-ah-le) is the enlargement of the thyroid gland.
67. Titrate (<u>ti</u>-trat) is to analyze a given solution component by adding a liquid reagent.
68. Turgor (<u>tur</u>-gor) is the condition of fullness; the expected resiliency of the skin.
69. Ativan (<u>at</u>-I-van) is the trade name for an anti-anxiety agent.
70. Axid (<u>ak</u>-sid) is the trade name for an antagonist for the treatment of gastric and duodenal ulcers.
71. Bumex (<u>bum</u>-eks) is the trade name for a loop diuretic.
72. Chem-7 (<u>kem</u>-7) is the trade name for a profile of seven different chemical laboratory tests.
73. Coumadin (<u>koo</u>-mah-din) is the trade name for an anticoagulant.
74. Demerol (<u>dem</u>-er-ol) is the trade name for a synthetic narcotic analgesic.
75. Dilantin (di-<u>lan</u>-tin) is the trade name for an anticonvulsant used to treat epilepsy.
76. Elavil (<u>el</u>-ah-vil) is the trade name for an antidepressant.
77. Hemoccult (<u>he</u>-mo-kult) is the trade name for a guaiac test for occult blood.
78. Humulin (<u>hu</u>-mu-lin) is the trade name for an antidiabetic.
79. Hytrin (<u>hi</u>-trin) is the trade name for an antihypertensive used in the treatment of benign-prostatic hyperplasia.
80. Indocin (<u>in</u>-do-sin) is the trade name for a nonsteroidal anti-inflammatory agent.
81. K-Dur (<u>ka</u>-dur) is the trade name for a potassium supplement.
82. Lopressor (lo-<u>pres</u>-or) is the trade name for an antihypertensive.
83. Macrobid (<u>mak</u>-ro-bid) is the trade name for an urinary bacteriostatic.

84. Maxzide (<u>mak</u>-sid) is the trade name for a diuretic and antihypertensive.
85. Metamucil (met-ah-<u>mu</u>-sil) is the trade name for a bulk laxative.
86. Naprosyn (nah-<u>pro</u>-sin) is the trade name for a nonsteroidal anti-inflammatory agent.
87. Norvasc (<u>nor</u>-vask) is the trade name for an antianginal and antihypertensive.
88. Paxil (<u>pa</u>-sil) is the trade name for an antidepressant.
89. Pepcid (<u>pep</u>-sid) is the trade name for an acid controller for heartburn and acid indigestion.
90. Prilosec (<u>pril</u>-o-sek) is the trade name for a gastric acid secretion inhibitor.
91. Procardia (pro-<u>kar</u>-de-ah) is the trade name for a coronary vasodilator.
92. Reglan (<u>reg</u>-lan) is the trade name for a gastrointestinal stimulent, antiemetic.
93. Ritalin (<u>rit</u>-ah-lin) is the trade name for a mild central nervous system stimulant and antidepressant.

94. Synthroid (<u>sin</u>-throid) is the trade name for a thyroid hormone.
95. Tenormin (<u>ten</u>-or-min) is the trade name for an antihypertensive.
96. Terramycin (<u>ter</u>-ah-mi-sin) is the trade name for an antibiotic.
97. Tigan (<u>ti</u>-gan) is the trade name for an antiemetic.
98. Timoptic (tim-<u>op</u>-tik) is the trade name for a beta-blocker, antiglaucoma agent.
99. Vasotec (<u>vah</u>-so-tek) is the trade name for an antihypertensive.
100. Versed (<u>ver</u>-sed) is the trade name for a short-acting benzodiazepine general anesthetic adjunct for preoperative sedation.
101. Zocor (zo-<u>kor</u>) is the trade name for a reductase inhibitor for hypercholesterolemia and coronary heart disease.

Part I / Activity 2
Spelling Medical Terms

Do you remember back in school when you had to write each spelling word ten times? Because you had to physically write each word, your mind and body were focused on the assignment and the method worked! Let's follow this successful method by reinforcing the spelling of selected terms and drugs found in the gastroenterology specialty through keyboarding drills.

Textbook Users
Launch your word processing package. On the open screen, read, mentally spell, and type each word in its sequence.
Save your work on your student disk.

1. adenomatous anastomosis arteriogram adenomatous anastomosis arteriogram
2. biliary cecum cholecystectomy biliary cecum cholecystectomy biliary cecum
3. colitis colonoscope colonoscopy colitis colonoscope colonoscopy colitis
4. colostomy creatinine cystocele colostomy creatinine cystocele colostomy
5. decubitus dysphagia electrolytes decubitus dysphagia electrolytes decubitus
6. emesis endoscopy erythema emesis endoscopy erythema emesis endoscopy
7. exacerbation folate formalin exacerbation folate formalin exacerbation folate
8. gastritis gastroesophageal gastrointestinal gastritis gastroesophageal gastrointestinal
9. gastroparesis gastrostomy hematemesis gastroparesis gastrostomy hematemesis
10. hematochezia heme hemicolectomy hematochezia heme hemicolectomy

11. heparin hepatosplenomegaly hydrocortisone heparin hepatosplenomegaly

12. icterus ketone labyrinthitis icterus ketone labyrinthitis icterus ketone labyrinthitis

13. laminectomy lidocaine lumen laminectomy lidocaine lumen laminectomy lidocaine

14. lymphadenopathy malaise meclizine lymphadenopathy malaise meclizine

15. melena motility myalgia melena motility myalgia melena motility myalgia melena

16. nitroglycerin nystagmus occult nitroglycerin nystagmus occult nitroglycerin

17. odynophagia pinna polyp odynophagia pinna polyp odynophagia pinna polyp

18. postprandial prednisone proctitis postprandial prednisone proctitis postprandial

19. prophylatic prostate pyridoxine prophylatic prostate pyridoxine prophylatic prostate

20. rectocele reflux retroflexion rectocele reflux retroflexion rectocele reflux retroflexion

21. sclera sigmoidoscope sigmoidoscopy sclera sigmoidoscope sigmoidoscopy sclera

22. stenosis stent thyromegaly stenosis stent thyromegaly stenosis stent thyromegaly

23. titrate turgor titrate turgor titrate turgor titrate turgor titrate turgor titrate turgor titrate

24. Ativan Axid Bumex Ativan Axid Bumex Ativan Axid Bumex Ativan Axid Bumex

25. Chem-7 Coumadin Demerol Chem-7 Coumadin Demerol Chem-7 Coumadin

26. Dilantin Elavil Hemoccult Dilantin Elavil Hemoccult Dilantin Elavil Hemoccult

27. Humulin Hytrin Indocin Humulin Hytrin Indocin Humulin Hytrin Indocin Humulin

28. K-Dur Lopressor Macrobid K-Dur Lopressor Macrobid K-Dur Lopressor Macrobid

29. Maxzide Metamucil Naprosyn Maxzide Metamucil Naprosyn Maxzide Metamucil

30. Norvasc Paxil Pepcid Norvasc Paxil Pepcid Norvasc Paxil Pepcid Norvasc Paxil

31. Prilosec Procardia Reglan Prilosec Procardia Reglan Prilosec Procardia Reglan

32. Ritalin Synthroid Tenormin Ritalin Synthroid Tenormin Ritalin Synthroid Tenormin

33. Terramycin Tigan Timoptic Terramycin Tigan Timoptic Terramycin Tigan Timoptic

34. Vasotec Versed Zocor Vasotec Versed Zocor Vasotec Versed Zocor Vasotec Versed

Part I / Activity 3
Transcribing Medical Sentences (9T-1)

Now you are ready to make the transition from keyboarding medical terms, which is a visual process, to transcribing medical terms, an aural process. You are going to use audiocassette tapes rather than printed material.

Textbook Users
Insert the audiocassette in your transcribing machine and find 9T-1.
You will be transcribing spelling words in sentence structure.
Insert your student disk in drive A or B. Ask your instructor for further assistance.
Launch your word processing software.
Use 1-inch left and right margins.
Listen carefully to each sentence on the audiocassette before transcribing.
Rewind and type (transcribe) the sentences.
After you have completed transcribing the sentences, save the file.
Refer to the answer key.

Part I / Check Your Progress

Let's pause a minute and see how well you are doing. This section will allow you to evaluate your mastery of keyboarding and spelling selected terms and drugs found in the gastroenterology specialty.

Textbook Users
Select the correctly spelled term that matches its definition.
Refer to the answer key for immediate feedback.
If you score below 90%, you are recommended to redo the *Part I Activities.*
If you score 90% or above, congratulations. You have mastered the material covered in Part I. If you wish, you can immediately move on to Part II.

Software Users
Click on *Chapter 9, Part I, Check Your Progress.*
Key the correctly spelled term that matches its definition.
When you are finished, click on *End Test.*
A pop-up screen will reveal your score.
If you score below 90%, you are recommended to redo the *Part I Activities.*
If you score 90% or above, congratulations. You have mastered the material covered in Part I. If you wish, you can immediately move on to Part II.

PART I / CHECK YOUR PROGRESS

Directions: Select the correctly spelled term that matches its definition.

1. The visual examination of the inner surface of the colon by means of a colonoscope:
   (a) colonscopy
   (b) colonoscopy
   (c) colostomy
   (d) colonstomy

2. To analyze a given solution component by adding a liquid reagent:
   (a) prostate
   (b) tirate
   (c) postate
   (d) titrate

3. Generic name for a vasodilator and is used to relieve certain types of pain:
   (a) meclizine
   (b) mecizine
   (c) nitroglycerin
   (d) nitoglycerin

4. Vomit blood indicating upper gastrointestinal bleeding:
   (a) hematemesis
   (b) hemetemesis
   (c) emasis
   (d) emesis

5. The tough white outer coat of the eyeball:
   (a) polyp
   (b) polpa
   (c) scera
   (d) sclera

6. The visual examination of the inner surface of the colon by means of a colonoscope:
   (a) colonscopy
   (b) colonoscopy
   (c) colostomy
   (d) colonstomy

7. The passage of bloody stools:
   (a) hematochezia
   (b) dysphagia
   (c) hemotachesia
   (d) dysphogia

8. A patient in a recumbant position:
   (a) decubitus
   (b) decubetus
   (c) icterus
   (d) ictreus

9. The surgical removal of the gallbladder:
   (a) hemicolectomy
   (b) hemacolectomy
   (c) cholecystectomy
   (d) colecystectomy

10. The examination of the interior of a canal or hollow viscus by means of endoscope:
    (a) endoscopy
    (b) sigmiodoscopy
    (c) endioscopy
    (d) sigmoidoscopy

11. The narrowing of a body passage or opening:
    (a) anastomosis
    (b) anastamosis
    (c) stenosis
    (d) stenasis

12. The oxygen-carrying, color-furnishing group of hemoglobin:
    (a) heme
    (b) cecum
    (c) hema
    (d) cecam

PART I / CHECK YOUR PROGRESS *continued*

13. The bending of an organ so that its top is thrust backward:
    (a) retroflexion
    (b) retroflesion
    (c) exacerbation
    (d) exacerbasion

14. The condition of fullness; the expected resiliency of the skin:
    (a) targor
    (b) turgor
    (c) malaise
    (d) malise

15. The cul-de-sac, about 6 cm in depth, lying below the terminal ileum forming the first part of the large intestine:
    (a) heme
    (b) cecum
    (c) hema
    (d) cecam

16. The direct examination of the interior of the sigmoid colon:
    (a) endoscopy
    (b) sigmiodoscopy
    (c) endioscopy
    (d) sigmoidoscopy

17. The establishment of an artificial opening into the colon:
    (a) colonscopy
    (b) colonoscopy
    (c) colostomy
    (d) colonstomy

18. Generic name for a local anesthetic; used as a cardiac antiarrhythmic:
    (a) heparin
    (b) lidocaine
    (c) heparen
    (d) lidacaine

19. Muscular pain:
    (a) myalgia
    (b) odynophagia
    (c) myelgia
    (d) oynophagia

20. One of the forms of vitamin B_6:
    (a) occult
    (b) ocult
    (c) pyridxine
    (d) pyridoxine

21. Burning, squeezing pain while swallowing:
    (a) myalgia
    (b) odynophagia
    (c) myelgia
    (d) oynophagia

22. Projecting part of the ear lying outside the head:
    (a) pinna
    (b) arterogram
    (c) pina
    (d) arteriogram

23. Redness of the skin due to capillary dilatation:
    (a) malena
    (b) erythema
    (c) melena
    (d) erthema

24. Relates to bile or the biliary tract:
    (a) bilary
    (b) biliary
    (c) motility
    (d) molity

25. Relates to both the stomach and the esophagus:
    (a) gastroesophageal
    (b) gasointestinal
    (c) gasoesophageal
    (d) gastrointestinal

PART I / CHECK YOUR PROGRESS *continued*

26. Relates to some types of glandular hyperplasia:
    (a) adenomatous
    (b) adenamatous
    (c) nistagmus
    (d) nystagmus

27. Relates to the stomach and the intestines:
    (a) gastroesophageal
    (b) gasointestinal
    (c) gasoesophageal
    (d) gastrointestinal

28. A 37% aqueous solution of formaldehyde:
    (a) forlate
    (b) formalen
    (c) formalin
    (d) forlaten

29. A backward or return flow:
    (a) stent
    (b) reflux
    (c) stant
    (d) refluxe

30. A normal component of urine:
    (a) keytone
    (b) ketone
    (c) creatine
    (d) creatinine

31. Generic name for a corticosteroid:
    (a) meclizane
    (b) meclazane
    (c) hydrocortsone
    (d) hydrocortisone

32. A gland in the male that surrounds the neck of the bladder and urethra:
    (a) prostate
    (b) tirate
    (c) postate
    (d) titrate

33. Enlargement of the thyroid gland:
    (a) hepatasplenmegaly
    (b) thyromegaly
    (c) hepatosplenomegaly
    (d) thyomegaly

34. A mold for keeping a skin graft in place:
    (a) stent
    (b) reflux
    (c) stant
    (d) refluxe

35. A radiographic record of an artery after injection of a contrast medium into it:
    (a) pinna
    (b) arterogram
    (c) pina
    (d) arteriogram

36. Ability to move spontaneously:
    (a) bilary
    (b) biliary
    (c) motility
    (d) molity

37. After a meal:
    (a) postprandial
    (b) prophylatic
    (c) posprandial
    (d) prophyacic

38. An agent that tends to ward off disease:
    (a) postprandial
    (b) prophylatic
    (c) posprandial
    (d) prophyacic

39. Generic name for an anticoagulant:
    (a) heparin
    (b) lidocaine
    (c) formalin
    (d) lidacaine

PART I / CHECK YOUR PROGRESS *continued*

40. Generic name for an anti-inflammatory and antiallergic agent:
    (a) prenisone
    (b) prednisone
    (c) lidocaine
    (d) lidocain

41. Generic name for an antinauseant:
    (a) meclizine
    (b) mecizine
    (c) nitroglycerin
    (d) nitoglycerin

42. An elongated endoscope, usually fiberoptic:
    (a) fiberscope
    (b) fiberoscope
    (c) colonoscope
    (d) colonscope

43. An endoscope for use in sigmoidoscopy:
    (a) sigmoidoscope
    (b) sigmiodoscope
    (c) colonoscope
    (d) colonscope

44. An increase in the severity of a disease or symptoms:
    (a) retroflexion
    (b) retroflesion
    (c) exacerbation
    (d) exacerbasion

45. An opening created by surgery, disease, or trauma between two or more organs or structures:
    (a) anastomosis
    (b) anastamosis
    (c) stenosis
    (d) stenasis

46. Any compound containing carbon oxide:
    (a) keytone
    (b) ketone
    (c) creatine
    (d) creatinine

47. Any growth or mass protruding from a mucous membrane:
    (a) polyp
    (b) polpa
    (c) scera
    (d) sclera

48. Any solution compound that conducts electricity:
    (a) lumen
    (b) lumin
    (c) electrilyte
    (d) electrolyte

49. Cavity or channel within a tube:
    (a) lumen
    (b) lumin
    (c) electrilyte
    (d) electrolyte

50. Darkening of the feces by blood pigments:
    (a) malena
    (b) erythema
    (c) melena
    (d) erthema

51. Difficulty in swallowing:
    (a) hematochezia
    (b) dysphagia
    (c) hemotachesia
    (d) dysphogia

52. Disease of the lymph nodes:
    (a) laminectomy
    (b) lymphadenopathy
    (c) lamenectomy
    (d) lympanopathy

PART I / CHECK YOUR PROGRESS *continued*

53. Enlargement of the liver and spleen:
    (a) hepatasplenmegaly
    (b) thyromegaly
    (c) hepatosplenomegaly
    (d) thyomegaly

54. Establishment of a new opening into the stomach:
    (a) gastriparesis
    (b) gastroparesis
    (c) gastristomy
    (d) gastrostomy

55. Feeling of uneasiness:
    (a) targor
    (b) turgor
    (c) malaise
    (d) malise

56. Folic acid:
    (a) folate
    (b) formalen
    (c) formalin
    (d) forlaten

57. Hernia of the bladder, usually into the vagina and introitus:
    (a) rectocele
    (b) recocele
    (c) cystocele
    (d) cestocele

58. Hernial protrusion of part of the rectum into the vagina:
    (a) rectocele
    (b) recocele
    (c) cystocele
    (d) cestocele

59. Inflammation of the colon:
    (a) colitis
    (b) colotis
    (c) proctitis
    (d) protitis

60. Inflammation of the otitis interna:
    (a) labrinithitis
    (b) gasritis
    (c) gastritis
    (d) labyrinthitis

61. Inflammation of the rectum:
    (a) colitis
    (b) colotis
    (c) proctitis
    (d) protitis

62. Inflammation of the stomach, especially the mucosal:
    (a) labrinithitis
    (b) gasritis
    (c) gastritis
    (d) labyrinthitis

63. Involuntary, rapid, rhythmic movement of the eyeball:
    (a) adenomatous
    (b) adenamatous
    (c) nistagmus
    (d) nystagmus

64. Jaundice:
    (a) decubitus
    (b) decubetus
    (c) icterus
    (d) ictreus

65. Removal of the right or left side of the colon:
    (a) hemicolectomy
    (b) hemacolectomy
    (c) cholecystectomy
    (d) colecystectomy

66. Slight degree of gastroparalysis:
    (a) gastriparesis
    (b) gastroparesis
    (c) gastristomy
    (d) gastrostomy

PART I / CHECK YOUR PROGRESS *continued*

67. Specimen hidden from view:
    (a) occult
    (b) ocult
    (c) pyridxine
    (d) pyridoxine

68. Surgical excision of the lamina:
    (a) laminectomy
    (b) lymphadenopathy
    (c) lamenectomy
    (d) lympanopathy

69. Trade name for an antihypertensive:
    (a) Tenormin
    (b) Tenorrmin
    (c) Terramycin
    (d) Teramycin

70. Trade name for an antibiotic:
    (a) Tenormin
    (b) Tenorrmin
    (c) Terramycin
    (d) Teramycin

71. Trade name for an antiemetic:
    (a) Timoptic
    (b) Tiggan
    (c) Timptic
    (d) Tigan

72. Trade name for a beta-blocker, antiglaucoma agent:
    (a) Timoptic
    (b) Tiggan
    (c) Timptic
    (d) Tigan

73. Trade name for an antihypertensive:
    (a) Vastec
    (b) Versed
    (c) Vasotec
    (d) Verse

74. Trade name for a short-acting benzodiazepine general anesthetic adjunct for preoperative sedation:
    (a) Vastec
    (b) Versed
    (c) Vasotec
    (d) Verse

75. Trade name for a reductase inhibitor for hypercholesterolemia and coronary heart disease:
    (a) Zoccor
    (b) Zokur
    (c) Zochor
    (d) Zocor

76. Trade name for an antihypertensive used in the treatment of benign prostatic hyperplasia:
    (a) Indocin
    (b) Indicin
    (c) Hitrin
    (d) Hytrin

77. Trade name for a nonsteroidal anti-inflammatory agent:
    (a) Indocin
    (b) Indicin
    (c) Hitrin
    (d) Hytrin

78. Trade name for a potassium supplement:
    (a) K-Dur
    (b) Lopressor
    (c) K-Dura
    (d) Lopresor

79. Trade name for an antihypertensive:
    (a) K-Dur
    (b) Lopressor
    (c) K-Dura
    (d) Lopresor

PART I / CHECK YOUR PROGRESS *continued*

80. Trade name for a urinary bacteriostatic:
    (a) Mazide
    (b) Maxzide
    (c) Macroid
    (d) Macrobid

81. Trade name for a diuretic and antihypertensive:
    (a) Mazide
    (b) Maxzide
    (c) Macroid
    (d) Macrobid

82. Trade name for a bulk laxative:
    (a) Metamacil
    (b) Naporsyn
    (c) Metamucil
    (d) Naprosyn

83. Trade name for a nonsteroidal anti-inflammatory agent:
    (a) Metamacil
    (b) Naporsyn
    (c) Metamucil
    (d) Naprosyn

84. Trade name for an antianginal and antihypertensive:
    (a) Paxil
    (b) Pasil
    (c) Norvasc
    (d) Norasc

85. Trade name for an antidepressant:
    (a) Paxil
    (b) Pasil
    (c) Norvasc
    (d) Norasc

86. Trade name for an acid controller for heartburn and acid indigestion:
    (a) Maxide
    (b) Pepcid
    (c) Maxzide
    (d) Pepid

87. Trade name for a gastric acid secretion inhibitor:
    (a) Priosec
    (b) Pepcid
    (c) Prilosec
    (d) Pepid

88. Trade name for a coronary vasodilator:
    (a) Regan
    (b) Procardia
    (c) Porcardia
    (d) Reglan

89. Trade name for a gastrointestinal stimulant, antiemetic:
    (a) Regan
    (b) Procardia
    (c) Porcardia
    (d) Reglan

90. Trade name for a mild central nervous system stimulant and antidepressant:
    (a) Ritalin
    (b) Ritilin
    (c) Synthroid
    (d) Synroid

91. Trade name for a thyroid hormone:
    (a) Ritalin
    (b) Ritilin
    (c) Synthroid
    (d) Synroid

PART I / CHECK YOUR PROGRESS *continued*

92. Trade name for an antianxiety agent:
    (a) Ativan
    (b) Atevan
    (c) Bumex
    (d) Bumix

93. Trade name for an antagonist for the treatment of gastric and duodenal ulcers:
    (a) Axid
    (b) Cheme-7
    (c) Chem-7
    (d) Axide

94. Trade name for a loop diuretic:
    (a) Ativan
    (b) Atevan
    (c) Bumex
    (d) Bumix

95. Trade name for a profile of seven different chemical laboratory tests:
    (a) Axid
    (b) Cheme-7
    (c) Chem-7
    (d) Axide

96. Trade name for an anticoagulant:
    (a) Demerol
    (b) Coumadin
    (c) Demirol
    (d) Doumaden

97. Trade name for a synthetic narcotic analgesic:
    (a) Demerol
    (b) Coumadin
    (c) Demirol
    (d) Doumaden

98. Trade name for an anticonvulsant used in the treatment of epilepsy:
    (a) Delantin
    (b) Dilantin
    (c) Elavil
    (d) Elevil

99. Trade name for an antidepressant:
    (a) Delantin
    (b) Dilantin
    (c) Elavil
    (d) Elevil

100. Trade name for a guaiac test for occult blood:
    (a) Humilin
    (b) Hemoccult
    (c) Humulin
    (d) Hemocult

101. Trade name for an antidiabetic:
    (a) Humilin
    (b) Hemoccult
    (c) Humulin
    (d) Hemocult

Pretest *(9T-2)*

Professional transcriptionists proofread their own work. Can you? Scoring 90% or better proves it!

Textbook Users

Launch your word processing package.

Insert the appropriate audiocassette in your transcribing machine and find dictation *9T-2*.

On the open screen, transcribe and proofread dictation *9T-2*. Identify and correct all errors.

Save your work on your student disk.

After completing the transcription, refer to the answer key.

Manually complete the error analysis and production for pay charts.

If you score below 90%, continue on to *Activities 4–7*.

If you score 90% or above, congratulations. If you wish, you can immediately move on to Part III.

Software Users

Click on *Chapter 9, Part II, Pretest (9T-2)*.

Insert the appropriate audiocassette in your transcribing machine and find dictation *9T-2*.

Click on *Start Watch*, then trascribe and proofread dictation *9T-2*.

Identify and correct all errors.

When you are finished, click on *Done*, then *Score Document:* to display your production for pay.

Click on *Display Error Analysis* to reveal your score and *View Errors* to see your errors.

Save your work (with errors showing) by clicking on *File*, then *Save As*.

If you score below 90%, continue on to *Activities 4–7*.

If you score 90% or above, congratulations. If you wish, you can immediately move on to Part III.

Part II / Activities 4–5
Proofreading Worksheet Exercises

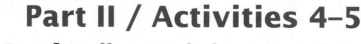

Finding and correcting your own errors is an essential skill. The worksheets in these activities will help develop your proofreading skills.

Textbook Users

Proofread and correct errors in the medical documents shown in *Activities 4–5*.

After completing the activities, refer to the answer key. Manually complete the error analysis chart for each document.

Software Users

Click on *Chapter 9, Part II, Activity 4*.

Proofread and correct errors in the medical document.

Click on *File*, then *Done*, then *Score Document* to reveal your score, and *View Errors* to see your errors.

Save your work (with errors showing) by clicking on *File*, then *Save As*.

Click on *File*, then *Exit*, to proceed.

Follow the same process to complete *Activity 5*.

PART II / ACTIVITY 4
PROOFREADING WORKSHEET EXERCISE

Directions: Proofread this medical document that contains multiple errors using full block, open punctuation, and all other formatting guidelines established in this textbook.

HISTORY AND PHYSICAL EXAMINATION

Patient Name: Schupp, Lacey

File Number: 00841

Date of Birth: November 2, 19xx

Examination Date: *current date*

Physician: Anna Bolism, MD

HISTORY:
CHEIF COMPLAINT: Melenic stools
HISTORY OF PRESSENT ILLNESS: The patient is a very pleasant 48 year old white male who I have previously saw for constipation that was due to a molity related disturbance as a complication of her polio. He has been taking Naporsyn on a chronic bases and over the last four-five days she has been having melenic stools. During the same time frame she has note progressive fatigue and weakness. A hemmoglobin study performed in Dr. Geiger's office showed that her hemmoglobin was in the six point five range and she was admitted to University Hospital. She denies any adbominal pain. There is know prior history of ulcer disease or hemotemesis. She has lost about three-5 pds. over this same time frame.

PAST MEDICAL HISTORY: She has numerous postpolio complications including a neurogenic bladder and constipation. She has had several back surgerys as well as a wrist operation. He does not smoke or drink..

MEDICATIONS:
Naporsyn.
Pasil.
Elevil.
Ativan.

FAMILY HISTORY: Noncontributory.
PHYSICAL EXAMINATION:
GENERAL: A pale white male who is in no a cute distress.

HEART: Negative.

LUNGS: Negative.
ABDOMEN: Negative.

PART II / ACTIVITY 4 *continued*

Page 2

RECTAL: A rectal exam showed know stool available for hemocult evaluation.

LABORATORY DATA: Lab studies show a BUN elevated at thirty three with a creatine of zero point four. His electrolites were normal as were her platelet count and co-agulation time. Hemmoglobin was six point nine.

IMPRESION: GI bleed. Its almost certainly upper GI bleeding due to nonsteroid use.

PLAN
Transfuse 2 units of packed sells.
Perform an upper endoescopy later this morning. We will make farther recomendations after the endoescopy.

_____

Anna Bolism

PART II / ACTIVITY 5
PROOFREADING WORKSHEET EXERCISE

Directions: Proofread this medical document that contains multiple errors using full block, open punctuation, and all other formatting guidelines established in this textbook.

OPERATIVE REPORT

Patient Name: Artemis, Jacob

File Number: 00864

Date of Birth: December 12, 1958

Preoperative Diagnosis: Hepatitis C and mildly elevated liver enzymes.

Postoperative Diagnosis: Hepatitis C and mildly elevated liver enzymes.

Operation: Percutaneous liver biopsy under ultrasound guidance.

PROCEDURE: The patient was counciled. Potential complications were explained. Concent was obtained. The patient was place supine on the exam table. Ultra-sound was used to scan in the midaxillary line. The liver margins were identified and the best location for the liver boipsy was selected along the mid axilary line at aproximately the tenth inter-coastal space. The skin was then preped and draped in the usual sterile manner. Lidocane one percent was used for tropical anesthesia of the skin sudcutaneous tissue and down to the inter-costal space. A number twenty two gauge spinal needel was used to sound the depth of the liver.

Because of the patients obesity the liver was found to be approximately five centimeters from the skin surface. The Klatskin needle was then attached to a glass syringe filled with sterile saline. The Clatskin needle was inserted into the intercostal space and then subsequently into the liver for a quick suction biopsy. The first past yielded only a five milimeters fragment of tissue. A second pass was therefore performed which yielded a much larger four centimeters peace of tan appearing liver. The liver biopsy was scent in a Formalen jar for pathological analyses. The skin was then dressed and tapped. The patient was then observed four four hours. No immediate complications were observed. Postbiopsy vital signs were normal. The patient tolerated the procedure well with out any complications.

IMPRESSION: Hepatitis C and mildly elevated liver enzymes.

_____

Kate Cobalamin Md.

Part II / Activities 6–7
Proofreading Transcription Exercises (9T-3, 9T-4)

Now you are ready to make the transition from simply proofreading printed material to both transcribing and proofreading dictated material. This is the time to concentrate on building your medical vocabulary, which ultimately will improve your speed and accuracy.

Textbook Users

Launch your word processing package.

Insert the appropriate audiocassette in your transcribing machine and find dictation *9T-3.*

Step 1: Listen to the entire dictation to gain an understanding of the medical concepts and terms involved. Rewind the tape to the beginning of the dictation and transcribe what you hear. Do not worry about formatting, style, or speed. Simply type what you hear being dictated, using correct punctuation, capitalization, and spelling. Stop as needed to look up words you do not understand or cannot spell. Adjust the speed control of the transcriber to a comfortable level and increase the speed as your accuracy improves.

Step 2: Rewind the tape again and using your created template, transcribe dictation *9T-3* again. Proofread the report. Identify and correct all errors. Save your work on your student disk. Refer to the answer key and manually complete the error analysis and the production for pay charts.

Repeat the same process for dictation *9T-4.*

Software Users

Click on *Chapter 9, Activity 6: Proofreading Transcription Exercise.*

Insert the appropriate audiocassette in your transcribing machine and find dictation *9T-3.*

Step 1: Listen to the entire dictation to gain an understanding of the medical concepts and terms involved. Rewind the tape to the beginning of the dictation, click *Start Watch,* and transcribe what you hear. Do not worry about formatting, style, or speed. Simply type what you hear being dictated, using correct punctuation, capitalization, and spelling. Stop as needed to look up words you do not understand or cannot spell. Adjust the speed control of the transcriber to a comfortable level and increase the speed as your accuracy improves. When you are finished, click on *Done,* then choose *Return to Main Menu.*

Step 2: Click on *Chapter 9, Activity 6* again. Rewind the tapes again, click on *Start Watch,* and transcribe dictation *9T-3.* Proofread the report. Identify and correct all errors. When you are finished, click on *Done,* then *Score Document:* to display your production for pay. Click on *Display Error Analysis* to reveal your score and then *View Errors* to see your errors. Save your work (with errors showing) by clicking on *File,* then *Save As.*

Follow the same process for dictation *9T-4.*

Part II / Check Your Progress (9T-2)

Let's pause a minute and see how well you are doing. This section will allow you to evaluate your success at transcribing and proofreading gastroenterology reports.

Textbook Users
Launch your word processing package.
Insert the appropriate audiocassette in your transcribing machine and find dictation *9T-2*.
On the open screen, transcribe and proofread dictation *9T-2*.
Identify and correct all errors.
Use formatting guidelines established in Chapter 2.
Save your work on your student disk.
After completing the transcription, refer to the answer key.
Manually complete the error analysis chart.
Manually complete the production for pay chart.
If you score below 90%, you are recommended to redo the Part II Activities.
If you score 90% or above, congratulations. You have mastered the material covered in Part II. If you wish, you can immediately move on to Part III.

Software Users
Click *on Chapter 9, Part II, Check Your Progress (9T-2)*.
Insert the appropriate audiocassette in your transcribing machine and find dictation *9T-2*.
Click on *Start Watch*, then transcribe and proofread dictation *9T-2*.
Identify and correct all errors.
When you are finished, click on *Done*, then *Score Document:* a pop-up window will display your production for pay.
Click on *Display Error Analysis* to reveal your score.
Click on *View Errors* to see the errors you made.
Save your work (with errors showing) on your student disk by clicking on *File*, then *Save As*.
If you score below 90%, you are recommended to redo the Part II Activities.
If you score 90% or above, congratulations. You have mastered the material covered in Part II. If you wish, you can immediately move on to Part III.

Pretest (9T-5, 9T-6)

Professional transcriptionists can transcribe and proofread their own work. Can you? Scoring 90% or better proves it!

Textbook Users

Launch your word processing package.

Insert the appropriate audiocassette in your transcribing machine and find dictation *9T-5*.

On the open screen, transcribe and proofread dictation *9T-5*.

Identify and correct all errors.

Use formatting guidelines established in Chapter 2.

Save your work on your student disk.

Follow the same process for dictation *9T-6*.

After completing the transcriptions, refer to the answer key.

Manually complete the error analysis chart for each document.

Manually complete the production for pay chart for each document.

If you score below 90%, continue with *Gastroenterology Transcription at FedDes Wellness Center*.

If you score 90% or above, congratulations. You have mastered the material covered in Part III. If you wish, you can immediately move on to the next chapter.

Software Users

Click on *Chapter 9, Part III, Pretest (9T-5)*.

Insert the appropriate audiocassette in your transcribing machine and find dictation *9T-5*.

Click on *Start Watch*, then transcribe and proofread dictation *9T-5*.

Identify and correct all errors.

When you are finished, click on *Done*, then *Score Document:* a pop-up window will display your production for pay.

Click on *Display Error Analysis* to reveal your score.

Click on *View Errors* to see the errors you made.

Save your work (with errors showing) on your student disk by clicking on *File*, then *Save As*.

Follow the same process for dictation *9T-6*.

If you score below 90%, continue with *Gastroenterology Transcription at FedDes Wellness Center*.

If you score 90% or above, congratulations. You have mastered the material covered in Part III. If you wish, you can immediately move on to the next chapter.

Gastroenterology Transcription at FedDes Wellness Center

You finally made it! You have been hired as a transcriptionist at FedDes Wellness Center in the Gastroenterology Division. Your supervisor has asked you to transcribe today's dictation.

Textbook Users

Launch your word processing package.

Insert the appropriate audiocassette in your transcribing machine and find dictation *9T-7*.

Create or use an existing template for the six types of reports.

On the open screen, transcribe and proofread dictation *9T-7*.

Identify and correct all errors.

Save your work on your student disk.

Follow the same process for dictations *9T-8* through *9T-15*.

After completing the transcriptions, refer to the answer key.

Manually complete the error analysis and production for pay charts for each document.

Software Users

Click on *Chapter 9, Part III, Gastroenterology Transcription at FedDes Wellness Center (9T-7).*

Insert the appropriate audiocassette in your transcribing machine and find dictation *9T-7*.

(Please note that you cannot utilize templates when using the software.)

Click on *Start Watch*, then transcribe and proofread dictation *9T-7*.

Identify and correct all errors.

When you are finished, click on *Done*, then *Score Document:* a pop-up window will display your production for pay.

Click on *Display Error Analysis* to reveal your score.

Click on *View Errors* to see the errors you made.

Save your work (with errors showing) on your student disk by clicking on *File*, then *Save As.*

Follow the same process for dictations *9T-8* and *9T-9*.

NOTE: Continue the medical documents *9T-10* through *9T-15* using your word processing package and manually complete the error analysis and production for pay charts.

Index of Dictations and Associated Transcription Tips

Please remember to follow the guidelines pertaining to capitalization, numbers, punctuation, abbreviations, measurements, symbols, and use of templates to create medical reports at FedDes Wellness Center. Review of this material can be found in Unit 1.

9T-7
Consultation Letter
Patient's Name: Alice Kier
Requesting Physician: Charles P. Davis, MD
Physician: Kate Cobalamin, MD

TRANSCRIPTION TIPS

- A hyphen is used between numbers and *year old.*
  You will hear the dictator say: Ms. Kier is a fifty nine year old woman
  You should transcribe as: Ms. Kier is a 59-year-old woman

- Quotation marks are used to indicate a direct quote.
  You will hear the dictator say: Her description of the discomfort is really quite vague stating that the pain jumps around her abdomen.
  You should transcribe as: Her description of the discomfort is really quite vague, stating that the pain "jumps around" her abdomen.

- The following medications are dictated in this letter:
  Synthroid: the trade name for a thyroid hormone
  hydrocortisone: the generic name for a corticosteroid
  K-Dur: the trade name for a potassium supplement
  Bumex: the trade name for a loop diuretic
  Lopressor: the trade name for an antihypertensive
  Vasotec: the trade name for an antihypertensive
  Dilantin: the trade name for an anticonvulsant used in the treatment of epilepsy
  Prilosec: the trade name a gastric secretion inhibitor
  Zocor: the trade name for a reductase inhibitor for hypercholesterolemia and coronary heart disease
  nitroglycerin paste: a generic name for a vasodilator and is used to relieve certain types of pain

- A hyphen is used to join two or more words when used as an adjective that proceeds a noun. The following word pairs are dictated in this report: well-appearing, heme-negative.

- Continuation pages for consultation letters must include a 3-line heading beginning at the 1-inch top margin, as shown below:
  Charles P. Davis, MD
  Current date
  Page 2

- An apostrophe is used to form the possessive of singular and plural nouns.
  You will hear the dictator say: Thank you for the opportunity of sharing in Ms. Keirs care.
  You should transcribe as: Thank you for the opportunity of sharing in Ms. Keir's care.

9T-8
Operative Report
Patient's Name: Raymond Dubin
Physician: Gwenn Maltase, MD

TRANSCRIPTION TIPS

- Figures are used for measurements and Latin terms. No period follows metric abbreviations unless the abbreviation ends a sentence.
  You will hear the dictator say: Sigmoidoscopy was completed to sixty centimeters into the descending colon.
  You should transcribe as: Sigmoidoscopy was completed to 60 cm into the descending colon.

- Numbers one through and including ten are spelled out when they do not refer to technical items and the sentence does not contain numbers over ten.
  You will hear the dictator say: a repeat colonoscopy is recommended in three years.

You should transcribe as: a repeat colonoscopy is recommended in three years.

9T-9
History and Physical Examination
Patient's Name: Chi Chen
Physician: Anna Bolism, MD

● **TRANSCRIPTION TIPS**
- The following abbreviations are dictated in this report:
  GI: gastrointestinal
  t.i.d.: three times a day
  RBC: red blood cell (count)
  WBC: white blood cell (count)

- The following medication is dictated in this report:
  Procardia: the trade name for a coronary vasodilator

- The following laboratory tests are dictated in this report:
  Chem-7: the trade name for a profile of seven different chemical laboratory tests. Partial thromboplastin time: the period of time that is required for clot formation in recalcified blood plasma after contact as well as the activation and the addition of platelet substitutes. This laboratory test is used to assess the pathways of coagulation.

9T-10
Operative Report
Patient's Name: Ronald Dubinsky
Physician: Gwenn Maltase, MD

● **TRANSCRIPTION TIPS**
- The following procedure is dictated in this report.
  For example: Olympus video sigmoidoscope

9T-11
Consultation Report
Patient's Name: Micah Landis
Requesting Physician: Matthew Sponch, MD
Physician: Anna Bolism, MD

9T-12
History and Physical Examination
Patient's Name: Manuelo Rodriquez
Physician: Gwenn Maltase, MD

● **TRANSCRIPTION TIPS**
- A hyphen is used to take the place of the words *to* or *through* to identify ranges. You will hear the dictator say: On questioning, the patient reports a three to four year history of solid food dysphagia. You should transcribe as: On questioning, the patient reports a 3-4 year history of solid food dysphagia.

- The following medications are dictated in this report: Reglan, insulin.

- A hyphen is used to join two or more words when used as an adjective that proceeds a noun. The following word pairs are dictated in this report: middle-aged, low-grade.

- Words beginning with *pre, re, post*, and *non* are generally not hyphenated.
  For example: nontender

- The following abbreviations are dictated in this report:
  CBC: complete blood count
  BUN: blood urea nitrogen bunion
  SGOT: serum glutamic oxaloacetic transaminase
  GI: gastrointestinal

9T-13
Consultation Report
Patient's Name: Alice Wonderland
Requesting Physician: Izzy Sertoli, MD
Physician: Kate Cobalamin, MD

● **TRANSCRIPTION TIPS**
- The following abbreviation is dictated in this report:
  PEG: percutaneous endoscopic gastrostomy

- Words beginning with *pre, re, post*, and *non* are generally not hyphenated: postinfarct.

- Capitalize eponyms. Eponyms are surnames teamed with a disease, instrument, or surgical procedure.

You will hear the dictator say: foley catheter

You should transcribe as: Foley catheter

- The number or pound sign (#) is used to abbreviate the word *number* followed by medical instrument or apparatus.

  You will hear the dictator say: The nurse placed a number twenty two French Foley catheter to keep the PEG tube tract open.

  You should transcribe as: The nurse placed a #22 French Foley catheter to keep the PEG tube tract open.

- A hyphen is used to join two or more words when used as an adjective that proceeds a noun. The following word pair is dictated in this report: fungal-appearing.

9T-14

History and Physical Examination
Patient's Name: Ahed Admad
Physician: Gwenn Maltase, MD

● **TRANSCRIPTION TIPS**

- The following medications are dictated in this report:

  Indocin: the trade name for a nonsteroidal anti-inflammatory agent

  Nitroglycerin: a generic name for a vasodilator and is used to relieve certain types of pain

  Metamucil: the trade name for a bulk laxative.

- Words beginning with *pre, re, post,* and *non* are generally not hyphenated:
  nonsmoker, nontender

- Figures and capital letters are used to refer to the vertebral column and spinal nerves.

  You will hear the dictator say: Cardiac exam reveals a regular rate and rhythm with a normal s one and s two.

  You should transcribe as: Cardiac exam reveals a regular rate and rhythm with a normal S1 and S2.

- The diagonal (/) is used to indicate the word *per* in laboratory values and respirations or the word *over* in blood pressure.

  You will hear the dictator say: There is a grade two over six systolic murmur at the apex.

  You should transcribe as: There is a grade II/VI systolic murmur at the apex.

- Roman numerals are used to express class, cranial leads (EKG), cranial nerves, limb leads (ECG), factor (blood clotting), grade, phase, pregnancy and delivery, stage, and type.

  You will hear the dictator say: There is a grade two over six systolic murmur at the apex.

  You should transcribe as: There is a grade II/VI systolic murmur at the apex.

- The following abbreviations are dictated in this report:
  ECG: electrocardiogram
  CBC: complete blood count
  WBC: white blood cell (count)

- The following diagnostic tests/procedures are dictated in this report:

  Prothrombin time: a test to measure the activity of factors I, II, V, VII, and X, which participate in the extrinsic pathway of coagulation

  Chem-7: the trade name for a profile of seven different chemical laboratory tests

9T-15

Consultation Report
Patient's Name: Ralph Norr
Physician: Anna Bolism, MD

● **TRANSCRIPTION TIPS**

- The following medications are dictated in this report:

  Pepcid: the trade name for an acid controller for heartburn and acid indigestion

  Tenormin: the trade name for an antihypertensive

  Prilosec: the trade name for a gastric acid secretion inhibitor

- Words beginning with *pre, re, post,* and *non* are generally not hyphenated:
  nonsteroidal

- A hyphen is used between two "like" vowels: anti-inflammatory.

- The following laboratory tests are dictated

in this report:

prothrombin time: a test to measure the activity of factors I, II, V, VII, and X, which participate in the extrinsic pathway of coagulation

partial thromboplastin time: the period required for clot formation in recalcified blood plasma after contact activation and the addition of platelet substitutes. It is used to assess the pathways of coagulation.

creatine kinase: the presence of this enzyme in the blood is strongly indicative of a recent myocardial infarction

lactic dehydrogenase: the presence of this enzyme occurs in elevated concentrations when these tissues are injured

- Capitalize eponyms. Eponyms are surnames teamed with a disease, instrument, or surgical procedure.
  You will hear the dictator say: barretts esophagus
  You should transcribe as: Barrett's esophagus

- The following abbreviation is dictated in this report:
  EGD: Esophagogastroduodenoscopy is an endoscopic examination of the interior of the esophagus, stomach, and initial portion of the duodenum.

Part III / Check Your Progress (9T-5, 9T-6)

Professional transcriptionists can transcribe and proofread their own work with speed and accuracy. Have you mastered the gastroenterology transcription rotation at FedDes Wellness Center?

Testbook Users

Launch your word processing package.

Insert the appropriate audiocassette in your transcribing machine and find dictation *9T-5*.

On the open screen, transcribe and proofread dictation *9T-5*.

Identify and correct all errors.

Save your work on your student disk. Follow the same process for dictation *9T-6*.

After completing the transcriptions, refer to the answer key.

Manually complete the error analysis chart for each document.

Manually complete the production for pay chart for each document.

If you score below 90%, you are recommended to repeat Part III.

If you score 90% or above, congratulations. You have mastered this chapter.

Software Users

Click on *Chapter 9, Part III, Check Your Progress (9T-5)*.

Insert the appropriate audiocassette in your transcribing machine and find dictation *9T-5*.

Click on *Start Watch*, then transcribe and proofread dictation *9T-5*.

Identify and correct all errors.

When you are finished, click on *Done*, then *Score Document* to display your production for pay.

Click on *Display Error Analysis* to reveal your score and *View Errors* to see your errors.

Save your work (with errors showing) by clicking on *File*, then *Save As*. Follow the same process for dictation *9T-6*.

If you score below 90%, you are recommended to repeat Part III.

If you score 90% or above, congratulations. You have mastered this chapter.

Chapter 10

Office Medical Transcription from the Cardiology Practice

OBJECTIVES

At the completion of Chapter 10, you should be able to do the following:

1. Match medical terms associated with the cardiology specialty with their definitions.

2. Spell medical terms associated with the cardiology specialty with their definitions.

3. Transcribe medical terms in sentence structure.

4. Proofread, edit, and correct medical documents associated with the cardiology specialty containing various errors.

5. Transcribe and proofread authentic medical documents associated with the cardiology specialty.

The Cardiology Rotation

The FedDes Wellness Center has three cardiologists, or specialists in cardiology, on staff. Cardiology is the study of the heart and vessels that carry blood throughout the body. The cardiologist assess the function of the heart by performing invasive and noninvasive testing.

Assessment of cardiovascular problems begin with the patient's abnormal vital signs. The cardiologist will note any bluish coloring around the lips and/or nail beds, which is an indication of decreased oxygen, and clubbing of the fingers, which is an indication of chronic oxygen deficiency. The cardiologist uses palpation to feel for the pulses and auscultation to listen for bruits or other abnormal sounds.

The physicians in FedDes cardiology division perform laboratory tests and procedures including chest x-rays, electrocardiogram (ECG), echocardiogram, and cardiac catheterization.

In this unit, you assume the role of a medical transcriptionist employed at FedDes Wellness Center. **Please remember to follow the guidelines per-** taining to capitalization, numbers, punctuation, abbreviations, measurements, symbols, and use of templates to create medical reports at FedDes Wellness Center. Review of this material can be found in Unit 1. A list of the patient's name and the type of report as well as associated transcription tips is included in this chapter.

You will work with the textbook, CD-ROM, and accompanying audiocassettes. Your mastery of cardiology transcription is assessed through worksheets, timed transcription exercises, the error analysis chart, and the Production for Pay summary.

All answer keys are found in the textbook and CD-ROM, providing immediate feedback. After transcribing a report, you will proofread your work and correct any errors. Then you will compare your proofread work against a master transcript, categorize all errors, and tabulate the errors on the error analysis chart. The Production for Pay summary correlates your production to the FedDes Wellness Center pay scale, which is based on industry compensation standards. The scale is also linked to your grade. This system allows you to assess your mastery of transcription skills in a real-world scenario.

PART I ▪ GETTING CLOSE TO THE REAL THING

Pretest

Let's find out if you can define and spell selected terminology and drugs of the cardiology specialty that are included in this chapter by scoring 90% or better.

Textbook Users
Select the correctly spelled term that matches its definition.
Refer to the answer key for immediate feedback.
After completing the pretest, refer to the answer key.
If you score below 90%, continue with *Activities 1–3*.
If you score 90% or above, congratulations. If you wish, you can immediately move on to Part II.

Software Users
Click on *Chapter 10, Part I, Pretest.*
Key the correctly spelled term that matches its definition.
When you are finished, click on *End Test*. A pop-up screen will appear to reveal your score.
If you score below 90%, continue with *Activities 1–3*.
If you score 90% or above, congratulations. If you wish, you can immediately move on to Part II.

PART I / PRETEST

Directions: Select the correctly spelled term that matches its definition.

1. Generic name for a cardiotonic agent:
   (a) dobutamine
   (b) dobitamine
   (c) cardiolite
   (d) cardialite

2. Generic name for a cardiotonic:
   (a) digixin
   (b) paroxysm
   (c) digoxin
   (d) paroxism

3. A condition of elevated lipid levels in the blood:
   (a) hyolipidemia
   (b) hyperlipidemia
   (c) hypokalemia
   (d) hyperkalemia

4. Generic name for a coronary vasodilator:
   (a) atrial
   (b) atrilae
   (c) diltiazem
   (d) diltazem

5. Generic name for a coronary vasodilator:
   (a) fibrilla
   (b) verapamil
   (c) fabrille
   (d) verpamil

6. The localized abnormal dilatation of the wall of a blood vessel:
   (a) verapemil
   (b) verpamil
   (c) aneurism
   (d) aneurysm

7. A sound or murmur heard in auscultation:
   (a) digoxin
   (b) digixin
   (c) bruit
   (d) briut

8. A triple cadence to the heart sounds:
   (a) gallop
   (b) galop
   (c) bruit
   (d) briut

9. An abnormal rapid heart rate:
   (a) tachycardia
   (b) tachicardia
   (c) bradicardia
   (d) bradycardia

10. Generic name for an antiarrhythmic agent used in the treatment of atrial flutter, atrial fibrillation, premature ventricular contractions, and tachycardia:
    (a) quindine
    (b) quinidine
    (c) nortrityline
    (d) nortriptyline

11. Generic name for an anticoagulant:
    (a) heparin
    (b) heperin
    (c) paroxysm
    (d) parxysim

12. Generic name for an antidepressant:
    (a) quindine
    (b) quinidine
    (c) nortrityline
    (d) nortriptyline

13. An increase in total red cell mass of blood:
    (a) polycythemia
    (b) pleura
    (c) polycyemia
    (d) pleuria

14. Cavity or channel:
    (a) guot
    (b) sinus
    (c) gout
    (d) sinnus

15. Characterized by low blood pressure or causing a reduction in blood pressure:
    (a) hypercholesterolemia
    (b) hypertensive
    (c) hypocholesterolemia
    (d) hypotensive

16. Continuous dry rattling in the throat due to a partial obstruction, heard on auscultation:
    (a) pectoralis
    (b) rhonchus
    (c) pectalis
    (d) rhionchus

17. Cramp-like pains in the calf; limping:
    (a) caudication
    (b) claudication
    (c) fibrilation
    (d) fibrillation

18. Dark bluish or purplish coloration of the skin due to deficient oxygenation of the blood:
    (a) cyanosis
    (b) diaphoresis
    (c) cyainosis
    (d) diaphorsis

19. Defective rhythm:
    (a) rhonchus
    (b) dysrhythmia
    (c) ronchus
    (d) dysrrhythmia

20. Device used to administer electrical shocks to the heart:
    (a) cardiomyopathy
    (b) cardioverter
    (c) cardomyopathy
    (d) cardoverter

21. Disease of unknown cause:
    (a) idiopathic
    (b) inotropic
    (c) idipathic
    (d) intropic

22. Disorder associated with an inborn error of uric acid metabolism that increases production or interferes with the excretion of uric acid:
    (a) guot
    (b) sinus
    (c) gout
    (d) sinnus

23. Exceedingly rapid contrations of muscular fibrils:
    (a) caudication
    (b) claudication
    (c) fibrilation
    (d) fibrillation

24. Failure to conduct an impulse down one division of the left bundle branch:
    (a) expiratory
    (b) expiratery
    (c) hemblock
    (d) hemiblock

25. Formation of a small depression:
    (a) pitting
    (b) iliac
    (c) piting
    (d) ilac

PART I / PRETEST *continued*

26. Greater than normal concentration of
    potassium ions in the blood:
    (a) hyolipidemia
    (b) hyperlipidemia
    (c) hypokalemia
    (d) hyperkalemia

27. Pertaining to the force of muscular
    contractions:
    (a) idiopathic
    (b) inotropic
    (c) idipathic
    (d) intropic

28. Decreased supply of oxygenated blood to a
    body part:
    (a) erythemia
    (b) erythema
    (c) ischema
    (d) ischemia

29. Mass of tissues and organs separating the
    sternum in front and the vertebral column
    behind:
    (a) mediastinum
    (b) venous
    (c) medastinum
    (d) veinous

30. Having a normal-sized head; mesocephalic:
    (a) atherosclerotic
    (b) atheriosclerotic
    (c) normocephalic
    (d) normiocephalic

31. Perspiration:
    (a) cyanosis
    (b) diaphoresis
    (c) cyainosis
    (d) diaphorsis

32. Pertains to a location situated below and to
    the side:
    (a) colleratal
    (b) inferolateral
    (c) coleratal
    (d) inferlateral

33. Pertains to the atrium:
    (a) afebrile
    (b) afebril
    (c) atrail
    (d) atrial

34. Pertains to the chest or breast:
    (a) pectoralis
    (b) rhonchus
    (c) pectalis
    (d) rhionchus

35. Pertains to the foot or feet:
    (a) pedal
    (b) padel
    (c) carotid
    (d) cariotid

36. Pertains to the muscular tissue of the heart:
    (a) myocardial
    (b) myocardal
    (c) thromosis
    (d) thrombosis

37. Pertains to the veins:
    (a) mediastinum
    (b) venous
    (c) medastinum
    (d) veinous

38. Radiograph of an artery after injecting a
    contrast medium in the bloodstream:
    (a) arthrography
    (b) artherography
    (c) arteriography
    (d) arterography

39. Radiographic visualization of blood vessels after injection of a contrast agent:
    (a) angiography
    (b) angography
    (c) athrography
    (d) atherography

40. Redness of the skin due to capillary dilatation:
    (a) erythemia
    (b) erythema
    (c) ischema
    (d) ischemia

41. Relates to exhalation:
    (a) expiratory
    (b) expiratery
    (c) hemblock
    (d) hemiblock

42. Relates to the duodenum, the first division of the small intestine:
    (a) intimal
    (b) intomal
    (c) doudenal
    (d) duodenal

43. Relates to the ilium:
    (a) pitting
    (b) iliac
    (c) piting
    (d) ilac

44. Relates to the inner coat of a vessel:
    (a) intimal
    (b) intomal
    (c) doudenal
    (d) duodenal

45. Relates to the principal artery of the neck:
    (a) pedal
    (b) padel
    (c) carotid
    (d) cariotid

46. Serous membrane investing the lungs and lining the walls of the thoracic cavity:
    (a) polycythemia
    (b) pleura
    (c) polycyemia
    (d) pleuria

47. A secondary or accessory blood pathway:
    (a) collateral
    (b) inferolateral
    (c) coleratal
    (d) inferlateral

48. Coughing or spitting of blood from the respiratory tract:
    (a) hemptysis
    (b) hemoptysis
    (c) epiphysis
    (d) epiphtysis

49. Sudden insufficiency of arterial or venous blood supply:
    (a) heparin
    (b) heperin
    (c) infarction
    (d) infartion

50. Sudden recurrence or increase in intensity of symptoms:
    (a) paroxysm
    (b) paroxism
    (c) aneurism
    (d) aneurysm

51. Surgical removal of the gallbladder:
    (a) cholecystectomy
    (b) endartertomy
    (c) cholcystectomy
    (d) endarterectomy

NAME _____   DATE _____

52. Temporary suspension of consciousness; fainting:
  (a) syncope
  (b) echocardiogram
  (c) synscope
  (d) echocardogram

53. Disease process of the heart muscle:
  (a) cardiomyopathy
  (b) cardioverter
  (c) cardomyopathy
  (d) cardoverter

54. The center for ossification of the proximal and distal ends of a long bone:
  (a) hemptysis
  (b) hemoptysis
  (c) epiphysis
  (d) epiphtysis

55. The formation of a blood clot within the vascular system:
  (a) myocardial
  (b) myocardal
  (c) thromosis
  (d) thrombosis

56. The loss of sight without the apparent lesion of the eye:
  (a) stensis
  (b) stenosis
  (c) amarosis
  (d) amaurosis

57. Hardening of an artery due to deposits of plaque within the vessel:
  (a) atherosclerotic
  (b) atheriosclerotic
  (c) normocephalic
  (d) normiocephalic

58. The narrowing or contraction of a body passage:
  (a) stensis
  (b) stenosis
  (c) amarosis
  (d) amaurosis

59. The presence of an abnormally large amount of cholesterol in the cells and plasma of the blood:
  (a) hypercholesterolemia
  (b) hypertensive
  (c) hypocholesterolemia
  (d) hypotensive

60. The slowness of the heartbeat:
  (a) tachycardia
  (b) tachicardia
  (c) bradicardia
  (d) bradycardia

61. The surgical procedure done to clear a blocked artery:
  (a) cholecystectomy
  (b) endartertomy
  (c) cholcystectomy
  (d) endarterectomy

62. A diagnostic procedure using ultrasound to study heart structure and motion:
  (a) syncope
  (b) echocardiogram
  (c) synscope
  (d) echocardogram

63. Variation from the normal rhythm of the heartbeat:
  (a) arhythmia
  (b) bruit
  (c) arrhythmia
  (d) bruite

PART I / PRETEST continued

64. Without fever:
    (a) afebrile
    (b) afebril
    (c) atrail
    (d) atrial

65. Trade name for an antihypertensive:
    (a) Capoten
    (b) Capatin
    (c) Zyloprim
    (d) Zylaprim

66. Trade name for myocardial perfusion agent for cardiac SPECT imaging:
    (a) Cardolite
    (b) Xanax
    (c) Cardiolite
    (d) Xanix

67. Trade name for a calcium channel blocker for atrial fibrillation:
    (a) Vasotec
    (b) Vasotic
    (c) Cardisem
    (d) Cardizem

68. Trade name for an anticoagulant:
    (a) Coumadim
    (b) Coumadin
    (c) Trentil
    (d) Trental

69. Trade name for a nonsteroidal anti-inflammatory drug used to prevent gastric ulcers:
    (a) Cycotec
    (b) Terramycin
    (c) Cytotec
    (d) Teramycin

70. Trade name for an analgesic, anti-inflammatory:
    (a) Ecotrin
    (b) Icotrin
    (c) Lasix
    (d) Laxis

71. Trade name for a nonsteroidal anti-inflammatory drug:
    (a) Indocin
    (b) Endocin
    (c) Lotensin
    (d) Lotinsen

72. Trade name for an antianginal:
    (a) Lescol
    (b) Lescil
    (c) Isordol
    (d) Isordil

73. Trade name for a potassium supplement:
    (a) Theo-Dur
    (b) K-Dur
    (c) T-Dur
    (d) Kheo-Dur

74. Trade name for an antiarrthymic, cardiotonic that increases cardiac output:
    (a) Lanoxin
    (b) Lanozin
    (c) Tenormin
    (d) Tenorrmin

75. Trade name for a diuretic:
    (a) Ecotrin
    (b) Icotrin
    (c) Lasix
    (d) Laxis

PART I / PRETEST continued

76. Trade name for a reductase inhibitor for hypercholesterolemia:
    (a) Lescol
    (b) Lescil
    (c) Isordol
    (d) Isordil

77. Trade name for an antihypertensive:
    (a) Indocin
    (b) Endocin
    (c) Lotensin
    (d) Lotinsen

78. Trade name for a reductase inhibitor for hypercholesterolemia:
    (a) Metavor
    (b) Mevacor
    (c) Synthroid
    (d) Syntoid

79. Trade name for a coronary vasodilator:
    (a) Persantine
    (b) Reglan
    (c) Presantine
    (d) Relan

80. Trade name for estrogen replacement therapy:
    (a) Provera
    (b) Prevera
    (c) Permarin
    (d) Premarin

81. Trade name for progestin for secondary amenorrhea and abnormal uterine bleeding:
    (a) Provera
    (b) Prevera
    (c) Permarin
    (d) Premarin

82. Trade name for an antiarrhythmic:
    (a) Quinidex
    (b) Senekot
    (c) Quindez
    (d) Senokot

83. Trade name for a gastrointestinal stimulant; antiemetic:
    (a) Persantine
    (b) Reglan
    (c) Presantine
    (d) Relan

84. Trade name for a laxative:
    (a) Quinidex
    (b) Senekot
    (c) Quindez
    (d) Senokot

85. Trade name for a thyroid hormone:
    (a) Metavor
    (b) Mevacor
    (c) Synthroid
    (d) Syntoid

86. Trade name for a beta-blocker; antihypertensive agent:
    (a) Lanoxin
    (b) Lanozin
    (c) Tenormin
    (d) Tenorrmin

87. Trade name for an antibiotic:
    (a) Cycotec
    (b) Terramycin
    (c) Cytotec
    (d) Teramycin

88. Trade name for a bronchodilator:
    (a) Theo-Dur
    (b) K-Dur
    (c) T-Dur
    (d) Kheo-Dur

89. Trade name for an oral hemorheologic drug:
    (a) Xanex
    (b) Zanax
    (c) Trentil
    (d) Trental

PART I / PRETEST *continued*

90. Trade name for an antihypertensive agent:
    (a) Vasotec
    (b) Vasotic
    (c) Zyloprim
    (d) Zyloprime

91. Trade name for an antianxiety agent:
    (a) Cardolite
    (b) Xanax
    (c) Cardiolite
    (d) Xanix

92. Trade name for an antigout agent:
    (a) Capoten
    (b) Capatin
    (c) Zyloprim
    (d) Zylaprim

Part I / Activity 1
Keyboarding Medical Terms and Definitions

Let's learn to spell and define selected terminology and drugs of the cardiology specialty that is included in this chapter. Keyboarding these terms is an innovative and fun way to improve your skills.

Textbook Users
Launch your word processing package.
On the open screen, read and key each word and its definition as shown above.
Save your work on your student disk.

1. Afebrile (a-feb-ril) is without fever.
2. Amaurosis (am-aw-ro-sis) is the loss of sight without the apparent lesion of the eye.
3. Aneurysm (an-u-rizm) is the localized abnormal dilatation of the wall of a blood vessel.
4. Angiography (an-je-og-rah-fe) is the radiographic visualization of a blood vessel after injecting a contrast agent
5. Arrhythmia (ah-rith-me-ah) is the variation from the normal rhythm of the heartbeat.
6. Arteriography (ar-te-re-og-rah-fe) is the radiographic visualization of an artery after injecting a contrast agent.
7. Atherosclerosis (ath-er-o-skle-ro-sis) is the hardening of an artery due to deposits of plaque within the vessel.
8. Atrial (a-tre-al) pertains to the atrium.

9. Bradycardia (bard-e-kar-de-ah) is the slowness of the heartbeat.
10. Bruit (broot) is a sound or murmur heard in auscultation.
11. Cardiomyopathy (kar-de-o-mi-op-ah-the) is a disease process of the heart muscle.
12. Cardioverter (kar-de-o-ver-ter) is a device that is used to administer electrical shocks to the heart.
13. Carotid (kah-rot-id) relates to the principal artery of the neck.
14. Cholecystectomy (ko-le-sus-tek-to-me) is the surgical removal of the gallbladder.
15. Claudication (klaw-di-ka-shun) is the cramplike pains in the calf; limping.
16. Collateral (ko-lat-er-al) is a secondary or accessory blood pathway.

17. Cyanosis (si-a-<u>no</u>-sis) is a dark bluish or purplish coloration of the skin due to deficient oxygenation of the blood.
18. Diaphoresis (di-a-fo-<u>re</u>-sis) is perspiration.
19. Digoxin (di-<u>jok</u>-sin) is a generic name for a cardiotonic.
20. Diltiazem (<u>dil</u>-ti-a-zem) is a generic name for a coronary vasodilator.
21. Dobutamine (do-<u>byu</u>-ta-men) is a generic name for a cardiotonic agent.
22. Duodenal (du-o-<u>de</u>-nal) relates to the duodenum, the first division of the small intestine.
23. Dysrhythmia (dis-<u>rith</u>-me-a) is a defective rhythm.
24. Echocardiogram (ek-o-<u>kar</u>-de-o-gram) is a diagnostic procedure using ultrasound to study heart structure and motion.
25. Endarterectomy (end-ar-ter-<u>ek</u>-to-me) is a surgical procedure that is performed to clear a blocked artery.
26. Epiphysis (e-<u>pif</u>-I-sis) is the center for ossification of the proximal and distal ends of a long bone.
27. Erythema (er-I-<u>the</u>-ma) is the redness of the skin due to capillary dilatation.
28. Expiratory (ek-<u>spi</u>-ra-to-re) relates to exhalation.
29. Fibrillation (fi-bri-<u>la</u>-shun) is the rapid, irregular, uncoordinated contractions of muscle fibers.
30. Gallop (<u>gal</u>-op) is a triple cadence to the heart sounds.
31. Gout (gowt) is a disorder associated with an inborn error of uric acid metabolism that increases production or interferes with the excretion of uric acid.
32. Hemiblock (<u>hem</u>-e-blok) is the failure to conduct an impulse down one division of the left bundle branch.
33. Hemoptysis (he-<u>mop</u>-ti-sis) is the coughing or spitting of blood from the respiratory tract.
34. Heparin (<u>hep</u>-a-rin) is a generic name for an anticoagulant.
35. Hypercholesterolemia (hi-per-ko-<u>les</u>-ter-ol-e-me-a) is the presence of an abnormally large amount of cholesterol in the cells and plasma of the blood.
36. Hyperkalemia (<u>hi</u>-per-kal-<u>e</u>-ma-a) is the greater than normal concentration of potassium ions in the blood.
37. Hyperlipidemia (<u>hi</u>-per-lip-I-<u>de</u>-me-a) is a condition of elevated lipid levels in the blood.
38. Hypotensive (<u>hi</u>-po-<u>ten</u>-siv) is characterized by low blood pressure or causing a reduction in blood pressure.
39. Idiopathic (<u>id</u>-e-o-<u>path</u>-ik) is a disease of unknown cause.
40. Iliac (<u>il</u>-e-ak) relates to the ilium.
41. Infarction (in-<u>fark</u>-shun) is the sudden insufficiency of arterial or venous blood supply.
42. Inferolateral (in-fer-o-<u>lat</u>-e-ral) pertains to a location situated below and to the side.
43. Inotropic (in-o-<u>trop</u>-ik) pertains to the force of muscular contractions.
44. Intimal (<u>in</u>-ti-mal) relates to the inner coat of a vessel.
45. Ischemia (is-<u>ke</u>-me-a) is the decreased supply of oxygenated blood to a body part.
46. Mediastinum (me-de-ah-<u>sti</u>-num) is the mass of tissues and organs separating the sternum in front and the vertebral column behind.
47. Myocardial (mi-o-<u>kar</u>-de-al) pertains to the muscular tissue of the heart.
48. Normocephalic (nor-mo-se-<u>fal</u>-ik) is having a normal-sized head; mesocephalic.
49. Nortriptyline (<u>nor</u>-trip-ti-lin) is a generic name for an antidepressant.
50. Paroxysm (<u>par</u>-ok-sim) is the sudden recurrence or increase in the intensity of symptoms.
51. Pectoralis (pek-to-<u>ra</u>-lis) pertains to the chest or breast.
52. Pedal (<u>ped</u>-al) pertains to the foot or feet.
53. Pitting (<u>pit</u>-ing) is the formation of a small depression.
54. Pleura (<u>ploo</u>-rah) is the serous membrane investing the lungs and lining the walls of the thoracic cavity.
55. Polycythemia (pol-e-si-<u>the</u>-me-ah) is an increase in the total red cell mass of the blood.
56. Quinidine (<u>kwin</u>-I-den) is a generic name for an antiarrhythmic agent used in the treatment of atrial flutter, atrial fibrillation, premature ventricular contractions, and tachycardias.
57. Rhonchus (<u>rong</u>-kus) is a continuous dry rattling in the throat or bronhcial tube due to a partial obstruction, heard on auscultation.
58. Sinus (<u>si</u>-nus) is a cavity or channel.
59. Stenosis (ste-<u>no</u>-sis) is the narrowing or contraction of a body passage.
60. Syncope (<u>sing</u>-ko-pe) is a temporary suspension of consciousness; fainting.

61. Tachycardia (tak-e-<u>kar</u>-de-ah) is an abnormal rapid heart rate.
62. Thrombosis (throm-<u>bo</u>-sis) is the formation of a blood clot within the vascular system.
63. Venous (<u>ve</u>-nus) pertains to the veins.
64. Verapamil (ver-ah-<u>pam</u>-il) is a generic name for a coronary vasodilator.
65. Capoten (<u>kap</u>-o-ten) is the trade name for an antihypertensive.
66. Cardiolite (<u>kar</u>-de-o-lit) is the trade name for myocardial perfusion agent for cardiac SPECT imaging.
67. Cardizem (<u>kar</u>-di-zem) is the trade name for a calcium channel blocker for atrial fibrillation.
68. Coumadin (<u>koo</u>-mah-din) is the trade name for an anticoagulant.
69. Cytotec: (si-to-<u>tek</u>) is the trade name for a nonsteroidal anti-inflammatory drug used to prevent gastric ulcers
70. Ecotrin (<u>ek</u>-o-trin) is the trade name for an analgesic, anti-inflammatory.
71. Indocin (<u>in</u>-do-sin) is the trade name for nonsteroidal anti-inflammatory drug.
72. Isordil (<u>I</u>-sor-dil) is the trade name for an antianginal.
73. K-Dur (Kay-dur) is the trade name for a potassium supplement.
74. Lanoxin (lah-<u>nok</u>-sin) is the trade name for an antiarrthymic, cardiotonic that is used to increase cardiac output.
75. Lasix (<u>la</u>-ziks) is the trade name for a diuretic.
76. Lescol (<u>le</u>-zkol) is the trade name for a reductase inhibitor for hypercholesterolemia.
77. Lotensin (<u>lo</u>-ten-sin) is the trade name for an antihypertensive.
78. Mevacor (mev-a <u>kor</u>) is the trade name for a reductase inhibitor for hypercholesterolemia.
79. Persantine (per-<u>san</u>-ten) is the trade name for a coronary vasodilator.
80. Premarin (<u>prem</u>-ah-rin) is the trade name for estrogen replacement therapy.
81. Provera (pro-<u>ver</u>-ah) is the trade name for progestin for secondary amenorrhea and abnormal uterine bleeding.
82. Quinidex (<u>kwin</u>-I-des) is the trade name for an antiarrhythmic.
83. Reglan (<u>reg</u>-lan) is the trade name for a gastrointestinal stimulant; antiemetic.
84. Senokot (se-<u>no</u>-kot) is the trade name for a laxative.
85. Synthroid (<u>sin</u>-throid) is the trade name for a thyroid hormone.
86. Tenormin (<u>ten</u>-or-min) is the trade name for a beta-blocker; antihypertensive agent.
87. Terramycin (<u>ter</u>-ah-mi-sin) is the trade name for an antibiotic.
88. Theo-Dur (<u>the</u>-o-dur) is the trade name for a bronchodilator.
89. Trental (<u>tren</u>-tal) is the trade name for an oral hemorheologic drug.
90. Vasotec (<u>vah</u>-o-tek) is the trade name for an antihypertensive agent.
91. Xanax (<u>zan</u>-aks) is the trade name for an antianxiety agent.
92. Zyloprim (<u>zi</u>-lo-prim) is the trade name for an antigout agent.

Part I / Activity 2
Spelling Medical Terms

Do you remember back in school when you had to write each spelling word ten times? Because you had to physically write each word, your mind and body were focused on the assignment and the method worked! Let's follow this successful method by reinforcing the spelling of selected terms and drugs found in the cardiology specialty through keyboarding drills.

Textbook Users
Launch your word processing package.
On the open screen, read, mentally spell, and type each word in its sequence.
Save your work on your student disk.

1. afebrile amaurosis aneurysm afebrile amaurosis aneurysm afebrile amaurosis aneurysm
2. angiography arrhythmia arteriography angiography arrhythmia arteriography angiography
3. atherosclerotic atrial bradycardia atherosclerotic atrial bradycardia atherosclerotic atrial
4. bruit cardiomyopathy cardioverter bruit cardiomyopathy cardioverter bruit cardiomyopathy
5. carotid cholecystectomy claudication carotid cholecystectomy claudication carotid
6. collateral cyanosis diaphoresis collateral cyanosis diaphoresis collateral cyanosis diaphoresis
7. digoxin diltiazem dobutamine digoxin diltiazem dobutamine digoxin diltiazem dobutamine
8. duodenal dysrhythmia echocardiogram duodenal dysrythmia echocardiogram duodenal
9. endarterectomy epiphysis erythema endarterectomy epiphysis erythema endarterectomy
10. expiratory fibrillation gallop expiratory fibrillation gallop expiratory fibrillation gallop
11. gout hemiblock hemoptysis gout hemiblock hemoptysis gout hemiblock hemoptysis gout
12. heparin hypercholesterolemia hyperkalemia heparin hypercholesterolemia hyperkalemia
13. hyperlipidemia hypotensive idiopathic hyperlipidemia hypotensive idiopathic hyperlipidemia
14. iliac infarction inferolateral iliac infarction inferolateral iliac infarction inferolateral iliac
15. inotropic ischemia intimal inotropic ischemia intimal inotropic ischemia intimal inotropic
16. mediastinum myocardial normocephalic mediastinum myocardial normocephalic
17. nortriptyline paroxysm pectoralis nortriptyline paroxysm pectoralis nortriptyline paroxysm
18. pedal pitting pleura pedal pitting pleura pedal pitting pleura pedal pitting pleura pedal pitting
19. polycythemia quinidine rhonchus polycythemia quinidine rhonchus polycythemia quinidine
20. sinus stenosis syncope sinus stenosis syncope sinus stenosis syncope sinus stenosis syncope
21. tachycardia thrombosis venous verapamil tachycardia thrombosis venous verapamil
22. Capoten Cardiolite Cardizem Capoten Cardiolite Cardizem Capoten Cardiolite Cardizem
23. Coumadin Cytotec Ecotrin Coumadin Cytotec Ecotrin Coumadin Cytotec Ecotrin Coumadin
24. Indocin Isordil K-Dur Indocin Isordil K-Dur Indocin Isordil K-Dur Indocin Isordil K-Dur
25. Lanoxin Lasix Lescol Lanoxin Lasix Lescol Lanoxin Lasix Lescol Lanoxin Lasix Lescol
26. Lotensin Mevacor Persantine Lotensin Mevacor Persantine Lotensin Mevacor Persantine
27. Premarin Provera Quinidex Premarin Provera Quinidex Premarin Provera Quinidex Premarin
28. Reglan Senokot Synthroid Reglan Senokot Synthroid Reglan Senokot Synthroid Reglan
29. Tenormin Terramycin Theo-Dur Tenormin Terramycin Theo-Dur Tenormin Terramycin
30. Trental Vasotec Xanax Zyloprim Trental Vasotec Xanax Zyloprim Trental Vasotec Xanax

Part I / Activity 3
Transcribing Medical Sentences (10T-1)

Now you are ready to make the transition from keyboarding medical terms, which is a visual process, to transcribing medical terms, an aural process. You are going to use audiocassette tapes rather than printed material.

Textbook Users

Launch your word processing package.

Insert the appropriate audiocassette in your transcribing machine and find dictation *10T-1*.

You will be transcribing spelling words in sentence structure.

Listen carefully to each sentence on the audiocassette before transcribing. Rewind and type (transcribe) the sentences.

Save your work on your student disk and refer to the answer key.

Part I / Check Your Progress

Let's pause a minute and see how well you are doing. This section will allow you to evaluate your mastery of keyboarding and spelling selected terms and drugs found in the cardiology specialty.

Textbook Users

Select the correctly spelled term that matches its definition.

If you score below 90%, you are recommended to redo the Part I Activities.

If you score 90% or above, congratulations. If you wish, you can immediately move on to Part II.

Software Users

Click on *Chapter 10, Part I, Check Your Progress.*

Key the correctly spelled term that matches its definition.

When you are finished, click on *End Test.*

A pop-up screen will reveal your score.

If you score below 90%, you are recommended to redo the Part I Activities.

If you score 90% or above, congratulations. If you wish, you can immediately move on to Part II.

PART I / CHECK YOUR PROGRESS

Directions: Select the correctly spelled term that matches its definition.

1. Without fever:
   (a) afebrile
   (b) afebril
   (c) atrail
   (d) atrial

2. Variation from the normal rhythm of the heartbeat:
   (a) arhythmia
   (b) bruit
   (c) arrhythmia
   (d) bruite

3. A diagnostic procedure using ultrasound to study heart structure and motion:
   (a) syncope
   (b) echocardiogram
   (c) synscope
   (d) dysrrhythmia

4. A surgical procedure done to clear a blocked artery:
   (a) cholecystectomy
   (b) endartertomy
   (c) cholcystectomy
   (d) endarterectomy

5. The slowness of the heartbeat:
   (a) tachycardia
   (b) tachicardia
   (c) bradicardia
   (d) bradycardia

6. The presence of an abnormally large amount of cholesterol in the cells and plasma of the blood:
   (a) hypercholesterolemia
   (b) hypertensive
   (c) hypocholesterolemia
   (d) hypotensive

7. The narrowing or contraction of a body passage:
   (a) stensis
   (b) stenosis
   (c) amarosis
   (d) amaurosis

8. The hardening of an artery from plaque deposits within the vessel:
   (a) atherosclerotic
   (b) atheriosclerotic
   (c) normocephalic
   (d) normiocephalic

9. The loss of sight without the apparent lesion of the eye:
   (a) stensis
   (b) stenosis
   (c) amarosis
   (d) amaurosis

10. The formation of a blood clot within the vascular system:
    (a) myocardial
    (b) myocardal
    (c) thromosis
    (d) thrombosis

11. The center for ossification of the proximal and distal ends of a long bone:
    (a) hemptysis
    (b) hemoptysis
    (c) epiphysis
    (d) epiphtysis

12. A disease process of the heart muscle:
    (a) cardiomyopathy
    (b) cardioverter
    (c) cardomyopathy
    (d) cardoverter

PART I / CHECK YOUR PROGRESS *continued*

13. Temporary suspension of consciousness; fainting:
    (a) syncope
    (b) echocardiogram
    (c) synscope
    (d) echocardogram

14. Surgical removal of the gallbladder:
    (a) cholecystectomy
    (b) endartertomy
    (c) cholcystectomy
    (d) endarterectomy

15. Sudden recurrence or increase in intensity of symptoms:
    (a) paroxysm
    (b) paroxism
    (c) aneurism
    (d) aneurysm

16. Sudden insufficiency of arterial or venous blood supply:
    (a) heparin
    (b) heperin
    (c) infarction
    (d) infartion

17. Coughing or spitting of blood from the respiratory tract:
    (a) hemptysis
    (b) hemoptysis
    (c) epiphysis
    (d) epiphtysis

18. A secondary or accessory blood pathway:
    (a) colleratal
    (b) inferolateral
    (c) coleratal
    (d) inferlateral

19. Serous membrane investing the lungs and lining the walls of the thoracic cavity:
    (a) polycythemia
    (b) pleura
    (c) polycyemia
    (d) pleuria

20. Relates to the principal artery of the neck:
    (a) pedal
    (b) padel
    (c) carotid
    (d) cariotid

21. Relates to the inner coat of a vessel:
    (a) intimal
    (b) intomal
    (c) doudenal
    (d) duodenal

22. Relates to the ilium:
    (a) pitting
    (b) iliac
    (c) piting
    (d) ilac

23. Relates to the duodenum, the first division of the small intestine:
    (a) intimal
    (b) intomal
    (c) doudenal
    (d) duodenal

24. Relates to exhalation:
    (a) expiratory
    (b) expiratery
    (c) hemblock
    (d) hemiblock

25. Redness of the skin due to capillary dilatation:
    (a) erythemia
    (b) erythema
    (c) ischema
    (d) ischemia

PART I / CHECK YOUR PROGRESS *continued*

26. Radiographic visualization of blood vessels after injection of a contrast agent:
    (a) angiography
    (b) angography
    (c) artheriography
    (d) atherography

27. Radiographic visualization of an artery after injecting a contrast agent:
    (a) arthrography
    (b) artherography
    (c) arteriography
    (d) artrography

28. Pertains to the veins:
    (a) mediastinum
    (b) venous
    (c) medastinum
    (d) veinous

29. Pertains to the muscular tissue of the heart:
    (a) myocardial
    (b) myocardal
    (c) thromosis
    (d) thrombosis

30. Pertains to the foot or feet:
    (a) pedal
    (b) padel
    (c) carotid
    (d) cariotid

31. Pertains to the chest or breast:
    (a) pectoralis
    (b) rhonchus
    (c) pectalis
    (d) rhionchus

32. Pertains to the atrium:
    (a) afebrile
    (b) afebril
    (c) atrail
    (d) atrial

33. Pertains to a location situated below and to the side:
    (a) colleratal
    (b) inferolateral
    (c) coleratal
    (d) inferlatral

34. Perspiration:
    (a) cyanosis
    (b) diaphoresis
    (c) cysainosis
    (d) diaphorsis

35. Having a normal-sized head; mesocephalic:
    (a) atherosclerotic
    (b) atheriosclerotic
    (c) normocephalic
    (d) normiocephalic

36. Mass of tissues and organs separating the sternum in front and the vertebral column behind:
    (a) mediastinum
    (b) venous
    (c) medastinum
    (d) veinous

37. Decreased supply of oxygenated blood to a body part:
    (a) erythemia
    (b) erythema
    (c) ischema
    (d) ischemia

38. Pertaining to the force of muscular contractions:
    (a) idiopathic
    (b) inotropic
    (c) idipathic
    (d) intropic

PART I / CHECK YOUR PROGRESS *continued*

39. Greater than normal concentration of potassium ions in the blood:
    (a) hypolipidemia
    (b) hyperlipidemia
    (c) hypokalemia
    (d) hyperkalemia

40. Formation of a small depression:
    (a) pitting
    (b) iliac
    (c) piting
    (d) ilac

41. Failure to conduct an impulse down one division of the left bundle branch:
    (a) expiratory
    (b) expiratery
    (c) hemblock
    (d) hemiblock

42. Exceedingly rapid contractions of muscular fibrils:
    (a) caudication
    (b) claudication
    (c) fibrilation
    (d) fibrillation

43. Disorder associated with an inborn error of uric acid metabolism that increases production or interferes with the excretion of uric acid:
    (a) guot
    (b) sinus
    (c) gout
    (d) sinnus

44. Disease of unknown cause:
    (a) idiopathic
    (b) inotropic
    (c) idipathic
    (d) intropic

45. Device used to administer electrical shocks to the heart:
    (a) cardiomyopathy
    (b) cardioverter
    (c) cardomyopathy
    (d) cardoverter

46. Defective rhythm:
    (a) rhonchus
    (b) dysrhythmia
    (c) ronchus
    (d) dysrrhythmia

47. Dark bluish or purplish coloration of the skin due to deficient oxygenation of the blood:
    (a) cyanosis
    (b) diaphoresis
    (c) cyainosis
    (d) diaphorsis

48. Cramp-like pains in the calf; limping:
    (a) caudication
    (b) claudication
    (c) fibrilation
    (d) fibrillation

49. Continuous dry rattling in the throat or bronchial tube due to a partial obstruction heard on auscultation:
    (a) pectoralis
    (b) rhonchus
    (c) pectalis
    (d) rhionchus

50. Characterized by low blood pressure or causing a reduction in blood pressure:
    (a) hypercholesterolemia
    (b) hypertensive
    (c) hypocholesterolemia
    (d) hypotensive

51. Cavity or channel:
    (a) guot
    (b) sinus
    (c) gout
    (d) sinnus

52. An increase in total red cell mass of blood:
    (a) polycythemia
    (b) pleura
    (c) polycyemia
    (d) pleuria

53. Generic name for an antidepressant:
    (a) quindine
    (b) quinidine
    (c) nortrityline
    (d) nortriptyline

54. Generic name for an anticoagulant:
    (a) heparin
    (b) heperin
    (c) paroxysm
    (d) parxysim

55. Generic name for an antiarrhythmic agent used in the treatment of atrial flutter, atrial fibrillation, premature ventricular contractions, and tachycardias:
    (a) quindine
    (b) quinidine
    (c) nortrityline
    (d) nortriptyline

56. An abnormal rapid heart rate:
    (a) tachycardia
    (b) tachicardia
    (c) bradicardia
    (d) bradycardia

57. A triple cadence to the heart sounds:
    (a) gallop
    (b) galop
    (c) bruit
    (d) briut

58. A sound or murmur heard in auscultation:
    (a) digoxin
    (b) digixin
    (c) bruit
    (d) briut

59. The localized abnormal dilatation of the wall of a blood vessel:
    (a) paroxysm
    (b) paroxism
    (c) aneurism
    (d) aneurysm

60. Generic name for a coronary vasodilator:
    (a) fibrilla
    (b) verapamil
    (c) fabrille
    (d) verpamil

61. Generic name for a coronary vasodilator:
    (a) dobutamine
    (b) dobitamine
    (c) diltiazem
    (d) diltazem

62. A condition of elevated lipid levels in the blood:
    (a) hypolipidemia
    (b) hyperlipidemia
    (c) hypokalemia
    (d) hyperkalemia

63. Generic name for a cardiotonic:
    (a) digixin
    (b) paroxysm
    (c) digoxin
    (d) paroxism

64. Generic name for a cardiotonic agent:
    (a) dobutamine
    (b) dobitamine
    (c) cardiolite
    (d) cardialite

PART I / CHECK YOUR PROGRESS *continued*

65. Trade name for an antihypertensive:
    (a) Capoten
    (b) Capatin
    (c) Zyloprim
    (d) Zylaprim

66. Trade name for myocardial perfusion agent for cardiac SPECT imaging:
    (a) Cardolite
    (b) Xanax
    (c) Cardiolite
    (d) Xanix

67. Trade name for a calcium channel blocker for atrial fibrillation:
    (a) Vasotec
    (b) Vasotic
    (c) Cardisem
    (d) Cardizem

68. Trade name for an anticoagulant:
    (a) Coumadim
    (b) Coumadin
    (c) Trentil
    (d) Trental

69. Trade name for a nonsteroidal anti-inflammatory drug used to prevent gastric ulcers:
    (a) Cycotec
    (b) Terramycin
    (c) Cytotec
    (d) Teramycin

70. Trade name for an analgesic, anti-inflammatory:
    (a) Ecotrin
    (b) Icotrin
    (c) Lasix
    (d) Laxis

71. Trade name for a nonsteroidal anti-inflammatory drug:
    (a) Indocin
    (b) Endocin
    (c) Lotensin
    (d) Lotinsen

72. Trade name for an antianginal:
    (a) Lescol
    (b) Lescil
    (c) Isordol
    (d) Isordil

73. Trade name for a potassium supplement:
    (a) Theo-Dur
    (b) K-Dur
    (c) T-Dur
    (d) Kheo-Dur

74. Trade name for an antiarrthymic, cardiotonic that is used to increase cardiac output:
    (a) Lanoxin
    (b) Lanozin
    (c) Tenormin
    (d) Tenorrmin

75. Trade name for a diuretic:
    (a) Ecotrin
    (b) Icotrin
    (c) Lasix
    (d) Laxis

76. Trade name for a reductase inhibitor for hypercholesterolemia:
    (a) Lescol
    (b) Lescil
    (c) Isordol
    (d) Isordil

77. Trade name for an antihypertensive:
    (a) Indocin
    (b) Endocin
    (c) Lotensin
    (d) Lotinsen

PART I / CHECK YOUR PROGRESS *continued*

78. Trade name for a reductase inhibitor for hypercholesterolemia:
    (a) Metavor
    (b) Mevacor
    (c) Synthroid
    (d) Syntoid

79. Trade name for a coronary vasodilator:
    (a) Persantine
    (b) Reglan
    (c) Presantine
    (d) Relan

80. Trade name for estrogen replacement therapy:
    (a) Provera
    (b) Prevera
    (c) Permarin
    (d) Premarin

81. Trade name for progestin for secondary amenorrhea and abnormal uterine bleeding:
    (a) Provera
    (b) Prevera
    (c) Permarin
    (d) Premarin

82. Trade name for an antiarrhythmic:
    (a) Quinidex
    (b) Senekot
    (c) Quindez
    (d) Senokot

83. Trade name for a gastrointestinal stimulant; antiemetic:
    (a) Persantine
    (b) Reglan
    (c) Presantine
    (d) Relan

84. Trade name for laxative:
    (a) Quinidex
    (b) Senekot
    (c) Quindez
    (d) Senokot

85. Trade name for a thyroid hormone:
    (a) Metavor
    (b) Mevacor
    (c) Synthroid
    (d) Syntoid

86. Trade name for a beta-blocker; antihypertensive agent:
    (a) Lanoxin
    (b) Lanozin
    (c) Tenormin
    (d) Tenorrmin

87. Trade name for an antibiotic:
    (a) Cycotec
    (b) Terramycin
    (c) Cytotec
    (d) Teramycin

88. Trade name for a bronchodilator:
    (a) Theo-Dur
    (b) K-Dur
    (c) T-Dur
    (d) Kheo-Dur

89. Trade name for an oral hemorheologic drug:
    (a) Xanax
    (b) Zanax
    (c) Trentil
    (d) Trental

90. Trade name for an antihypertensive agent:
    (a) Vasotec
    (b) Vasotic
    (c) Zyloprim
    (d) Zyloprime

PART I / CHECK YOUR PROGRESS *continued*

91. Trade name for an antianxiety agent:
    (a) Cardolite
    (b) Xanax
    (c) Cardiolite
    (d) Xanix

92. Trade name for an antigout agent:
    (a) Capoten
    (b) Capatin
    (c) Zyloprim
    (d) Zylaprim

PART II ▪ PROOFREADING AND ERROR ANALYSIS

Pretest *(10T-2)*

Professional transcriptionists proofread their own work. Can you? Scoring 90% or better proves it!

Textbook Users
Launch your word processing package.
Insert the appropriate audiocassette in your transcribing machine and find dictation *10T-2*.
On the open screen, transcribe and proofread dictation *10T-2*. Identify and correct all errors.
Save your work on your student disk.
After completing the transcription, refer to the answer key.
Manually complete the error analysis and production for pay charts.
If you score below 90%, continue on to *Activities 4–7*.
If you score 90% or above, congratulations. If you wish, you can immediately move on to Part III.

Software Users
Click on *Chapter 10, Part II, (10T-2)*.
Insert the appropriate audiocassette in your transcribing machine and find dictation 10T-2.
Click on *Start Watch*, then transcribe and proofread dictation *10T-2*. Identify and correct all errors.
When you are finished, click on *Done*, then *Score Document* to display your production for pay.
Click on *Display Error Analysis* to reveal your score and *View Errors* to see your errors.
Save your work (with errors showing) by clicking on *File*, then *Save As*.
If you score below 90%, continue on to *Activities 4–7*.
If you score 90% or above, congratulations. If you wish, you can immediately move on to Part III.

Part II / Activities 4–5
Proofreading Worksheet Exercises

Finding your own errors and correcting them is not easy, but it is an essential skill for your success as a medical transcriptionist. The worksheets in this activity will help you to develop your proofreading skills.

Textbook Users
Proofread and correct errors in the medical documents shown in *Activities 4–5.*
After completing the activities, refer to the answer key.
Manually complete the error analysis chart for each document.

Software Users
Click on *Chapter 10, Part II, Activity 4.*
Proofread and correct errors found in the medical document.
Click on *File,* then *Done* and a pop-up window will appear.
Click on *Score Document* to reveal your score.
Click on *View Errors* to see the errors you made.
Save your work (with errors showing) on your student disk by clicking on *File,* then *Save As.*
Click on *File,* then *Exit,* to proceed.
Follow the same process to complete *Activity 5.*

PART II / ACTIVITY 4
PROOFREADING WORKSHEET EXERCISE

Directions: Proofread this medical document that contains multiple errors using full block, open punctuation, and all other formatting guidelines established in this textbook.

FedDes Wellness Center
Cardiology Division, Suite 413
101 Wellness Way Drive
New York, NY 10036

Current date

Charles P. Davis, MD
FedDes Wellness Center
Family Practice Division, Suite 300
101 Wellness Way Drive
New York, NY 10036
Re: George Niehls
Date of Birth: January 16, 19xx

Dear Dr. Davis

George Niehls is a 62 year old man who was admitted for a cystectomy because of carcinoma of the bladder. She has a history of intermitent visual bluring. A routine physical examination revealed a right carotid bruit. A carotid sonagram was obtained which suggested high grade stenosis of the left internal carotid. He is a long time cigarette smoker and has moderate exertional dispnea. There has been no definite angina pectis nor definite symptoms related to his right carotide lession. There is a long history of hypotension but drug therapy was discontined in 1990.

Physical examination show a blood pressure of 180 over 100 and a pulse of 80 and regular. Venous pulses are unremarkable. There is a long left carotid bruitt. Ocassional rhonchus are present in the chest and there is a moderately slightly prolonged expiratery phrase. The heart is not inlarged. Thier are no significant murmur or gallops. The adbomen contains no mases and no bruits. There is no periferal edema.

Mr. Neihls would appear to have high grade carotid artery stensis. With contemplated major surgery this should presumably be repaired pre-operatively despite it's essentially assymptomatic state. In addition combined coronary arterography with cerebral angography would be apropriate. With his long history of hypertension it would seem reasonable to also perform a renal arterogram during the same procedure.

We will arrange these studies and subsequent recomendations will be based on the results of the diagnostic findings. We appreciate the opportunity to participate in her car.

PART II / ACTIVITY 4 *continued*

Page 2
Sincerely,

Lucas Site MD

xx

PART II / ACTIVITY 5
PROOFREADING WORKSHEET EXERCISE

Directions: Proofread this medical document that contains multiple errors using full block, open punctuation, and all other formatting guidelines established in this textbook.

HISTORY AND PHYSICAL EXAMINATION

Patient Name: Rolf, Nathan

File Number: 59025
Date of Birth: February 21, 19xx

Examination Date: *current date*

Physician: Adam Valence, MD

HISTORY:

CHIEF COMPLAINT: Shortness of breathe.
HISTORY OF PRESENT ILLNESS: Nathan Rolfe is a 35 year old with documented idopathic cardiomypathy. She became symptomatic in 1995 and a subsequent cardiac catheterization was performed in 1997 at which time an ejection faction of 25 was documented. His symptoms have progressed and she was recently hospitalized several weeks ago for intravenous Dobutamine therapy. He symptomatically improvedbut in the past week he developed increasing dispnea and orthipnea.

PHYSICAL EXAMINATION
VITAL SIGNS: Physical examination shows a blood pressure of one hundred thirty over seventy three and a pulse of 112 and irregular.

NECK: Jugular venus pulse is slightly prominent.
CHEST The chest is fairly clear.

HEART: The heart is moderate inlarged with an S three gallop. No significant murmurs.

IMPRESSION: Mr. Rolf has severe cardiomyopathy. Parental enotropic agents will again be employ. Presumably his gastrointestinal symptoms is also indicative of congestive heart failure but a complicating factors needs to be included as well.
Plan Admit to University's Hospital due to her increasing dispnea and orthipnea. He will again be assesed for a possible cardiac transplantation.

_____

Adam Valence

Part II / Activities 6–7
Proofreading Transcription Exercises *(10T-3, 10T-4)*

Now you are ready to make the transition from simply proofreading printed material to both transcribing and proofreading dictated material.

Textbook Users

Launch your word processing package.

Insert the appropriate audiocassette in your transcribing machine and find dictation *10T-3*.

Step 1: Listen to the entire dictation to gain an understanding of the medical concepts and terms involved. Rewind the tape to the beginning of the dictation and transcribe what you hear. Do not worry about formatting, style, or speed. Simply type what you hear being dictated, using correct punctuation, capitalization, and spelling. Stop as needed to look up words you do not understand or cannot spell. Adjust the speed control of the transcriber to a comfortable level and increase the speed as your accuracy improves.

Step 2: Rewind the tape again and using your created template, transcribe dictation *10T-3* again, including correct spacing and formatting. Proofread the report. Identify and correct all errors. Save your work. Refer to the answer key and manually complete the error analysis and the production for pay charts.

Repeat the same process for dictation *10T-4*.

Software Users

Click on *Chapter 10, Activity 6: Proofreading Transcription Exercise*.

Insert the appropriate audiocassette in your transcribing machine and find dictation *10T-3*.

Step 1: Listen to the entire dictation to gain an understanding of the medical concepts and terms involved. Rewind the tape to the beginning of the dictation, click *Start Watch*, and transcribe what you hear. Do not worry about formatting, style, or speed. Simply type what you hear being dictated, using correct punctuation, capitalization, and spelling. Stop as needed to look up words you do not understand or cannot spell. Adjust the speed control of the transcriber to a comfortable level and increase the speed as your accuracy improves. When you are finished, click on *Done*, then choose *Return to Main Menu*.

Step 2: Click on *Chapter 10, Activity 6* again. Rewind the tapes again, click on *Start Watch*, and transcribe dictation *10T-3* again, including correct spacing and formatting. Proofread the report. Identify and correct all errors. When you are finished, click on *Done*, then *Score Document* to display your production for pay. Click on *Display Error Analysis* to reveal your score and then *View Errors* to see your errors. Save your work (with errors showing) by clicking on *File*, then *Save As*.

Follow the same process for dictation *10T-4*.

Part II / Check Your Progress (10T-2)

Let's pause a minute and see how well you are doing. This section will allow you to evaluate your success at transcribing and proofreading cardiology reports.

Textbook Users

Launch your word processing package.

Insert the appropriate audiocassette in your transcribing machine and find dictation *10T-2.*

On the open screen, transcribe and proofread dictation *10T-2.*

Identify and correct all errors.

Use formatting guidelines established in Chapter 2.

Save your work on your student disk.

After completing the transcription, refer to the answer key.

Manually complete the error analysis chart.

Manually complete the production for pay chart.

If you score below 90%, you are recommended to redo the Part II Activities.

If you score 90% or above, congratulations. You have mastered the material covered in Part II. If you wish, you can immediately move on to Part III.

Software Users

Click on *Chapter 10, Part II, Check Your Progress (10T-2).*

Insert the appropriate audiocassette in your transcribing machine and find dictation *10T-2.*

Click on *Start Watch,* then transcribe and proofread dictation *10T-2.*

Identify and correct all errors.

When you are finished, click on *Done,* then *Score Document:* a pop-up window will display your production for pay.

Click on *Display Error Analysis* to reveal your score.

Click on *View Errors* to see the errors you made.

Save your work (with errors showing) on your student disk by clicking on *File,* then *Save As.*

If you score below 90%, you are recommended to redo the Part II Activities.

If you score 90% or above, congratulations on your mastery of the material covered in Part II. If you wish, you can immediately move on to Part III.

Pretest *(10T-5, 10T-6)*

Professional transcriptionists can transcribe and proofread their own work. Can you? Scoring 90% or better proves it!

Textbook Users

Launch your word processing package.

Insert the appropriate audiocassette in your transcribing machine and find dictation *10T-5.*

On the open screen, transcribe and proofread dictation *10T-5.*

Identify and correct all errors.

Use formatting guidelines established in Chapter 2.

Save your work on your student disk.

Follow the same process for dictation *10T-6.*

After completing the transcriptions, refer to the answer key.

Manually complete the error analysis chart for each document.

Manually complete the production for pay chart for each document.

If you score below 90%, continue with *Cardiology Transcription at FedDes Wellness Center.*

If you score 90% or above, congratulations. You have mastered the material covered in Part III. If you wish, you can immediately move on to the next chapter.

Software Users

Click on *Chapter 10, Part III, Pretest (10T-5).*

Insert the appropriate audiocassette in your transcribing machine and find dictation *10T-5.*

Click on *Start Watch,* then transcribe and proofread dictation *10T-5.*

Identify and correct all errors.

When you are finished, click on *Done,* then *Score Document* to display your production for pay.

Click on *Display Error Analysis* to reveal your score.

Click on *View Errors* to see the errors you made

Save your work (with errors showing) on your student disk by clicking on *File,* then *Save As.*

Follow the same process for dictation *10T-6.*

If you score below 90%, continue with *Cardiology Transcription at FedDes Wellness Center.*

If you score 90% or above, congratulations. You have mastered the material covered in Part III. If you wish, you can immediately move on to the next chapter.

Cardiology Transcription at FedDes Wellness Center

You finally made it! You have been hired as a transcriptionist at FedDes Wellness Center in the Cardiology Division. Your supervisor has asked you to transcribe today's dictation.

Textbook Users

Launch your word processing package.

Insert the appropriate audiocassette in your transcribing machine and find dictation *10T-7*.

Create or use an existing template for the six types of reports.

On the open screen, transcribe and proofread dictation *10T-7*. Identify and correct all errors.

Save your work on your student disk. Follow the same process for dictations *10T-8* through *10T-12*.

After completing the transcriptions, refer to the answer key.

Manually complete the error analysis and production for pay charts for each document.

Software Users

Click on *Chapter 10, Part III, Cardiology Transcription at FedDes Wellness Center*.

Insert the appropriate audiocassette in your transcribing machine and find dictation *10T-7*.

Click on *Start Watch*, then transcribe and proofread dictation *10T-7*.

Identify and correct all errors.

When you are finished, click on *Done*, then *Score Document* to display your production for pay.

Click on *Display Error Analysis* to reveal your score and *View Errors* to see the errors you made.

Save your work (with errors showing) by clicking on *File*, then *Save As*.

Follow the same process for dictations *10T-8* and *10T-9*.

NOTE: Continue the medical documents *10T-10* through *10T-12* using your word processing package and manually complete the error analysis and production for pay charts.

Index of Dictations and Associated Transcription Tips

Please remember to follow the guidelines pertaining to capitalization, numbers, punctuation, abbreviations, measurements, symbols, and use of templates. Review of this material is found in Unit 1.

10T-7
Consultation Report
Patient's Name: Naomi Isiaba
Requesting Physician: Izzy Sertoli, MD
Physician: Adam Valence, MD

● **TRANSCRIPTION TIPS**
• A hyphen is used between numbers and *year old*.

You will hear the dictator say: Naomi Isiaba is a 19 year old Asian female.
You should transcribe as: Naomi Isiaba is a 19-year-old Asian female.

• The following abbreviation is dictated in this report:
DVT: deep vein thrombsis

• The following test is dictated in this report:
Doppler study: an ultrasound flowmeter that is used in assessing intermittent claudiation, thrombus obstruction of deep veins, and several other abnormalities of blood flow in the major arteries and veins

10T-8
History and Physical Examination
Patient's Name: Samuel Whitehead
Physician: Adam Valence, MD

● **TRANSCRIPTION TIPS**

- Capitalize the name of specific departments or sections in a hospital or institution.
  You will hear the dictator say: He presented to the university hospital emergency room
  You should transcribe as: He presented to the University Hospital Emergency Room

- The following abbreviations are dictated in this report:
  ECG: electrocardiogram
  WBC: white blood count

- Figures are used for age, weight, height, blood pressure, pulse, and respiration. The diagonal (/) is used to indicate the word *over* in blood pressure.
  You will hear the dictator say: B P one hundred over sixty
  You should transcribe as: BP 100/60

- Capital letters are used for electrocardiographic leads, waves, and segments. Chest leads are indicated with a *V* for the central terminal, an Arabic number for the chest electrode, and a letter for right or left arm or foot. The leads are *V1* through *V6* and *aVL, aVR,* and *aVF.* Waves include P, Q, R, S, T, and U and their combinations.
  You will hear the dictator say: peaked tees laterally
  You should transcribe as: peaked Ts laterally

- Roman numerals are used for standard leads and intercostal space positions.
  You will hear the dictator say: There is reciprocal depression in leads one and two
  You should transcribe as: There is reciprocal depression in leads I and II

- A period is used to replace the word *point.*
  You will hear the dictator say: WBC twenty point two hemoglobin fifteen point two

You should transcribe as: WBC 20.2, hemoglobin 15.2

- The following laboratory test is dictated in this report:
  GUSTO trial: Global utilization of streptokinase and tissue plasminogen activator for occluded coronary arteries

- Words beginning with *non, re, pre,* and *post* are not hyphenated.
  For example: nontender

10T-9
History and Physical Examination
Patient's Name: Clifford Gallette
Physician: A. B. Doner, MD

● **TRANSCRIPTION TIPS**

- The following drugs are dictated in this report:
  Lotensin: trade name for an antihypertensive
  Terramycin: trade name for an antibiotic
  Beta blocker: a generic name for a drug that blocks the action of epinephrine at beta-adrenergic receptors on the cells of effector organs. Beta blockers are used to treat angina pectoralis, hypertension, and cardia arrhythmias.
  Aspirin: generic name for an analgesic, antipyretic, anti-inflammatory; antirheumatic
  Heparin: generic name for an anticoagulant

- Capital letters are used for electrocardiographic leads, waves and segments. Chest leads are indicated with a *V* for the central terminal, an Arabic number for the chest electrode, and a letter for the right or left arm or foot. The electrocardiographical leads are *V1* through *V6* and *aVL, aVR,* and *aVF.* Waves include P, Q, R, S, T, and U and their combinations.
  You will hear the dictator say: There is one millimeter of s t segment depression in leads two three and a v f
  You should transcribe as: There is 1 mm of ST segment depression in leads II, III, and aVF

- The diagonal (/) is used to indicate the word *per* in laboratory values and respirations or the word *over* in blood pressure.
  You will hear the dictator say: his blood pressure is one hundred forty four over eighty eight with a pulse of eighty respiratory rate is sixteen per minute.
  You should transcribe as: His blood pressure is 144/88 with a pulse of 80. Respiratory rate is 16/min.

- Words beginning with *non, re, pre,* or *post* are not hyphenated.
  For example: nonsmoker, nondrinker, noncontributory

10T10

History and Physical Examination
Patient's Name: Lorraine Sosa
Physician: Erica Purkinje, MD

● **TRANSCRIPTION TIPS**
- The following abbreviations are dictated in this report:
  ICU: intensive care unit
  MI: myocardial infarction
  COPD: chronic obstructive pulmonary disease

- A hyphen is used to join two or more words when used as an adjective that proceeds a noun.
  The following word pairs are dictated in this report: two-month, two-pack-a-day.

- Quotation marks are used to indicate a direct quote.
  You will hear the dictator say: She describes as an ache in her left upper chest.
  You should transcribe this sentence as follows: She describes as "an ache in her left upper chest."

- The following drugs are dictated in this report:
  Vasotec: trade name for an angiotensin-converting enzyme inhibitor
  Diltiazem: generic name for a coronary vasodilator
  Pepcid: trade name for an acid controller for heartburn and acid indigestion
  Lasix: trade name for a diuretic

- The degree (°) sign is not used in describing temperature if the word *degree* is not dictated or not represented on the keyboard.
  You will hear the dictator say: There is no visible neck vein distension at forty five degrees.
  You should transcribe as: There are no visible neck vein distension at 45 degrees.

- Figures and capital letters are used with electrocardiographic waves.
  You will hear the dictator say: heart reveals a regular rhythm with an s four
  You should transcribe as: heart reveals a regular rhythm with an S4

- Figures are used with the + or − symbols.
  You will hear the dictator say: She has four plus pitting edema of her lower extremities.
  You should transcribe as: She has 4+ pitting edema of her lower extremities.

- Words beginning with *non, re, pre,* or *post* are not hyphenated.
  For example: nontender

10T-11

History and Physical Examination
Patient's Name: Michael Fellows
Physician: Lucas Site, MD

● **TRANSCRIPTION TIPS**
- The following drugs are dictated in this report:
  vitamin E: vitamin E supplement; topical emollient
  vitamin C: ascorbic acid, anticorbutic, urinary acidifier
  Trental: trade name for an oral hemorheologic drug
  beta carotene: ultraviolet screen; vitamin A precursor
  Centrum Silver: trade name for a geriatric vitamin and mineral supplement
  Zyloprim: trade name for a xanthine oxidase inhibitor
  heparin: generic name for an anticoagulant

Coumadin: trade name for an anticoagulant

- Plurals of numbers are formed by adding the letter *s*.
  You will hear the dictator say: His heart rate is in the seventies and regular.
  You should transcribe as: His heart rate is in the 70s and regular.

- The following abbreviation is dictated in this report:
  PERRL: pupils equal, round, reactive to light and accommodation

- Words beginning with *non, re, pre,* and *post* are not hyphenated: nonfocal.

 10T-12
Consultation Letter
Patient's Name: Marie Monyet
Requesting Physician: J. Thomas Geiger, MD
Physician: Erica Purkinje, MD

● **TRANSCRIPTION TIPS**
- The following abbreviations are dictated in this report:
  MRI: magnetic resonance imaging
  ECG: electrocardiogram

- The percent sign (%) is used with words and figures.
  You will hear the dictator say: a recent m r I angiogram showing a fifty percent right internal carotid artery stenosis
  You should transcribe as: recent MRI angiogram showing a 50% right internal carotid artery stenosis

- Capital letters are used for electrocardiographic leads, waves, and segments. Waves include P, Q, R, S, T, and U and their combinations.
  You will hear the dictator say: abnormal electrocardiogram with anterior t wave abnormalities and a q wave in lead three.
  You should transcribe as: abnormal electrocardiogram with anterior T-wave abnormalities and a Q-wave in lead III.

- The following diagnostic tests are dictated in this report:
  dobutamine stress test: a generic name for a synthetic catecholamine administered parenterally for inotropic support in short-term treatment of adults with cardiac decompensation
  liver function test: a series of laboratory procedures that measure some aspect of liver functions, including serum protein electrophoresis and one-stage prothrombin time

- A hyphen is used between two "like" vowels: anti-inflammatories.

- The following drugs are dictated in this report:
  Tenormin: trade name for a beta-blocker
  Indocin: trade name for nonsteroidal anti-inflammatory drug
  Cytotec: trade name for the prevention of nonsteroidal anti-inflammatory drug induced gastric ulcers

- Words beginning with *non, re, pre,* or *post* are not hyphenated: nonocclusive, nonsteroidal.

Part III / Check Your Progress
(10T-5, 10T-6)

Professional transcriptionists can transcribe and proofread their own work with speed and accuracy. Have you mastered the cardiology transcription rotation at FedDes Wellness Center?

Textbook Users

Launch your word processing package.

Insert the appropriate audiocassette in your transcribing machine and find dictation *10T-5*.

On the open screen, transcribe and proofread dictation *10T-5*.

Identify and correct all errors.

Use formatting guidelines established in Chapter 2.

Save your work on your student disk.

Follow the same process for dictation *10T-6*.

After completing the transcriptions, refer to the answer key.

Manually complete the error analysis chart for each document.

Manually complete the production for pay chart for each document.

If you score below 90%, you are recommended to repeat Part III.

If you score 90% or above, congratulations. You have mastered the material covered in this chapter.

Software Users

Click on *Chapter 10, Part III, Check Your Progress (10T-5)*.

Insert the appropriate audiocassette in your transcribing machine and find dictation *10T-5*.

Click on *Start Watch*, then transcribe and proofread dictation *10T-5*.

Identify and correct all errors.

When you are finished, click on *Done*, then *Score Document:* a pop-up window will display your production for pay.

Click on *Display Error Analysis* to reveal your score.

Click on *View Errors* to see the errors you made

Save your work (with errors showing) on your student disk by clicking on *File*, then *Save As*.

Follow the same process for dictation *10T-6*.

If you score below 90%, you are recommended to repeat Part III.

If you score 90% or above, congratulations. You have mastered the material covered in this chapter.

Chapter 11

Office Medical Transcription from the Diagnostic Imaging Practice

OBJECTIVES

At the completion of Chapter 11, you should be able to do the following:

1. Match medical terms associated with the diagnostic imaging specialty with their definitions.

2. Spell medical terms associated with the diagnostic imaging specialty with their definitions.

3. Transcribe medical terms in sentence structure.

4. Proofread, edit, and correct medical documents associated with the diagnostic imaging specialty containing various errors.

5. Transcribe and proofread authentic medical documents associated with the diagnostic imaging specialty.

What's Ahead

The Diagnostic Imaging Rotation

The FedDes Wellness Center has four radiologists, or specialists in diagnostic radiology, on staff. Diagnostic radiology is the field of medicine concerned with the use of roentgen rays and other forms of energy in the diagnosis and treatment of diseases. The diagnostic radiologist uses a variety of techniques, including x-rays, computed tomography, magnetic resonance imaging, ultrasound, and nuclear medicine, to evaluate the anatomy of interest. Patients are often referred to a hospital or diagnostic imaging center for their medical imaging study. A contracted or staff radiologist associated with the facility interprets the images and may also perform the exam with the assistance of a registered radiologic technologist.

The physicians in FedDes diagnostic and imaging division perform and interpret sophisticated imaging such as MRI, CT scans, ultrasounds, PET (position emission tomography) scans, DSA (digital subtraction angiography) scans, and nuclear medicine studies. Transcribed reports may be sent back to the referring physician in a letter format or in a more informal x-ray report format. Radiologists often dictate in the present tense because they are interpreting the findings as they view the films. As a general rule, the history is past tense and the findings are present tense.

In this unit, you assume the role of a medical transcriptionist employed at the Diagnostic Imaging Division of the FedDes Wellness Center. **Please remember to follow the guidelines pertaining to capitalization, numbers, punctuation, abbreviations, measurements, symbols, and use of templates to create medical reports at FedDes Wellness Center. Review of this material can be found in Unit 1.** A list of the patient's name and the type of report as well as associated transcription tips are included in this chapter.

You will work with the textbook, CD-ROM, and accompanying audiocassettes. Your mastery of diagnostic imaging transcription is assessed through worksheets, timed transcription exercises, the error analysis chart, and the Production for Pay summary.

All the answer keys are found in the textbook and CD-ROM, providing immediate feedback. After transcribing a report, you will proofread your work and correct any errors. Then you will compare your proofread work against a master transcript, categorize all errors, and tabulate the errors on the error analysis chart. The Production for Pay summary correlates your production to the FedDes Wellness Center pay scale, which is based on industry compensation standards. The scale is also linked to your grade. This system allows you to assess your mastery of transcription skills in a real-world scenario.

Pretest

Let's find out if you can define and spell selected terminology and drugs of the diagnostic imaging specialty that are included in this chapter by scoring 90% or better.

Textbook Users

Select the correctly spelled term that matches its definition.

Refer to the answer key for immediate feedback.

If you score below 90%, continue on to *Activities 1–3*.

If you score 90% or above, congratulations on your mastery of the material covered in Part I. If you wish, you can immediately move on to Part II.

Software Users

Click on *Chapter 11, Part I, Pretest*.

Select the correctly spelled term that matches its definition.

When you are finished, click on *End Test*.

A pop-up screen will reveal your score.

If you score below 90%, continue on to *Activities 1–3*.

If you score 90% or above, congratulations on your mastery of the material covered in Part I. If you wish, you can immediately move on to Part II.

PART I / PRETEST

Directions: Select the correctly spelled term that matches its definition.

1. Set limits or boundaries:
   (a) demarcated
   (b) structure
   (c) demacated
   (d) stricture

2. Stone:
   (a) calulus
   (b) calculus
   (c) amorphous
   (d) amorphus

3. Pertaining to the cricoid cartilage and the pharynx:
   (a) cricoidpharyngeal
   (b) Pasavant's cusion
   (c) cricopharyngeal
   (d) Passavant's cushion

4. A ridge appearing on the posterior wall of the pharynx during swallowing due to contraction of the palatopharyngeal sphincter:
   (a) cricoidpharyngeal
   (b) Pasavant's cusion
   (c) cricopharyngeal
   (d) Passavant's cushion

5. Herniation of an abdominal organ through the esophageal opening of the diaphragm:
   (a) haitus hernai
   (b) hiatus hernia
   (c) hydronephrosis
   (d) hydronphrosis

6. Backward flow:
   (a) reflux
   (b) refluxe
   (c) reflex
   (d) reflax

7. Articulation between the acromial process of the scapula and the clavicle:
   (a) perarticular
   (b) acromiocalvicular
   (c) acromioclavicular
   (d) periarticular

8. Abnormal forward tilting of an organ:
   (a) antiverted
   (b) adnixa
   (c) anteverted
   (d) adnexa

9. Abnormal narrowing of a duct or passage:
   (a) demarcated
   (b) structure
   (c) demacated
   (d) stricture

10. Fluid around the gallbladder:
    (a) periocholecystic
    (b) periartecular
    (c) periarticular
    (d) pariochelecystic

11. Lacking similar form or relationship of parts:
    (a) asymmetry
    (b) asites
    (c) ascites
    (d) asymetry

12. The escape and accumulation of serous fluid in the abdominal cavity:
    (a) asymmetry
    (b) asites
    (c) ascites
    (d) asymetry

PART I / PRETEST *continued*

13. Partial dislocation:
    (a) infarction
    (b) infaction
    (c) sublixation
    (d) subluxation

14. Pharmaceutical given to the patient to allow radiographic visualization of a body structure:
    (a) centrum semiovale
    (b) contrast medium
    (c) contast medium
    (d) centram semvale

15. The functional elements of an organ as distinguished from its structure:
    (a) parenchyma
    (b) pareshyma
    (c) paresthesia
    (d) parenchyesia

16. Behind the peritoneum:
    (a) criopharyngeal
    (b) crioperitoneal
    (c) retroperitoneal
    (d) retraperitoneal

17. Joint spaces between the carpal and metacarpal bones:
    (a) carpametacarpal
    (b) carpocarpal
    (c) carpometacarpal
    (d) carpacarpeal

18. Situated around a joint:
    (a) periocholecystic
    (b) periartecular
    (c) periarticular
    (d) pariochelecystic

19. A decrease in bone mass below the norm:
    (a) ischemic
    (b) osteopenia
    (c) iscemia
    (d) ostepenic

20. Disease of the lymph nodes:
    (a) lymphadenopathy
    (b) lymphadepathy
    (c) etiology
    (d) etoilogy

21. A device that translates one form of energy to another:
    (a) transducer
    (b) lacsnar
    (c) lacunar
    (d) transducar

22. Within the liver:
    (a) intrehepatic
    (b) ischemic
    (c) intrahepatic
    (d) ischamic

23. Distention of the renal pelvis and calices with urine:
    (a) calculus
    (b) calulus
    (c) hydronephrosis
    (d) hydrophrosis

24. Second section of the small intestine:
    (a) jejunum
    (b) jejum
    (c) joint mouse
    (d) jont mose

25. The causes or origin of a disease or disorder:
    (a) lymphadenopathy
    (b) lymphadepathy
    (c) etiology
    (d) etoilogy

26. Having no definite form:
    (a) asymmetry
    (b) amorphous
    (c) asymetry
    (d) amorphus

PART I / PRETEST *continued*

27. A factor that makes it undesirable to treat a patient in the usual manner:
    (a) contraindicate
    (b) contradicate
    (c) contradiction
    (d) contrandicate

28. Both sides:
    (a) bileteral
    (b) vertex
    (c) bilateral
    (d) vertix

29. A small cavity within or between other body structures:
    (a) transducer
    (b) lacsna
    (c) lacuna
    (d) transducar

30. Lack of blood in a body part:
    (a) intrehepatic
    (b) ischemic
    (c) intrahepatic
    (d) ischamic

31. Loose bodies in synovial joints:
    (a) jejunum joint
    (b) jejum jonte
    (c) joint mouse
    (d) jonte mose

32. The top or crown of the head:
    (a) centrum semiovale
    (b) vertex
    (c) vertix
    (d) centrum semivale

33. Formation of a blood clot:
    (a) thrombosis
    (b) thrombasis
    (c) hydronephrosis
    (d) hydronphrosis

34. The white matter of the cerebral hemispheres that has an almost oval shape:
    (a) centrum semiovale
    (b) vertex
    (c) vertix
    (d) centrum semivale

35. The death of a tissue due to lack of blood flow to the area:
    (a) sublaxation
    (b) infartion
    (c) subluxation
    (d) infarction

36. Sensation of tingling and numbness:
    (a) osteopania
    (b) osteopenia
    (c) paresthesia
    (d) peresthesia

37. Trade name for a drug used in restoring hormonal imbalance:
    (a) Provera
    (b) Synthroid
    (c) Synthoid
    (d) Provira

38. Trade name for a drug used as a replacement in decreased or absent thyroid function:
    (a) Provera
    (b) Synthroid
    (c) Synthoid
    (d) Provira

39. Trade name for a drug that decreases LDL cholesterol:
    (a) Isovue
    (b) Isovae
    (c) Liscol
    (d) Lescol

40. Trade name for a drug used as a contrast medium:
    (a) Isovue
    (b) Isovae
    (c) Liscol
    (d) Lescol

Part I / Activity 1
Keyboarding Medical Terms and Definitions

Let's learn to spell and define selected terminology and drugs of the diagnostic imaging specialty that are included in this chapter. Keyboarding these terms is an innovative and fun way to improve your skills.

Textbook Users
Launch your word processing package.
On the open screen, read and type each word and its definition. Save your work on your student disk.

1. Acromioclavicular (ah-kro-me-o-klah-vik-u-lar) describes the articulation between the acromial process of the scapula and the clavicle.
2. Amorphous (ah-mor-fus) is having no definite form, or shapeless.
3. Anteverted (an-te-vert-ed) is the abnormal forward tilting of an organ.
4. Ascites (ah-si-teez) is the effusion and the accumulation of serous fluid within the abdominal cavity.
5. Asymmetry (a-sim-e-tre) is without symmetry, lacking similar form or relationship of parts.
6. Bilateral (bi-lat-er-al) is affecting both sides.
7. Calculus (kal-ku-lus) is a stone.
8. Carpometacarpal (kar-po-met-ah-kar-pal) is the joint spaces between the carpal and metacarpal bones.
9. Centrum semiovale (sen-trum sem-i-o-val) is the white matter of the cerebral hemispheres that has an almost oval shape.
10. Contraindicate (kon-trah-in-di-kate) is a factor that makes it undesirable to treat a patient in the usual manner.
11. Contrast medium (kon-trast med-e-um) is the pharmaceutical given to the patient to allow radiographic visualization of a body structure.
12. Cricopharyngeal (kri-ko-fah-rin-je-al) is pertaining to the cricoid cartilage and the pharynx.
13. Demarcated (de-mar-ka-ted) is set limits or boundaries.
14. Etiology (e-te-ol-oj-e) is the science concerned with the causes or origin of a disease or disorder.
15. Hiatus hernia (hi-a-tus her-ne-ah) is the herniation of an abdominal organ through the esophageal opening of the diaphragm.
16. Hydronephrosis (hi-dro-ne-fro-sis) is the distention of the renal pelvis and calices with urine, often as a result of an obstructed ureter.

17. Infarction (in-farkt-shun) is the death of a tissue due to lack of blood flow to the area.
18. Intrahepatic (in-trah-he-pat-ik) is within the liver.
19. Ischemic (is-ke-mek) is the lack of blood in a body part.
20. Jejunum (je-joo-num) is the second section of the small intestine.
21. Joint mouse (joint mows) is the loose bodies in synovial joints.
22. Lacuna (lah-ku-nah) is the small cavity within or between other body structures.
23. Lymphadenopathy (lim-fad-e-nop-ah-the) is the disease of the lymph nodes.
24. Osteopenia (os-te-o-pe-ne-ah) is the decrease in bone mass below the normal.
25. Parenchyma (pah-reng-ki-mah) is the general anatomical term to describe the functional elements of an organ, as distinguished from its structure.
26. Paresthesia (par-es-the-ze-ah) is the sensation of tingling and numbness.
27. Passavant's cushion (pas-a-vants koosh-un) is a ridge appearing on posterior wall of pharynx during swallowing due to contraction of palatopharyngeal sphincter.
28. Periarticular (per-e-ar-tici-u-lar) is situated around a joint.
29. Pericholecystic fluid (per-I-ko-le-sis-tic) is a coined term, meaning fluid around the gallbladder.
30. Reflux (re-fluks) is a backward flow.
31. Retroperitoneal (ret-ro-per-i-to-ne-al) is behind the peritoneum.
32. Stricture (strik-chor) is an abnormal narrowing of a duct or passage.
33. Subluxation (sub-luk-sa-shun) is a partial dislocation.
34. Thrombosis (throm-bo-sis) is a formation of a blood clot.
35. Transducer (trans-doo-ser) is a device that translates one form of energy to another; in sonography it transforms a sound wave into electronically displayed image.
36. Vertex (ver-teks) is the top or crown of the head.
37. Isovue (is-o-vu) is the trade name for a drug used as a contrast medium.
38. Lescol (les-kol) is the trade name for a drug that decreases LDL cholesterol.
39. Provera (pro-ver-ah) is the trade name for a drug used in restoring hormonal imbalance.
40. Synthroid (sin-troid) is the trade name for a drug used as a replacement in decreased or absent thyroid function.

Part I / Activity 2
Spelling Medical Terms

Do you remember back in school when you had to write each spelling word ten times? Because you had to physically write each word, your mind and body were focused on the assignment and the method worked! Let's follow this successful method by reinforcing the spelling of selected terms and drugs found in the diagnostic imaging specialty through keyboarding drills.

Textbook Users
Launch your word processing package.
On the open screen, read, mentally spell, and type each word in its sequence.
Save your work on your student disk.

1. acromioclavicular adnexa amorphous acromioclavicular adnexa amorphous acromioclavicular

2. anteverted ascites asymmetry anteverted ascites asymmetry anteverted ascites asymmetry

3. bilateral calculus carpometacarpal bilateral calculus carpometacarpal bilateral calculus

4. centrum semiovale contrast medium centrum semiovale contrast medium centrum semiovale

5. contraindicate cricopharyngeal demarcated contraindicate cricopharyngeal demarcated

6. etiology hiatus hernia hydronephrosis etiology hiatus hernia hydronephrosis etiology

7. infarction intrahepatic ischemic infarction intrahepatic ischemic infarction intrahepatic

8. jejunum joint mouse lacuna jejunum joint mouse lacuna jejunum joint mouse lacuna

9. lymphadenopathy parenchyma paresthesia lymphadenopathy parenchyma paresthesia

10. Passavant's cushion periarticular reflux Passavant's cushion periarticular reflux periarticular

11. pericholecystic fluid osteopenia pericholecystic fluid osteopenia pericholecystic fluid

12. retroperitoneal stricture subluxation retroperitoneal stricture subluxation retroperitoneal

13. thrombosis transducer vertex thrombosis transducer vertex thrombosis transducer vertex

14. Isovae Lescol Provera Synthroid Isovae Lescol Provera Synthroid Isovue Lescol Provera

Part I / Activity 3
Transcribing Medical Sentences *(11T-1)*

Now you are ready to make the transition from keyboarding medical terms, which is a visual process, to transcribing medical terms, an aural process. You are going to use audiocassette tapes rather than printed material.

Textbook Users
Launch your word processing software.
Insert the audiocassette in your transcribing machine and find dictation *11T-1.*
You will be transcribing spelling words in sentence structure.
Listen carefully to each sentence on the audiocassette before transcribing.
Rewind and type (transcribe) the sentences.
Save your work on your student disk.
Refer to the answer key.

Part I / Check Your Progress

Let's pause a minute and see how well you are doing. This section will allow you to evaluate your mastery of keyboarding and spelling selected terms and drugs found in the diagnostic imaging specialty.

Textbook Users
Select the correctly spelled term that matches its definition.
Refer to the answer key for immediate feedback.
If you score below 90%, you are recommended to redo the Part I activities.
If you score 90% or above, congratulations on your mastery of the material covered in Part I. If you
    wish, you can immediately move on to Part II.

Software Users
Click on *Chapter 11, Part I, Check Your Progress.*
Key the correctly spelled term that matches its definition.
When you are finished, click on *End Test.*
A pop-up screen will reveal your score.
If you score below 90%, you are recommended to redo the Part I activities.
If you score 90% or above, congratulations on your mastery of the material covered in Part I. You
    can immediately move on to Part II.

PART I / CHECK YOUR PROGRESS

Directions: Select the correctly spelled term that matches its definition.

1. A decrease in the bone mass below the normal:
   (a) ischemic
   (b) osteopenia
   (c) iscemia
   (d) ostepenic

2. A device that translates one form of energy to another:
   (a) transducer
   (b) lacsna
   (c) lacuna
   (d) transducar

3. A factor that makes it undesirable to treat a patient in the usual manner:
   (a) contraindicate
   (b) contradicate
   (c) contradiction
   (d) contrandicate

4. A small cavity within or between other body structures:
   (a) transducer
   (b) lacsna
   (c) lacuna
   (d) transducar

5. Abnormal narrowing of a duct or passage:
   (a) demarcated
   (b) structure
   (c) demacated
   (d) stricture

6. Both sides:
   (a) bileteral
   (b) vertex
   (c) bilateral
   (d) vertix

7. A ridge appearing on the posterior wall of the pharynx during swallowing due to contraction of the palatopharyngeal sphincter:
   (a) cricoidpharyngeal
   (b) Pasavant's cusion
   (c) cricopharyngeal
   (d) Passavant's cushion

8. Abnormal forward tilting of an organ:
   (a) antiverted
   (b) adnixa
   (c) anteverted
   (d) adnexa

9. Articulation between the acromial process of the scapula and the clavicle:
   (a) perarticular
   (b) acromiocalvicular
   (c) acromioclavicular
   (d) periarticular

10. Backward flow:
    (a) reflux
    (b) refluxe
    (c) reflex
    (d) reflax

11. Behind the peritoneum:
    (a) criopharyngeal
    (b) crioperitoneal
    (c) retroperitoneal
    (d) retraperitoneal

12. Disease of the lymph nodes:
    (a) lymphadenopathy
    (b) lymphadepathy
    (c) etiology
    (d) etoilogy

PART I / CHECK YOUR PROGRESS *continued*

13. Distention of the renal pelvis and calices with urine:
    (a) calculus
    (b) calulus
    (c) hydronephrosis
    (d) hydrophrosis

14. Fluid around the gallbladder:
    (a) periocholecystic
    (b) periartecular
    (c) periarticular
    (d) pariochelecystic

15. Formation of a blood clot:
    (a) thrombosis
    (b) thrombasis
    (c) hydronephrosis
    (d) hydronphrosis

16. Having no definite form:
    (a) asymmetry
    (b) amorphous
    (c) asymetry
    (d) amorphus

17. Herniation of an abdominal organ through the esophageal opening of the diaphragm:
    (a) haitus hernai
    (b) hiatus hernia
    (c) hydronephrosis
    (d) hydronphrosis

18. Joint spaces between the carpal and metacarpal bones:
    (a) carpametacarpal
    (b) carpocarpal
    (c) carpometacarpal
    (d) carpacarpeal

19. Lack of blood in a body part:
    (a) intrehepatic
    (b) ischemic
    (c) intrahepatic
    (d) ischamic

20. Lacking similar form or relationship of parts:
    (a) asymmetry
    (b) asites
    (c) ascites
    (d) asymetry

21. Loose bodies in synovial joints:
    (a) jejunum joint
    (b) jejum jonte
    (c) joint mouse
    (d) jonte mose

22. Partial dislocation:
    (a) infarction
    (b) infaction
    (c) sublixation
    (d) subluxation

23. Pertaining to the cricoid cartilage and the pharynx:
    (a) cricoidpharyngeal
    (b) Pasavant's cusion
    (c) cricopharyngeal
    (d) Passavant's cushion

24. Pharmaceutical given to the patient to allow radiographic visualization of a body structure:
    (a) centrum semiovale
    (b) contrast medium
    (c) contast medium
    (d) centram semvale

25. Second section of the small intestine:
    (a) jejunum
    (b) jejum
    (c) joint mouse
    (d) jont mose

26. Sensation of tingling and numbness:
    (a) osteopania
    (b) osteopenia
    (c) paresthesia
    (d) peresthesia

PART I / CHECK YOUR PROGRESS *continued*

27. Set limits or boundaries:
    (a) demarcated
    (b) structure
    (c) demacated
    (d) stricture

28. Situated around a joint:
    (a) periocholecystic
    (b) periartecular
    (c) periarticular
    (d) pariochelecystic

29. Stone:
    (a) calulus
    (b) calculus
    (c) amorphous
    (d) amorphus

30. The causes or origin of a disease or disorder:
    (a) lymphadenopathy
    (b) lymphadepathy
    (c) etiology
    (d) etoilogy

31. The death of a tissue due to lack of blood flow to the area:
    (a) sublaxation
    (b) infartion
    (c) subluxation
    (d) infarction

32. The escape and accumulation of serous fluid in the abdominal cavity:
    (a) asymmetry
    (b) asites
    (c) ascites
    (d) asymetry

33. The functional elements of an organ as distinguished from its structure:
    (a) parenchyma
    (b) pareshyma
    (c) paresthesia
    (d) parenchyesia

34. The top or crown of the head:
    (a) centrum semiovale
    (b) vertex
    (c) vertix
    (d) centrum semivale

35. The white matter of the cerebral hemispheres that has an almost oval shape:
    (a) centrum semiovale
    (b) vertex
    (c) vertix
    (d) centrum semivale

36. Within the liver:
    (a) intrehepatic
    (b) ischemic
    (c) intrahepatic
    (d) ischamic

37. Trade name for a drug that decreases LDL cholesterol:
    (a) Isovue
    (b) Isovae
    (c) Liscol
    (d) Lescol

38. Trade name for a drug used as a contrast medium:
    (a) Isovue
    (b) Isovae
    (c) Liscol
    (d) Lescol

PART I / CHECK YOUR PROGRESS *continued*

39. Trade name for a drug used as a replacement in decreased or absent thyroid function:
    (a) Provera
    (b) Synthroid
    (c) Synthoid
    (d) Provira

40. Trade name for a drug used in restoring hormonal imbalance:
    (a) Provera
    (b) Synthroid
    (c) Synthoid
    (d) Provira

PART II ▪ PROOFREADING AND ERROR ANALYSIS

Pretest *(11T-2)*

Professional transcriptionists proofread their own work. Can you? Scoring 90% or better proves it!

Textbook Users
Launch your word processing package.
Insert the appropriate audiocassette in your transcribing machine and find dictation *11T-2*.
On the open screen, transcribe and proofread dictation *11T-2*. Identify and correct all errors.
Save your work on your student disk.
After completing the transcription, refer to the answer key.
Manually complete the error analysis and production for pay charts.
If you score below 90%, continue with *Activities 4–7*.
If you score 90% or above, congratulations on your mastery of Part II. If you wish, you can immediately move on to Part III.

Software Users
Click on *Chapter 11, Part II, Pretest (11T-2)*.
Insert the appropriate audiocassette tape in your transcribing machine and find dictation *11T-2*.
Click on *Start Watch*, then transcribe and proofread dictation *11T-2*.
Identify and correct all errors.
When you are finished, click on *Done*, then *Score Document* to display your production for pay.
Click on *Display Error Analysis* to reveal your score and *View Errors* to see your errors.
Save your work (with errors showing) by clicking on *File*, then *Save As*.
If you score below 90%, continue with *Activities 4–7*.
If you score 90% or above, congratulations on your mastery of Part II. If you wish, you can immediately move on to Part III.

Part II / Activities 4–5
Proofreading Worksheet Exercises

Finding your own errors and correcting them is not easy, but it is an essential skill for your success as a medical transcriptionist. The worksheets in this activity will help you to develop your proofreading skills.

Textbook Users

Proofread and correct errors in the medical documents shown in *Activities 4–5.*
After completing the activities, refer to the answer key.
Manually complete the error analysis chart for each document.

Software Users

Click on *Chapter 11, Part II, Activity 4.*
Proofread and correct errors found in the medical document.
Click on *File,* then *Done* and a pop-up window will appear.
Click on *Score Document* to reveal your score.
Click on *View Errors* to see the errors you made.
Save your work (with errors showing) on your student disk by clicking on *File,* then *Save As.*
Click on *File,* then *Exit,* to proceed.
Follow the same process to complete *Activity 5.*

PART II / ACTIVITY 4
PROOFREADING WORKSHEET EXERCISE

Directions: Proofread this medical document that contains multiple errors using full block, open punctuation, and all other formatting guidelines established in this textbook.

FedDes Wellness Center
Diagnostic Imaging Division, Suite 157
101 Wellness Way Drive
New York, NY 10036

current date

P.H. Waters, MD
FedDes Wellness Center
Family Practice Division, Suite 300
101 Wellness Way Drive
New York, NY 10036

RE: Robin Hatherode
       Date of Birth: 12/19/53
       Examination: LEFT WRIST ARITHROGRAM

Dear Dr. Waters

Scout films are unremarkable.

Following appropriate preparation of the skin a 22 gage needle was inserted into the radioavicular joint and 2 cc. of iodinated contast media was injected. Films were then obtained after minimal manipulation of the wrist. A additional group of films was obtained following further manipulation of the wrist. Contrast is present in the distal radioulnar joint indicating a tear of triangular fibrocartilage.

There is no evidence of contrast in the midcarpal joints to suggest the presence of a ligamentus tear. No additional findings of significance are seen.

IMPRESSION: Findings consistent with a tear of the triangular fibrocartilage.

Thank you for referring this patient to us.

Yours Truly,

Hounsfield T. Scanner, MD/xx

PART II / ACTIVITY 5
PROOFREADING WORKSHEET EXERCISE

Directions: Proofread this medical document that contains multiple errors using full block, open punctuation, and all other formatting guidelines established in this textbook.

FedDes Wellness Center
Diagnostic Imaging Division, Suite 157
101 Wellness Way Drive
New York, NY 10036

current date
Ida Gundrum, MD
Railroad Station Health Center
321 Trainmaster Boulevard
Reading, PA 19604

RE: Tonya Guerrero
      Date of Birth: 5/24/81
      Examination: CT ADBOMEN AND PELVIS
Dear Dr. Gundrun

Computerized tomography was performed from the diafragm to the symphysis pubus with the use of oral and intravenous contast medium.

The liver and spleen are normal. I see no visible gallstones or pericholecystic fluid. There is no pancreatic mast or calcifications. The kidneys are both functional and inobstructed. There is no retropertoneal lymphadenpathy or pelvic lymphadenpathy. The uterus is mid line. There is some slight fullness in the right adnuxa. An ultrasound was performed on June 9 20xx that showed no adnuxal pathology. Asymetry is therefore probably due to the supine position of unopacified bowl over the adnexa. No other pelvic abnormality is seen.

IMPRESSION: Negative exam.

Thank you for refering this patient to us.

Yours Truly,

Hounsfield T. Scanner, MD/xx

Part II / Activities 6–7
Proofreading Transcription Exercises *(11T-3, 11T-4)*

Now you are ready to make the transition from simply proofreading printed material to both transcribing and proofreading dictated material. This is the time to concentrate on building your medical vocabulary, which ultimately, will improve your speed and accuracy.

Textbook Users

Launch your word processing package.

Insert the appropriate audiocassette in your transcribing machine and find dictation *11T-3*.

Step 1: Listen to the entire dictation to gain an understanding of the medical concepts and terms involved. Rewind the tape to the beginning of the dictation and transcribe what you hear. Do not worry about formatting, style, or speed. Simply type what you hear, using correct punctuation, capitalization, and spelling. Stop as needed to look up words you do not understand or cannot spell. Adjust the speed control of the transcriber to a comfortable level and increase the speed as your accuracy improves.

Step 2: Rewind the tape again and using your created template, transcribe dictation *11T-3*. Proofread the report and correct all errors. Save your work. Refer to the answer key and manually complete the error analysis and the production for pay charts.

Repeat the same process for dictation *11T-4*.

Software Users

Click on *Chapter 11, Activity 6, Proofreading Transcription Exercise.*

Insert the appropriate audiocassette in your transcribing machine and find dictation *11T-3*.

Step 1: Listen to the entire dictation to gain an understanding of the medical concepts and terms involved. Rewind the tape to the beginning of the dictation, click *Start Watch*, and transcribe what you hear. Do not worry about formatting, style, or speed. Simply type what you hear, using correct punctuation, capitalization, and spelling. Stop as needed to look up words you do not understand or cannot spell. Adjust the speed control of the transcriber to a comfortable level and increase the speed as your accuracy improves. When you are finished, click on *Done*, then choose *Return to Main Menu.*

Step 2: Click on *Chapter 11, Activity 6* again. Rewind the tapes again, click on *Start Watch*, and transcribe *11T-3*. Proofread the report and correct all errors. When you are finished, click on *Done*, then *Score Document* to display your production for pay. Click on *Display Error Analysis* to reveal your score and then *View Errors* to see your errors. Save your work (with errors showing) by clicking on *File*, then *Save As.*

Follow the same process for dictation *11T-4*.

Part II / Check Your Progress (11T-2)

Let's pause a minute and see how well you are doing. This section will allow you to evaluate your success at transcribing and proofreading diagnostic imaging reports.

Textbook Users

Launch your word processing package.

Insert the appropriate audiocassette in your transcribing machine and find dictation *11T-2*.

On the open screen, transcribe and proofread dictation *11T-2*.

Identify and correct all errors.

Use formatting guidelines established in Chapter 2.

Save your work on your student disk.

After completing the transcription, refer to the answer key.

Manually complete the error analysis chart.

Manually complete the production for pay chart.

If you score below 90%, you are recommended to redo the Part II Activities.

If you score 90% or above, congratulations. If you wish, you can immediately move on to Part III.

Software Users

Click on *Chapter 11, Part II, Check Your Progress (11T-2)*

Insert the appropriate audiocassette in your transcribing machine and find dictation *11T-2*.

Click on *Start Watch,* then transcribe and proofread dictation *11T-2.*

Identify and correct all errors.

When you are finished, click on *Done,* then *Score Document:* a pop-up window will display your production for pay.

Click on *Display Error Analysis* to reveal your score.

Click on *View Errors* to see the errors you made.

Save your work (with errors showing) on your student disk by clicking on *File,* then *Save As.*

If you score below 90%, you are recommended to redo the Part II Activities.

If you score 90% or above, congratulations. If you wish, you can immediately move on to Part III.

Pretest *(11T-5, 11T-6)*

Professional transcriptionists can transcribe and proofread their own work. Can you? Scoring 90% or better proves it!

Textbook Users

Launch your word processing package.

Insert the appropriate audiocassette in your transcribing machine and find dictation *11T-5.*

On the open screen, transcribe and proofread dictation *11T-5.*

Identify and correct all errors.

Use formatting guidelines established in Chapter 2.

Save your work on your student disk.

Follow the same process dictation *11T-6.*

After completing the transcriptions, refer to the answer key.

Manually complete the error analysis and production for pay charts for each document.

If you score below 90%, continue with *Diagnostic Imaging Transcription at FedDes Wellness Center.*

If you score 90% or above, congratulations. You have mastered the material covered in Part III.

Software Users

Click on *Chapter 11, Part III, Pretest (11T-5).*

Insert the appropriate audiocassette in your transcribing machine and find dictation *11T-5.*

Click on *Start Watch,* then transcribe and proofread dictation *11T-5.*

Identify and correct all errors.

When you are finished, click on *Done,* then *Score Document* to display your production for pay.

Click on *Display Error Analysis* to reveal your score.

Click on *View Errors* to see the errors you made.

Save your work (with errors showing) by clicking on *File,* then *Save As.*

Follow the same process for dictation *11T-6.*

If you score below 90%, continue with *Diagnostic Imaging Transcription at FedDes Wellness Center.*

If you score 90% or above, congratulations. You have mastered the material covered in Part III.

Diagnostic Imaging Transcription at FedDes Wellness Center

You finally made it! You have been hired as a transcriptionist at FedDes Wellness Center in the Diagnostic Imaging Division. Your supervisor has asked you to transcribe today's dictation.

Textbook Users
Launch your word processing package.
Insert the appropriate audiocassette in your transcribing machine and find dictation *11T-7*.
Create or use an existing template for the six types of reports.
Transcribe and proofread dictation *11T-7*. Identify and correct all errors.
Save your work on your student disk.
Follow the same process for dictations *11T-8* through *11T-19*.
After completing the transcriptions, refer to the answer key.
Manually complete the error analysis and production for pay charts for each document.

Software Users
Click on *Chapter 11, Part III, Diagnostic Imaging Transcription at FedDes Wellness Center (11T-7)*.
Insert the appropriate audiocassette in your transcribing machine and find dictation *11T-7*.
Click on *Start Watch*, then transcribe and proofread dictation *11T-7*.
Identify and correct all errors.
Click on *Done*, then *Score Document* to display your production for pay.
Click on *Display Error Analysis* to reveal your score and *View Errors* to see your errors.
Save your work (with errors showing) by clicking on *File*, then *Save As*.
Follow the same process for dictations *11T-8* and *11T-9*.
NOTE: Continue the medical documents *11T-10* through *11T-19* using your word processing package and manually complete the error analysis and production for pay charts.

Index of Dictations and Associated Transcription Tips

Please remember to follow the guidelines pertaining to capitalization, numbers, punctuation, abbreviations, measurements, symbols, and use of templates. Review of this material can be found in Unit 1.

Radiologists often dictate in the present tense because they are interpreting the findings as they view the films. As a general rule, the history is past tense and the findings are present tense.

11T-7
Right Breast Sonogram
Patient's Name: Stephanie D. Vaughn
Referring Physician: David Campella, MD
Physician: William C. Roentgen, MD

● **TRANSCRIPTION TIPS**
- The letter *x* is used to abbreviate the words *by* and *times* when it precedes a number or another abbreviation.
  You hear the dictator say: Eighteen by eight by twenty millimeters
  You should transcribe as: 18 x 8 x 20 mm

- The expression *o'clock* is used to refer to points on a circular surface.
  You hear the dictator say: Twelve o'clock position
  Transcribe as: 12 o'clock position

- The hyphen is used to take the place of the word *to* to identify ranges.

You hear the dictator say: breast projecting six to seven millimeters from the nipple
You should transcribe as: breast projecting 6-7 mm from the nipple

- A hyphen is used when two or more words are viewed as a single word: well-demarcated.

11T-8
IVP
Patient's Name: Helen Mac Bride
Referring Physician: J. Thomas Geiger
Physician: William C. Roentgen, MD

● TRANSCRIPTION TIPS
- The plural form of the word calculus is *calculi.*

- Words beginning with *pre, re, post,* and *non* are generally not hyphenated.
  For example: nonobstructing, postvoid, prevoid

- The following studies are dictated in this report:
  Postvoid film: a film of the bladder area taken after the patient has emptied the bladder
  Prevoid film: a film of the bladder area taken before the patient has emptied the bladder

- Figures with capital letters are used to refer to the vertebral column and spinal nerves.
  You will hear the dictator say: slight ureteral narrowing is noted at the L three level
  You transcribe as: slight ureteral narrowing is noted at the L3 level

- The following abbreviation is dictated in this report:
  IVP: intravenous pyelogram

11T-9
Video Esophagram and GI Series; Flat Plate of the Abdomen
Patient's Name: Elizabeth Nicholas
Referring Physician: Matthew D. Sponch
Physician: William C. Roentgen, MD

● TRANSCRIPTION TIPS
- The following abbreviation is dictated in this report:
  GI: gastrointestinal

- A hyphen is used to join two or more words when used as an adjective that proceeds a noun. The following word pairs are dictated in this report: stop-frame, pharyngeal-prevertebral.

- The following are new terms: nasopharynx, epiglottis, diverticulum, esophagogastric, mucosal.

- Quotation marks indicate a direct quote. You will hear the dictator say: elderly patient who complains of food getting stuck in her throat when she eats and difficulty swallowing
  You should transcribe as: elderly patient who complains of food "getting stuck in her throat" when she eats and "difficulty swallowing"

11T-10
Bilateral Hands and Wrist
Patient's Name: Terresa Rosario
Referring Physician: J. Thomas Geiger, MD
Physician: Scott E. Film, MD
Copy to Leslie Albert, MD, Orchard Hills Rheumatology Associates

11T-11
Bone Density Scan
Patient's Name: Cathy Evanson
Referring Physician: Matthew D. Sponch, MD
Physician: Scott E. Film, MD

● TRANSCRIPTION TIPS
- Hyphens are used between numbers and *year old.*
  You will hear the dictator say: The patient is a seventy three year old postmenopausal white female.
  You should transcribe as: The patient is a 73-year-old postmenopausal white female.

- Words beginning with *pre, re, post,* and *non* are generally not hyphenated:
  postmenopausal

- A hyphen is used with words beginning with *ex* and *self*.
  For example: self-history

- The following drugs are dictated:
  Synthroid: the trade name for a drug used as a replacement in decreased or absent thyroid function; classification as a thyroid
  Lesco: the trade name for a drug that decreases LDL cholesterol; classification as an antihyperlipoproteinemic

- The percent sign (%) is used with words and figures.
  You will hear the dictator say: a total bone mineral density of ninety nine percent
  You should transcribe as: a total bone mineral density of 99%

- The term *young normals* is dictated. Bone density is measured by several methods to determine bone mass loss. The bone mass loss is expressed as a percentage of the standard deviation, such as 99%.
  You hear the dictator say: Bone mineral density of ninety nine percent compared to young normals which is zero point one three standard deviations below the mean.
  You should transcribe this sentence as: Bone mineral density of 99% compared to young normals which is 0.13 standard deviations below the mean.

- The following standard deviations below the mean are dictated in this report:
  Dictated: one point three two. Transcribed: 1.32.
  Dictated: two point one nine. Transcribed: 2.19.
  Dictated: zero point three nine. Transcribed: 0.39.

- Figures with capital letters are used to refer to the vertebral column and spinal nerves.
  You will hear the dictator say: It is noted that L one and L two were eliminated from analysis.
  You should transcribe this sentence as: It is noted that L1 and L2 were eliminated from analysis.

11T-12
Pelvic Sonogram
Patient's Name: Nancy Spangler
Referring Physician: Ms. Pamela S. Bartholin, MA, RN, CRNP
Physician: Potter T. Bucky, MD

TRANSCRIPTION TIPS
- The following diagnostic test is dictated in this report:
  Real-time ultrasound: a rapid imaging system that produces a video display of organ motion

- The following abbreviation is dictated in this report:
  AP: anterior-posterior

11T-13
Bone Density Scan
Patient's Name: Eileen Bunny
Referring Physician: Charles Davis, MD
Physician: William C. Roentgen, MD

TRANSCRIPTION TIPS
- Words beginning with *pre, re, post,* and *non* are generally not hyphenated: postmenopausal

- A hyphen is used with words beginning with *ex* and *self*: self-history.

- Capitalize words that express the name of a particular people: Caucasian.

- The following drugs are dictated in this report:
  Estrace: the trade name of an estrogen; classification as an antineoplastic
  Provera: the trade name for a drug used in restoring hormonal imbalance; classification as a Progestin, antineoplastic

- The percent sign (%) is used with words and figures.
  You will hear the dictator say: a total bone mineral density of seventy one percent
  You should transcribe as: a total bone mineral density of 71%

- The following standard deviations below the mean are dictated in this report.
  Dictated: two point seven nine. Transcribed: 2.79.

Dictated: three point zero nine. Transcribed: 3.09.

- A hyphen is used to join two or more words when used as an adjective that proceeds a noun. The following word pair is dictated in this report: follow-up.

- A hyphen is used to take the place of the word *to* or *through* to identify ranges.
  You will hear the dictator say: placing the patient on one thousand to fifteen hundred milligrams of calcium and four hundred to eight hundred of vitamin D per day
  You should transcribe as: placing the patient on 1000-1500 mg of calcium and 400-800 of vitamin D per day

11T-14

Abdominal Sonogram (Real-Time Imaging)
Patient's Name: Donald Nathan Helix
Referring Physician: Matthew D. Sponch, MD
Physician: Potter T. Bucky, MD

TRANSCRIPTION TIPS

- A hyphen is used when two or more words are viewed as a single word: real-time.

- A hyphen is used between two "like" vowels: intra-abdominal.

11T-15

Mammography
Patient's Name: Laura Dobbins
Referring Physician: P. H. Waters, MD
Physician: Potter T. Bucky, MD

TRANSCRIPTION TIPS

- For mammography sonograms, the radiologists at FedDes Wellness Center include two paragraphs before closing sentence. These paragraphs should be transcribed in all capitals as shown.
  NOTE: IT SHOULD BE NOTED THAT THERE IS A 10% FALSE-NEGATIVE RATE IN MAMMOGRAPHIC DETECTION OF BREAST CARCINOMA. MANAGEMENT OF A PALPABLE ABNORMALITY SHOULD BE BASED ON CLINICAL GROUNDS.
  A NEGATIVE REPORT SHOULD NOT DELAY BIOPSY IF A CLINICALLY PALPABLE OR SUSPICIOUS MASS IS PRESENT.

- The mammography section at FedDes Wellness Center is accredited by the American College of Radiology. The statement below is included after the "false-negative" disclaimer and before the closing sentence: Our mammography facilities are accredited by the American College of Radiology.

11T-16

Upper GI Series
Patient's Name: Allison McBeal
Referring Physician: Kate Cobalamin, MD
Physician: Hounsfield T. Scanner, MD

TRANSCRIPTION TIPS

- A hyphen is used in the dictation to take the place of the words *to* or *through* to identify ranges.
  You will hear the dictator say: After an interval of approximately twenty to twenty five minutes the stomach emptied in normal fashion.
  You should transcribe this sentence as follows: After an interval of approximately 20-25 minutes, the stomach emptied in normal fashion.

11T-17

Upper GI Series; Flat Plate of the Abdomen
Patient's Name: Timothy Lavage
Referring Physician: Anna Bolism, MD
Physician: Scott E. Film, MD

TRANSCRIPTION TIPS

- The following abbreviation is dictated in this report:
  GI: gastrointestinal

- Ordinal numbers first through ninth are spelled out.
  You will hear the dictator say: The second third and fourth portions of the duodenum

You should transcribe as: The second, third, and fourth portions of the duodenum

11T-18
Barium Enema; KUB
Patient's Name: Barbara Whitefelter
Referring Physician: Gwenn Maltase, MD
Physician: Scott E. Film, MD

● **TRANSCRIPTION TIPS**
- Figures are used to express metric measurements. No period follows metric abbreviations unless the abbreviation ends a sentence.
  You will hear the dictator say: two point three by zero point eight centimeters
  You will transcribe as: 2.3 x 0.8 cm

- Words beginning with *pre, re, post,* and *non* are generally not hyphenated: postevacuation

11T-19
Doppler Study of the Deep Veins of the Right Leg
Patient's Name: Sarah Fleb
Referring Physician: Helen Loop, MD
Physician: Scott E. Film, MD

● **TRANSCRIPTION TIPS**
- The following procedure is dictated in this report:
  Doppler scanning: a technique used in sonography to image and analyze the behavior of a moving substance such as blood flow or a beating heart

- A hyphen is used when two or more words are viewed as a single word.
  For example: real-time, color-flow

Part III / Check Your Progress
(11T-5, 11T-6)

Professional transcriptionists can transcribe and proofread their own work with speed and accuracy. Have you mastered the diagnostic imaging transcription rotation at FedDes Wellness Center?

Textbook Users

Launch your word processing package.

Insert the appropriate audiocassette in your transcribing machine and find dictation *11T-5.*

On the open screen, transcribe and proofread dictation *11T-5.*

Identify and correct all errors.

After completing the transcriptions, refer to the answer key.

Manually complete the error analysis chart for each document.

Manually complete the production for pay chart for each document.

If you score below 90%, you are recommended to repeat Part III.

If you score 90% or above, congratulations. You have mastered the material covered in this chapter.

Software Users

Click on *Chapter 11, Part III, Check Your Progress (11T-5).*

Insert the appropriate audiocassette in your transcribing machine and find dictation *11T-5.*

Click on *Start Watch,* then transcribe and proofread dictation *11T-5.*

Identify and correct all errors.

When you are finished, click on *Done,* then *Score Document* to display your production for pay.

Click on *Display Error Analysis* to reveal your score.

Click on *View Errors* to see the errors you made.

Save your work (with errors showing) on your student disk by clicking on *File,* then *Save As.*

Follow the same process for dictation *11T-6.*

If you score below 90%, you are recommended to repeat Part III.

If you score 90% or above, congratulations. You have mastered the material covered in this chapter.

Error Analysis Chart

The error analysis chart was developed as a tool to categorize and track undetected errors. A transcription error analysis chart for each document will help you and your instructor prescribe a remedy for each error. Observing the occurrence of repeated mistakes through charting will improve your transcription skills.

The chart is divided into two major categories, Medical Language and English Language, as shown in the error analysis chart. The medical language errors are weighted heavier. Because medication and allergy errors and incorrect patient identification adversely affect patient care, medical transcriptionists are heavily penalized if such errors are found during quality assurance audits. Some institutions strip incentive pay no matter when the error is discovered—even if it is discovered weeks later. An error follows you!

ERROR ANALYSIS CHART

NAME _____   DOCUMENT NO. _____

TYPE OF ERROR	ERROR VALUE	NUMBER OF ERRORS	*TOTAL ERROR VALUE
Medical Language			
Add/omit word(s)			
Misspelled word(s)			
Incorrect date(s) or number(s)			
Total Medical Language Errors	3 ×	=	
English Language			
Add/omit word(s)			
Misspelled word(s)			
Grammatical error(s)			
Punctuation error(s)			
Total English Language Errors	1 ×	=	
Total Language Errors			

*To compute total error value, multiply the number of errors by error value (number of errors × error value = total error value).

Production for Pay Summary

In medical transcription, the transcriber's salary is often based on the amount of work produced rather than a regular monthly salary. The character is the preferred method of measuring productivity and has been supported by several national allied health organizations. A character is any letter, number, symbol, or function key necessary for the final appearance and content of a document including the space bar, enter key, underscore, bold, and any character contained within a macro, header, or footer. Typically, the industry calculates five characters as one word.

The Production for Pay Summary demonstrates the way a transcriber's wage is determined for documents transcribed in this textbook. The summary includes the total number of words produced, total production time, and total number of errors to compute the net production pay. A $0.15 per minute per net production word rate is used to compute wages.

PRODUCTION FOR PAY SUMMARY

Document No.	
Total Word Count	
Total Production Time	
Words per Minute (Total Word Count ÷ Total Production Time)	
Total Error Value (Error Analysis Chart)	
Net Production (Words per Minute − Total Error Value)	
Production for Pay ($.15 × Net Production)	

Anatomic Illustrations and Medical Images

Directional terms and planes of the body: Figure C-1

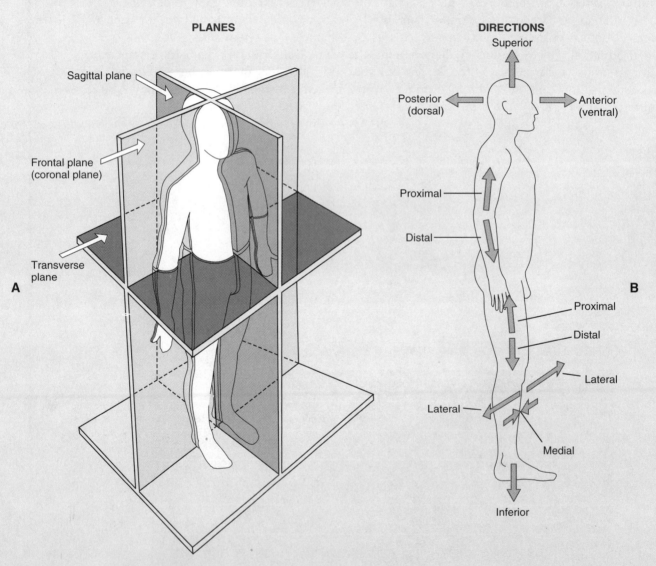

FIGURE C-1 **A,** Planes of the body. **B,** Directional terms. (From Leonard PC: *Building a medical vocabulary*, ed 4, Philadelphia, 1997, WB Saunders.)

Muscular system: Figures C-2 to C-5

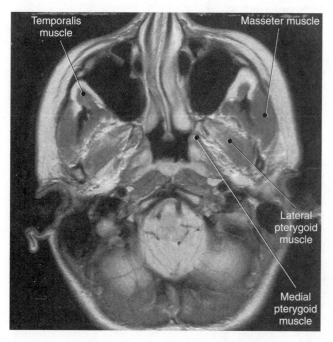

FIGURE C-2 Axial MR scan of neck with muscles of mastication. (From Kelley LL, Petersen CM: *Sectional anatomy for imaging professionals,* St Louis, 1996, Mosby.)

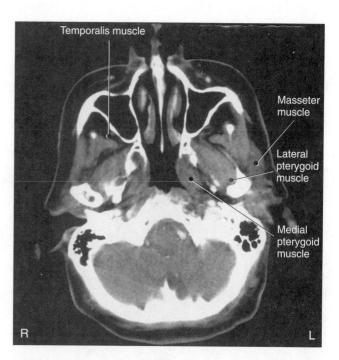

FIGURE C-3 Axial CT scan of neck with muscles of mastication.

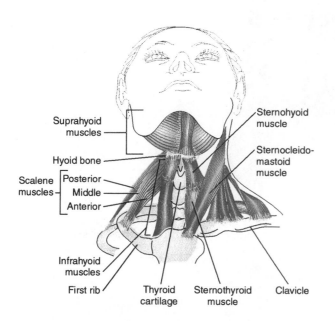

FIGURE C-4 Anterior view of the neck muscles.

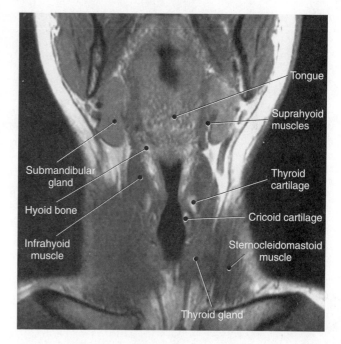

FIGURE C-5 Coronal MR scan of anterior neck muscles. (From Kelley LL, Petersen CM: *Sectional anatomy for imaging professionals,* St Louis, 1996, Mosby.)

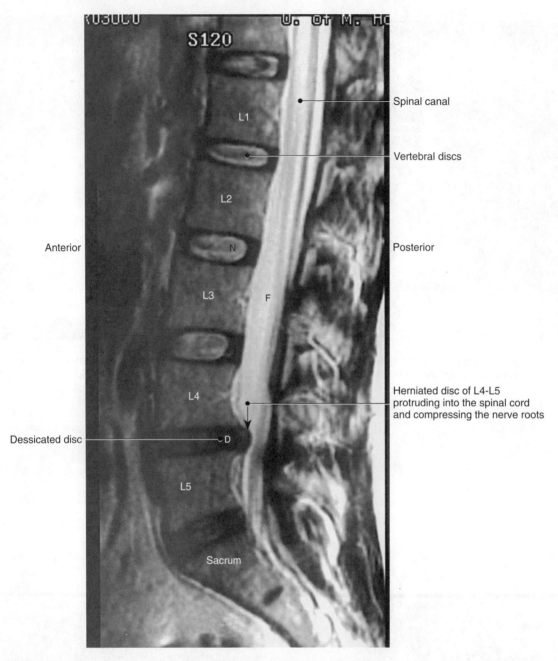

S120

Spinal canal

Vertebral discs

Anterior

Posterior

L1

L2

N

L3

F

L4

Herniated disc of L4-L5 protruding into the spinal cord and compressing the nerve roots

Dessicated disc

D

L5

Sacrum

FIGURE C-6 Lumbar spine. (From Ballinger PW, Frank ED: *Merrill's atlas of radiographic positions and radiologic procedures*, ed 9, St Louis, 1999, Mosby.)

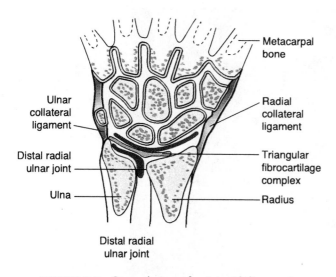

FIGURE C-7   Coronal view of wrist with ligaments.

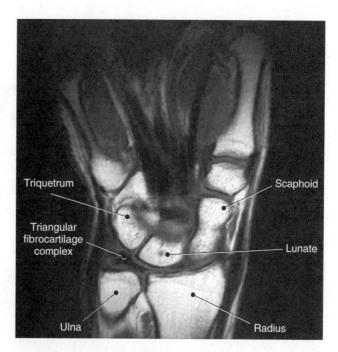

FIGURE C-8   Coronal MR scan of wrist. (From Kelley LL, Petersen CM: *Sectional anatomy for imaging professionals,* St Louis, 1996, Mosby.)

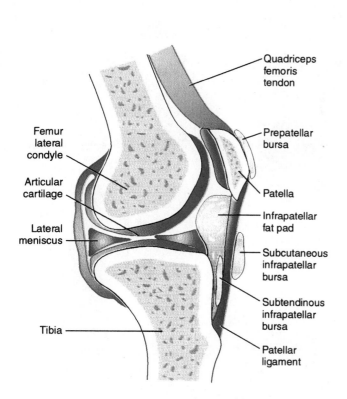

FIGURE C-9A   Sagittal view of knee.

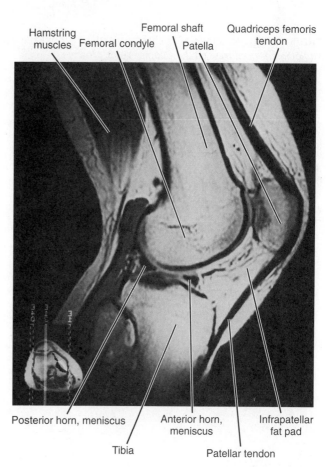

FIGURE C-9B   Sagittal MR scan of knee. (From Kelley LL, Petersen CM: *Sectional anatomy for imaging professionals,* St Louis, 1996, Mosby.)

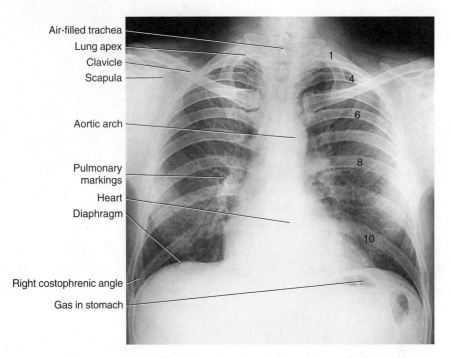

Air-filled trachea
Lung apex
Clavicle
Scapula
Aortic arch
Pulmonary markings
Heart
Diaphragm
Right costophrenic angle
Gas in stomach

1
4
6
8
10

FIGURE C-10 Posteroanterior chest projection. (From Ballinger PW, Frank ED: *Merrill's atlas of radiographic positions and radiologic procedures,* ed 9, St Louis, 1999, Mosby.)

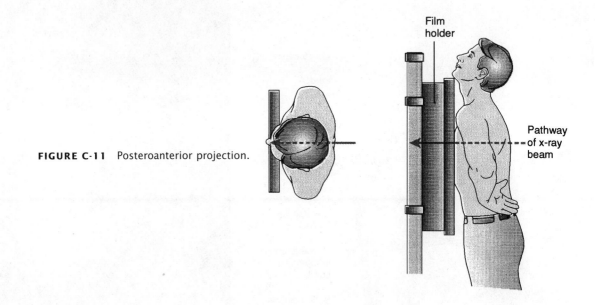

Film holder

Pathway of x-ray beam

FIGURE C-11 Posteroanterior projection.

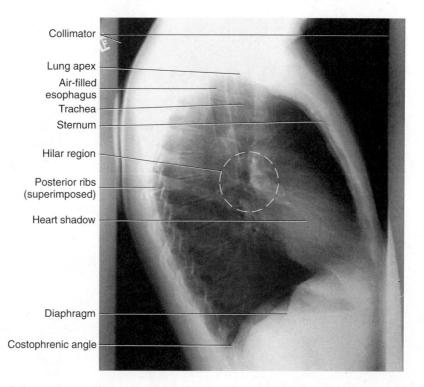

Collimator

Lung apex

Air-filled
esophagus

Trachea

Sternum

Hilar region

Posterior ribs
(superimposed)

Heart shadow

Diaphragm

Costophrenic angle

FIGURE C-12 Left lateral chest. (From Ballinger PW, Frank ED: *Merrill's atlas of radiographic positions and radiologic procedures,* ed 9, St Louis, 1999, Mosby.)

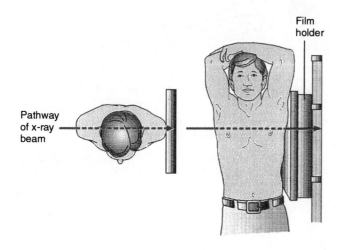

Film
holder

Pathway
of x-ray
beam

FIGURE C-13 Patient in an erect, left lateral position resulting in a lateral x-ray projection.

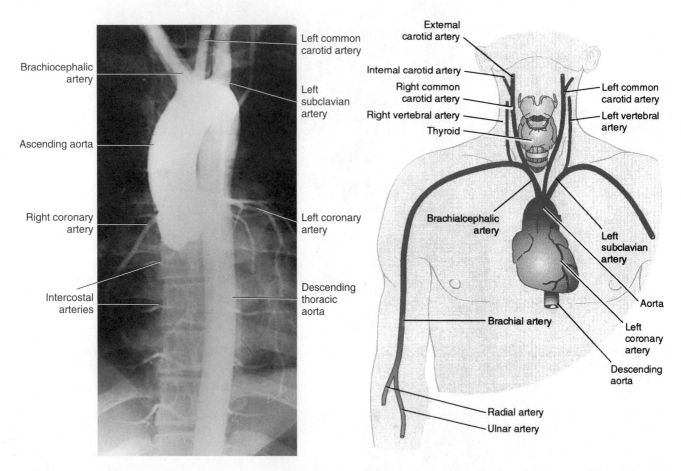

FIGURE C-14 AP thoracic aorta that also demonstrates right and left coronary arteries. (From Ballinger PW, Frank ED: *Merrill's atlas of radiographic positions and radiologic procedures,* ed 9, St Louis, 1999, Mosby.)

FIGURE C-15 Major arteries of the upper chest, neck, and arm.

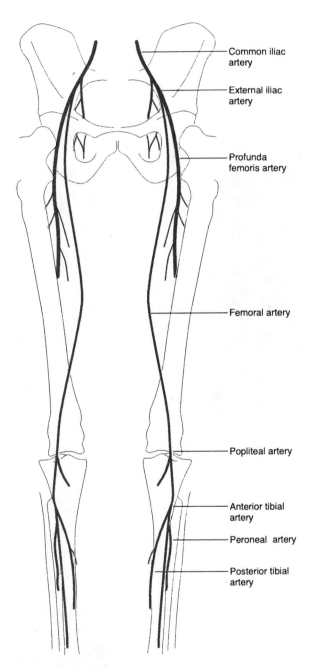

FIGURE C-16 Arteries of the lower extremities.

Common iliac
artery

External iliac
artery

Profunda
femoris artery

Femoral artery

Popliteal artery

Anterior tibial
artery

Peroneal artery

Posterior tibial
artery

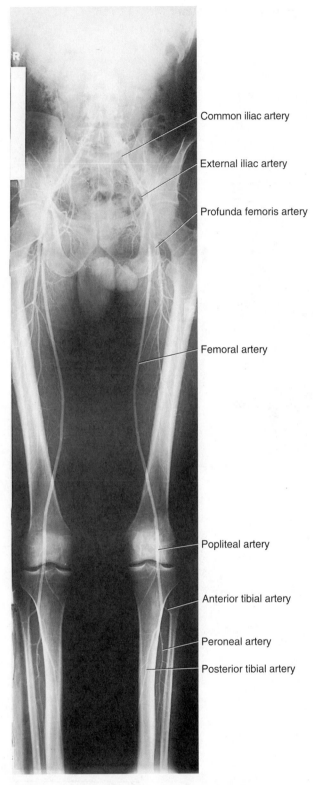

Common iliac artery

External iliac artery

Profunda femoris artery

Femoral artery

Popliteal artery

Anterior tibial artery

Peroneal artery

Posterior tibial artery

FIGURE C-17 Normal aortofemoral arteriogram in late arterial phase. (From Ballinger PW, Frank ED: *Merrill's atlas of radiographic positions and radiologic procedures,* ed 9, St Louis, 1999, Mosby.)

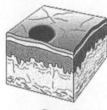

MACULE
Flat, circumscribed

Example: Freckles

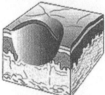

PAPULE
Small, solid elevation

Example: Warts

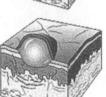

VESICLE OR BLISTER
Thin wall, raised, fluid filled

Example: Second degree burn

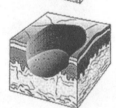

ULCER
Cavity in tissue

Example: Bedsore or pressure sore

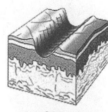

EXCORIATION
Epidermis missing, exposing dermis

Example: Scratch

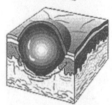

PUSTULE
Raised, often with a "head," filled with exudate or "pus"

Example: Acne

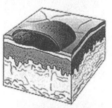

PLAQUE
Slightly elevated, flat, "scale"-like lesion

Example: Psoriasis

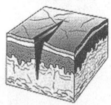

FISSURE
Cracks in tissue

Example: Athlete's foot

FIGURE C-18 Common skin lesions.

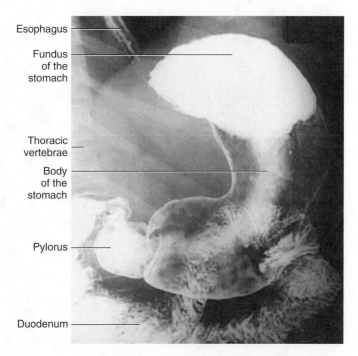

FIGURE C-19 Double contrast x-ray of the stomach in the left posterior oblique position (LPO). (From Ballinger PW, Frank ED: *Merrill's atlas of radiographic positions and radiologic procedures,* ed 9, St Louis, 1999, Mosby.)

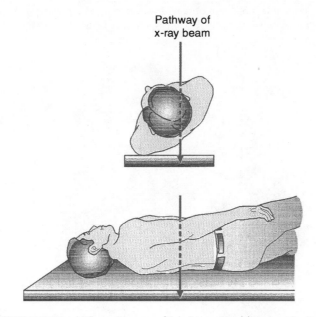

FIGURE C-20 LPO position resulting in an AP oblique projection.

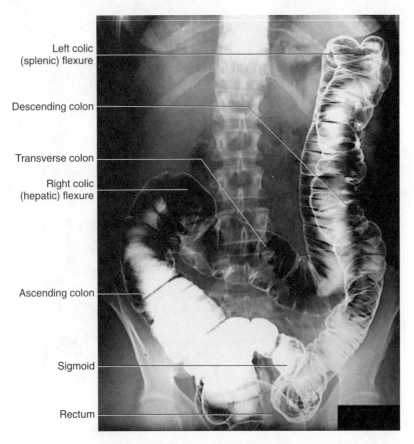

Left colic
(splenic) flexure

Descending colon

Transverse colon

Right colic
(hepatic) flexure

Ascending colon

Sigmoid

Rectum

FIGURE C-21 Double-contrast PA large intestine. Film obtained with patient in a prone position. (From Ballinger PW, Frank ED: *Merrill's atlas of radiographic positions and radiologic procedures,* ed 9, St Louis, 1999, Mosby.)

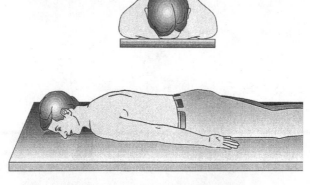

FIGURE C-22 Prone body position.

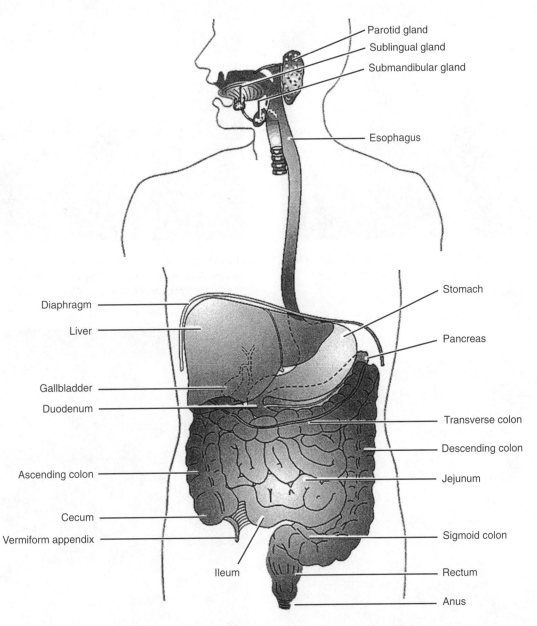

Parotid gland

Sublingual gland

Submandibular gland

Esophagus

Diaphragm

Liver

Gallbladder

Duodenum

Ascending colon

Cecum

Vermiform appendix

Ileum

Stomach

Pancreas

Transverse colon

Descending colon

Jejunum

Sigmoid colon

Rectum

Anus

FIGURE C-23 The human digestive system (anterior view).

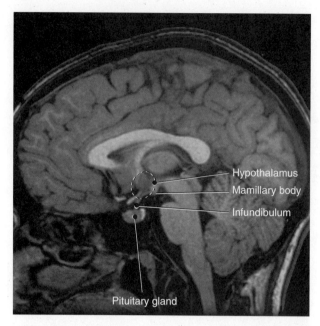

FIGURE C-24 Midsagittal MR scan of hypothalamus. (From Kelley LL, Petersen CM: *Sectional anatomy for imaging professionals*, St Louis, 1996, Mosby.)

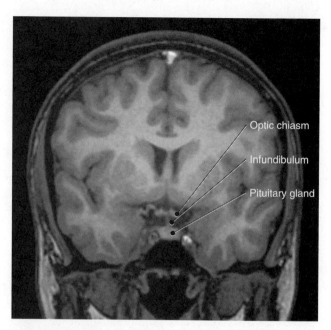

FIGURE C-25 Coronal MR scan of pituitary gland and optic chiasm. (From Kelley LL, Petersen CM: *Sectional anatomy for imaging professionals*, St Louis, 1996, Mosby.)

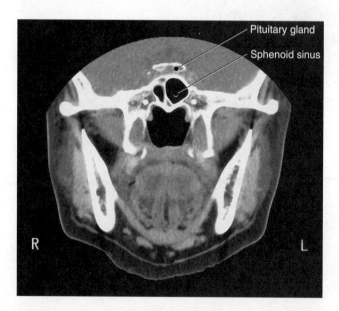

FIGURE C-26 Coronal scan of pituitary gland. (From Kelley LL, Petersen CM: *Sectional anatomy for imaging professionals*, St Louis, 1996, Mosby.)

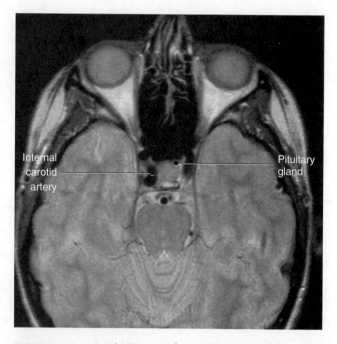

FIGURE C-27 Axial MR scan of pituitary gland. (From Kelley LL, Petersen CM: *Sectional anatomy for imaging professionals*, St Louis, 1996, Mosby.)

Nervous system: Figure C-28 *A, B*

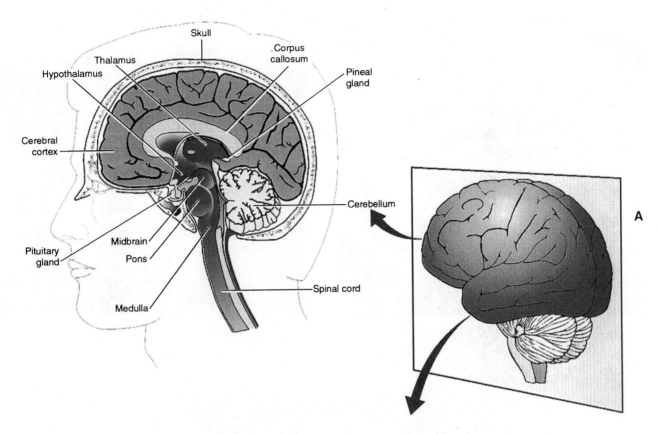

FIGURE C-28a Sagittal section of brain and spinal cord.

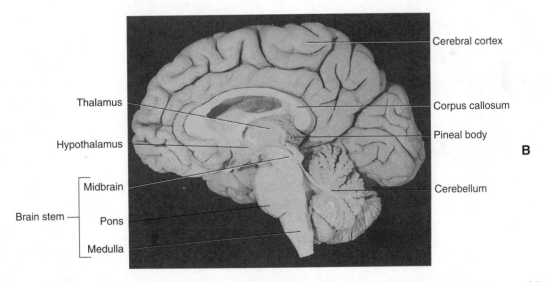

FIGURE C-28b Cadaver section of brain. (From Thibodeau GA, Patton KT: *The human body in health and disease*, ed 2, St Louis, 1997, Mosby.)

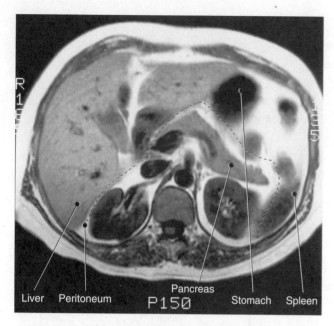

FIGURE C-29 Axial MR scan of peritoneal and retroperitoneal structures (separated by dotted line). (From Kelley LL, Petersen CM: *Sectional anatomy for imaging professionals*, St Louis, 1996, Mosby.)

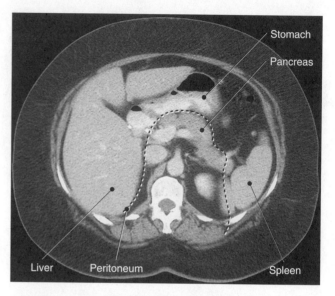

FIGURE C-30 Axial CT scan of peritoneal and retroperitoneal structures (separated by dotted line). (From Kelley LL, Petersen CM: *Sectional anatomy for imaging professionals*, St Louis, 1996, Mosby.)

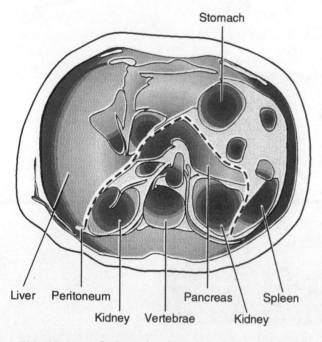

FIGURE C-31 Peritoneal and retroperitoneal structures.

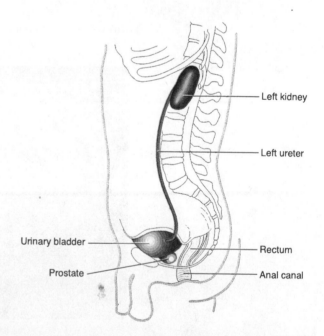

FIGURE C-32 Sagittal view of the male urinary system in relation to surrounding structures. Note the retroperitoneal location of kidney.

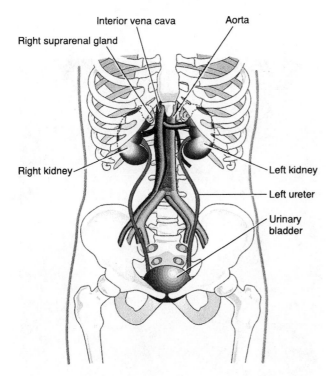

Interior vena cava Aorta
Right suprarenal gland

Right kidney   Left kidney

                                                Left ureter

                                                Urinary
                                                bladder

FIGURE C-33 Anterior aspect of urinary system in relation to surrounding structures.

FIGURE C-34 AP urogram. (From Ballinger PW, Frank ED: *Merrill's atlas of radiographic positions and radiologic procedures,* ed 9, St Louis, 1999, Mosby.)

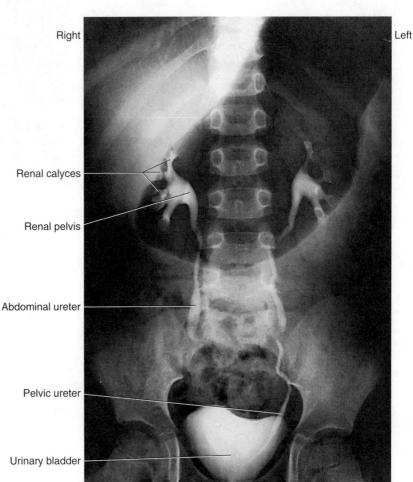

Right   Left

Renal calyces

Renal pelvis

Abdominal ureter

Pelvic ureter

Urinary bladder

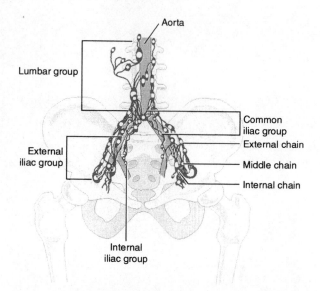

FIGURE C-35 Iliopelvic-aortic lymphatic system. Anterior projection.

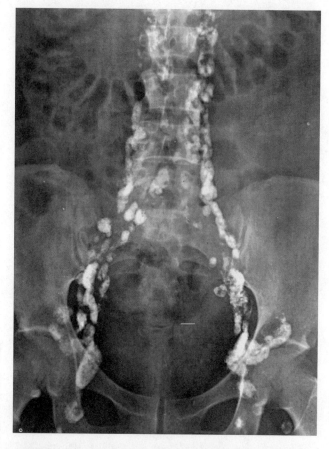

FIGURE C-36 AP projection of iliopelvic-abdominoaortic lymph nodes. (From Ballinger PW, Frank ED: *Merrill's atlas of radiographic positions and radiologic procedures,* ed 9, St Louis, 1999, Mosby.)

Reproductive system: Figures C-37 to C-40

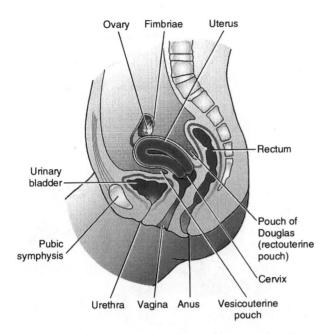

FIGURE C-37 Sagittal view of female reproductive system.

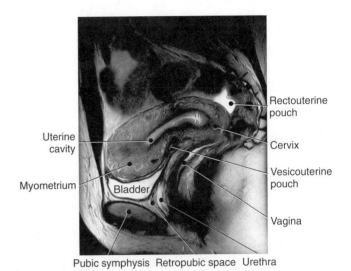

FIGURE C-38 Sagittal MR scan of female reproductive system. (From Kelley LL, Petersen CM: *Sectional anatomy for imaging professionals*, St Louis, 1996, Mosby.)

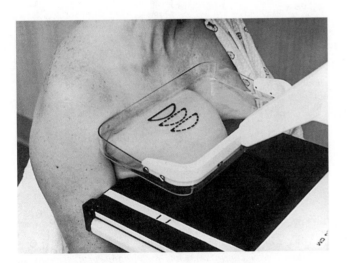

FIGURE C-39 Patient positioned for craniocaudal projection of breast. (From Ballinger PW, Frank ED: *Merrill's atlas of radiographic positions and radiologic procedures*, ed 9, St Louis, 1999, Mosby.)

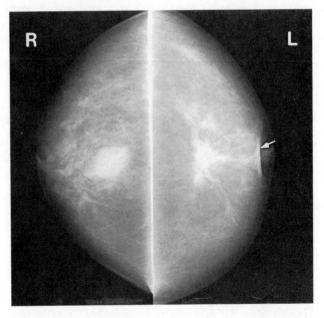

FIGURE C-40 Craniocaudal projection of bilateral breast masses. (From Ballinger PW, Frank ED: *Merrill's atlas of radiographic positions and radiologic procedures*, ed 9, St Louis, 1999, Mosby.)

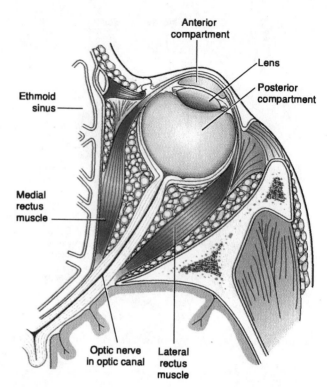

FIGURE C-41   Axial view of orbit.

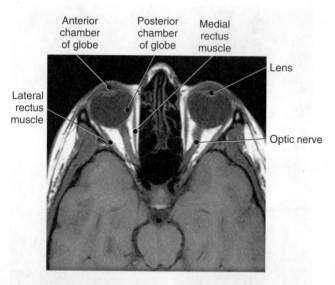

FIGURE C-42   Axial MR scan of orbit. (From Kelley LL, Petersen CM: *Sectional anatomy for imaging professionals,* St Louis, 1996, Mosby.)

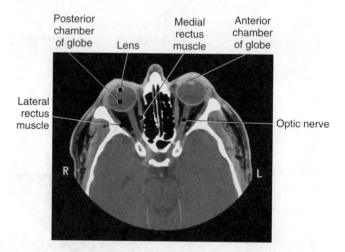

FIGURE C-43   Axial CT scan of orbit. (From Kelley LL, Petersen CM: *Sectional anatomy for imaging professionals,* St Louis, 1996, Mosby.)

Appendix D

FedDes Style Manual

FedDes Wellness Center Physician's Directory

The FedDes Wellness Center is located at 101 Wellness Way Drive, New York, NY 10036. Providers on site include 24 physicians, a physical therapist, and a certified nurse practitioner.

Family Practice Division, Suite 300
Charles P. Davis, MD
J. Thomas Geiger, MD
Matthew D. Sponch, MD
Izzy Sertoli, MD
P. H. Waters, MD
Melissa A. Anconeus, MA, PT
Pamela S. Barthonin, MA, RN, CRNP

Orthopaedic Division, Suite 133
David Treppe, MD
James P. Osseous, MD
Harry A. Medulla, MD

Urology Division, Suite 237
Helen Loop, MD
Theodore Trigone, MD
Benjamin Keytone, MD

Pulmonary Medicine Division, Suite 451
Allan Bolus, MD
Neal Alveoli, MD
Douglas Sputum, MD

Gastroenterology Division, Suite 279
Gwenn Maltase, MD
Kate Cobalamin, MD
Anna Bolism, MD

Cardiology Division, Suite 413
Erica Purkinje, MD
Lucas Site, MD
A. B. Doner, MD
Adam Valence, MD

Diagnostic Imaging Division, Suite 157
William C. Roentgen, MD
Hounsfield T. Scanner, MD
Potter T. Bucky, MD
Scott E. Film, MD

Formatting Guidelines

F-1
All medical reports and letters use the blocked style format with 1-inch margins. No tabulation appears in the document.

F-2
All medical reports and letters use open punctuation. No punctuation marks follow the salutation and complimentary closing.

F-3
The complete headings, topics, and subtopics are always used. These are keyed in all capital letters followed by a colon and separated by a blank line.

F-4
The dictated words *current date* must be transcribed as the actual month, day, and year.

F-5
Identifying statistical data must be included on medical reports. FedDes Wellness Center uses the following format for consistency:
Chart notes using the SOAP and/or history and physical format styles require the patient's statistical data on the first and succeeding pages to include the patient's full name (surname, first name), date of birth, and examination date as shown:
For example: CHART NOTE
Patient Name: Felter, Michael
Date of Birth: July 3, 1954
Examination Date: *current date*

History and physical examination reports, diagnostic imaging reports, and procedure reports require the patient's statistical data for first and succeeding pages to include the patient's name, file number or social security number, date of birth, examination date, physician's name, and type of examination (keyed in all capital letters).
For example: HISTORY AND PHYSICAL EXAMINATION REPORT
Patient Name: Doe, Jane
File Number: 1235678
Date of Birth: January 3, 1950
Examination Date: Current date
Physician: Charles P. Davis, MD

For example: X-RAY REPORT
Patient Name: Doe, Jane
File Number: 1235678
Date of Birth: January 3, 1950

Examination Date: Current date
Ordering Physician: Izzy Sertoli, MD
Examination: MAMMOGRAM

For example: PROCEDURE REPORT
Patient Name: Doe, Jane
File Number: 1235678
Date of Birth: January 3, 1950
Examination Date: Current date
Ordering Physician: Izzy Sertoli, MD
Procedure: EXERCISE STRESS TEST

For example: CONSULTATION REPORT
Patient Name: Doe, Jane
File Number: 1235678
Date of Birth: January 3, 1950
Examination Date: Current date
Requesting Physician: Izzy Sertoli, MD

F-6
All medical documents formatted as a letter are
    transcribed on letterhead stationary, as
    shown:
FedDes Wellness Center
Name of the Division, Suite No.
101 Wellness Way Drive
New York, NY 10036

F-7
All medical documents formatted as a letter will in-
    clude a reference line above the salutation
    line as shown:
Re: Betty Williams
Date of Birth: February 2, 1949
Examination: RIGHT BREAST SONOGRAM

Dear Dr. Davis

F-8
Continuation pages for all medical reports must in-
    clude the patient's statistical data and page
    number beginning at the 1-inch top margin.
    The word *continued* appears at the left margin
    at the bottom of the previous page.
HISTORY AND PHYSICAL EXAMINATION
Patient Name: Doe, Jane
File Number: 1235678
Date of Birth: January 3, 1950
Examination Date: *current date*

Physician: Charles P. Davis, MD
Page 2

F-9
Continuation pages for letters must include a 3-line
    heading beginning at the 1-inch top margin
    as shown:
Charles P. Davis, MD
Current date
Page 2

F-10
The signature line includes the physician's name
    followed by the transcriptionist's initials on
    the third or fourth line below the last entry as
    shown.
For example: Charles P. Davis, MD/xx

Usage Guidelines

U-1
When the age of the patient is mentioned within the
    body of the transcript, the patient's year of
    birth is not provided, and the student will
    need to calculate this date.

U-2
All dates are spelled out in medical documents re-
    gardless of where the date appears on a re-
    port or letter.
For example: The patient was seen in this office on
    Monday, January 12, 20xx.

U-3
A comma separates each vital sign.
For example: BP 108/72, pulse 78 and regular, res-
    pirations 20/min.

U-4
Drug allergies are underscored.
For example: Tetracycline

U-5
Drug dosages are expressed in Latin abbreviations
    and transcribed in lowercase letters with pe-
    riods and no internal spaces.
For example: The patient was started on
    Keflex, 250 mg q.i.d.

U-6

Measurements of tumors are expressed in metric terms.

For example: The tumor measured 12 × 12 × 6 mm.

U-7

Fractions are converted to the decimal equivalent. Place a zero *before* a decimal that lacks a whole number.

For example: The lesion measured 0.75 × 1 cm.

U-8

Mixed numbers are transcribed in figures.

For example: The 5 ½-year-old female was seen at 1:00 p.m.

U-9

Numbers one through ten are spelled out when they do not refer to technical items and the sentence does not contain numbers over ten.

For example: The patient will be seen again in three weeks.

U-10

Figures are used for numbers greater than ten.

For example: The diarrhea has been less frequent over the last 12 hours.

U-11

If a sentence contains numbers under and over ten, use figures for all.

For example: The patient smokes 2 packs per day and has done so for 24 years.

U-12

Figures are used in lists.

For example: IMPRESSION:

1. Acute appendicitis.
2. Rule out ureteral calculus.

U-13

Figures and the pound sign (#) are used for suture materials.

For example: The subcutaneous tissues were closed with interrupted #3-0 plain catgut.

U-14

Figures are used for ranges and ratios.

For example: She has vomited 4-5 times in the past 24 hours, mostly a bile-colored, watery liquid.

U-15

Ordinal numbers are spelled out.

Example: He kicked a chair, suffering an injury to the base of the fifth metatarsal of the right foot.

U-16

Do not use superscripts and subscripts when expressing electrocardiographic leads, vertebral columns, chemical compounds, and so on.

For example: The leads are V1 through V6.
We used distilled H2O.

U-17

Do not use the degree symbol when expressing temperature. The word *degree* is included only if dictated. Fahrenheit or Celcuis is included only if dictated and expressed as a capital letter F or C.

For example: Her temperature was 98.6 F.

U-18

The letter *x* is used to abbreviate the words *by* or *times* when it precedes a number of another abbreviation.

For example: The lesion is 1.5 x 1 cm on her leg.
The patient was prescribed
Augmentin 500 mg p.o. t.i.d. × 2 weeks.

U-19

A hyphen is used between numbers and *year old*.

For example: The patient was a 26-year-old female.

U-20

A hyphen is used between two "like" vowels.

For example: We will plan to see the patient in three weeks for re-evaluation.

U-21

A hyphen is used to take the place of the word *to* or *through* to identify ranges.

For example: The last time he vomited was 4-5 hours ago.

U-22

A diagonal (/) is used to indicate the word *per* in laboratory values and respirations or the word *over* in blood pressure.

For example: BP 120/80, pulse 106 and regular, temperature 37.2 C, respirations 14/min.

U-23
The number or pound (#) symbol is used to abbreviate the word *number* when followed by a medical instrument or apparatus.
For example: The small piece of metal was removed with a #25 gauge needle.

U-24
The names of specific departments or sections of a hospital, such as Intensive Care, are capitalized.
For example: After surgery, the patient was sent to City Hospital Intensive Care.

U-25
Nouns preceding Roman numbers are not capitalized unless the noun begins a sentence.
For example: The patient is gravida I, para I.

FedDes Wellness Center Approved Abbreviation List

AB	abortion
ABG	arterial blood gas
ACTH	Aderenocorticotropic hormone
A&D	ascending and descending
ADL	activities of daily living
AP	anteroposterior, apical pulse
A&P	auscultation and percussion
ARD	acute respiratory distress
ASAP	as soon as possible
ASCVD	atherosclerotic cardiovascular disease
AU	each ear, both ears
AV	atrioventricular
BCC	basal cell carcinoma
BE	barium enema
BLE	both lower extremities
BLT	bilateral tubal ligation
BM	bowel movement
BP	blood pressure
BPH	benign prostatic hypertrophy
BS	blood sugar, bowel sounds
BUN	blood urea nitrogen
BUS	Bartholin urethral and Skene (glands)
C&S	culture and sensitivity

CABG	coronary artery bypass graft surgery
CAD	coronary artery disease
CBC	complete blood count
CHF	congestive heart failure
CNS	central nervous system
COPD	chronic obstructive pulmonary disease
CPR	cardiopulmonary resuscitation
CR	cardiorespiratory
CVA	cerebrovascular accident
CT	computerized tomography
D&C	dilation and curettage
DJD	degenerative joint disease
DOE	dyspnea on exertion
DPT	diphteria-pertussis-tetanus
DTR	deep tendon reflexes
DVT	deep vein thrombosis
EAC	external auditory canal
ECG	electrocardiogram
EGD	esophagogastroduodenoscopy
EKG	electrocardiogram
EOM	extraocular movements
EOMI	extraocular movements intact
ER	emergency room
ESR	erythrocyte sedimentation rate
FB	foreign body
FBS	fasting blood sugar
FUO	fever of unknown origin
GB	gallbladder
GI	gastrointestinal
GYN	gynecology/gynecologist
HCG	human chorionic gonadotropin
H&P	history and physical
HPI	history of present illness
I&D	incision and drainage
IM	intramuscular
INR	International Normalized Ratio
IV	intravenous
IVP	intravenous pyelogram
KUB	kidneys, ureters, bladder
L&A	light and accommodation
LLQ	lower left quadrant
LMP	last menstrual period
LUQ	left upper quadrant
MI	myocardial infarction
MM	mucous membrane
NKA	no known allergies
NOS	not otherwise specified
NPH	no previous history

NSAID	nonsteroidal antiinflammatory drug	SOB	shortness of breath
NSR	normal sinus rhythm	STD	sexually transmitted disease
NTP	normal temperature and pressure	T&A	tonsillectomy and adenoidectomy
OB-GYN	obstetrics and gynecology	TAB	therapeutic abortion
OS	left eye	TM	tympanic membrane
PA	posteroanerior	TPR	temperature, pulse, respiration
P&A	percussion and auscultation	TUR	transurethral resection
PERL	pupils equal, reactive to light	TURP	transurethral resection of the prostate
PERLA	pupils equal and reactive to light and accommodation	UA	urinalysis
PERRLA	pupils equal, round, reactive to light, and accommodation	URI	upper respiratory infection
		UTI	urinary tract infection
PID	pelvic inflammatory disease	UV	ultraviolet
PIP	proximal interphalangeal	VPB	ventricular premature beat
PSA	picryl sulfonic acid	VS	vital signs
RBC	red blood cell count	V&T	volume and tension
RLQ	right lower quadrant	WBC	white blood cell count
ROM	range of motion	WF	white female
RUQ	right upper quadrant	WM	white male
SGOT	serum glutamic oxaloacetic transaminase	WNL	within normal limits

Appendix E /Answer Key

CHAPTER 2 / PRETEST

1. False: four
2. True
3. True
4. True
5. True
6. False: templates are frequently used
7. True
8. False: high
9. False: paragraphs
10. True
11. True
12. True
13. False: initials should be avoided
14. True
15. True
16. False: sentence fragments are used
17. False: two
18. True
19. False: social history
20. True
21. False: history of present illness
22. False: include type of examination
23. False
24. False: two
25. True
26. d
27. b
28. c
29. c
30. b
31. a
32. b
33. c
34. d
35. b
36. d
37. d
38. c
39. d
40. c
41. a
42. b
43. a
44. a
45. d
46. c
47. a
48. a
49. a
50. b

CHAPTER 2 / ACTIVITY 1

1. True
2. True
3. True
4. False: neurologic
5. False: outpatient
6. True
7. True
8. False: abbreviations/ phrases are used
9. False: statistical data appear on all pages
10. True
11. True
12. True
13. False: can include many headings
14. True
15. True
16. False: past medical history
17. True
18. False: history of present illness
19. True
20. True
21. True
22. True
23. True
24. False: months spelled out
25. True
26. c
27. d
28. b
29. a
30. b
31. c
32. b
33. c
34. d
35. a

CHAPTER 2 / ACTIVITY 2

1. False: subjective
2. False: more
3. True
4. True
5. True
6. True
7. False: x-ray
8. True
9. False: high
10. True
11. False: not all the time
12. True
13. True
14. True
15. True
16. True
17. True
18. True
19. False
20. False: SSN
21. True
22. False: as-sessment
23. True
24. True
25. False: chest
26. b
27. a
28. b
29. d
30. a
31. d
32. c
33. d
34. b
35. c

CHAPTER 2 / CHECK YOUR PROGRESS

1. True
2. True
3. True
4. True
5. False: easy
6. True
7. False
8. True
9. True
10. False
11. True
12. False: narrow margins
13. True
14. False: plan
15. True
16. False: negative
17. True
18. False: neck
19. False: above
20. False: below
21. True
22. True
23. True
24. False: low levels
25. True
26. True
27. True
28. True
29. False
30. True
31. True
32. True
33. True
34. b
35. c
36. c
37. c
38. b
39. c
40. c
41. d
42. b
43. d
44. d
45. b
46. c
47. b
48. a
49. b
50. c

CHAPTER 2 / ACTIVITIES 3–5

Please refer to Figure 2.2 (Activity 3), Figure 2.4 (Activity 4), and Figure 2.6 (Activity 5) in your textbook.

CHAPTER 3

Pretest 1: See *Check Your Progress 1.*
Pretest 2: See *Check Your Progress 2.*
Pretest 3: See *Check Your Progress 3.*

CHAPTER 3 / ACTIVITY 1

All errors are indicated in bold and italics. Margins are formatted at 1 inch.
CHART NOTE
Double space
Patient Name: Bernshaw, Sue

Date of **B**irth: ***September 12, 1965***

Examination Date: *Current date*
Double space
SUBJECTI**VE**: Removal of sutures placed ***ten*** days ago.

OBJECTI**VE**: The wound on the lateral ***as***pect of the left knee **looks** well healed. The ***#5-0*** nylon sutures were removed without difficulty.

ASSESSMENT: Laceration of ***left*** knee, well healed.

PLAN: Advised applying vitamin ***E*** to the area.

Harry A. Medulla, MD/xx

CHART NOTE

Patient Name: Gapolli, Rachi

Date of Birth: February 3, 1969

Examination Date: *Current date*

SUBJECTIVE: Patient complains of sensitive pimple-like bump on right posterior shoulder area.

OBJECTIVE: A mole, approximately 1 cm in diameter, is visible. It is uniformly brown in color with no irregular borders. Patient denies pain or discharge, although she does admit that the area is quite sensitive for the past three days.

ASSESSMENT: Nevus.

PLAN: I am referring the patient to a dermatologist for its removal and biopsy.

_____

Charles Davis, MD/xx

CHART NOTE

Patient Name: Brodrick, Heather

Date of Birth: April 19, 1989

Examination Date: *Current date*

SUBJECTIVE: Patient complains of warts on palm of right hand that are becoming bothersome.

OBJECTIVE: Examination of both hands reveals a 3 mm growth over the dorsum of the distal fourth and fifth metacarpals of the right hand.

ASSESSMENT: Verruca.

PLAN: The warts were frozen with liquid nitrogen without incident. Recheck in 2-3 weeks if problem not resolved.

_____

Charles Davis, MD/xx

All errors are indicated in bold and italics. Margins are formatted at 1 inch.

CHART NOTE
Double space
Patient Name: Wright, Nathan

Date of Birth: November 30, 1983

Examination Date: Current date
Double space
SUBJECTIVE: Patient presents with typical ***flu-like*** symptoms of fever, muscular ***aches*** and pains**,** shaking chills, ***headache,*** and ***weakness.***

OBJECTIVE: Bilateral tympanic membranes are clear. ***Oropharynx*** is not ***in***jected. No neck nodes detected. Chest is clear to percussion and auscultation. Temperature ***102.3 F.***

ASSESSMENT: *Influenza.*

PLAN: Symptomatic therapy. **A**cetaminophen ***p.r.n.*** for fever and pain. Recheck in ***5-12*** days if not improving.

_____

Charles Davis, MD/***xx***

HISTORY AND PHYSICAL EXAMINATION

Patient Name: Monahan, Esther

File Number: 2348901

Date of Birth: September 10, 19xx

Examination Date: *Current date*

Physician: Harry A. Medulla, MD

HISTORY

HISTORY OF PRESENT ILLNESS: This 88-year-old lady was admitted to a nursing home with an extensive cellulitis involving the right side of the abdomen and the chest. She had been living at home with her daughter, but had become increasingly unable to eat. She developed hyponatremia and dehydration along with the cellulitis. The cause of the cellulitis was never clearly determined. It was felt ultimately to be due to cracks in the skin from her poor condition and then an infection starting. She received six days of Ancef, was put on Keflex for follow up. There is some suggestion of possible alcohol use involved, and she did receive some Thiamine.

PAST MEDICAL HISTORY: Otherwise fairly benign. Dr. Peebody had provided most of her care.

SOCIAL HISTORY: As above.

FAMILY HISTORY: No pertinent data.

REVIEW OF SYSTEMS: Left hip has bothered her from a hip fracture 12 years ago with pinning. Other medical problems include GI bleed, which occurred back in February. Decision was made by the daughter and the patient not to investigate further. She had been on aspirin at the time, and it was stopped. It sounds like a lower GI bleed rather than an upper at that time.

PHYSICAL EXAMINATION:

GENERAL: Elderly woman who is a little hard of hearing. Her vision is poor. Vital signs are good.

HEENT: No jaundice. Mouth and pharynx are unremarkable.

NECK: Supple. Carotids are equal. No JVD.

LUNGS: Clear to percussion and auscultation.

- begin page 2* -

HEART: Regular rhythm. No murmurs, no gallops.

BREASTS: Atrophic.

ABDOMEN: Soft without organomegaly. The right side of the abdomen and chest, particularly underneath the breast, is still a bit irritated and red, but clearly much better than had been previously described.

EXTREMITIES: Ankles show 3+ edema up to the knee.

IMPRESSION:
1. Resolving cellulitis of the right side of abdomen and chest. Continue antibiotics.
2. Ankle edema attributed to CHF. Prescribed Lotensin, 5 mg daily along with brief regimen of diuretics. Will monitor progress.
3. Right hip pain.
4. Questionable alcohol abuse versus dementia.

———————————————————
Harry A. Medulla, MD/xx

---

*A dotted line is used to indicate page breaks in multi-page documents. Refer to Chapter 2 for formatting guidelines for continuation pages in medical documents and letters.

CHAPTER 3 / ACTIVITY 6

Current date

Dr. Katherine Davis
Medical Practice Ltd.
312 Main Street
New York, NY 10010

Re: Kevin Schlitz
    Date of Birth: October 29, 1936

Dear Dr. Davis

I had the opportunity to examine Mr. Schlitz in my office on *(current date)* in regards to his slow-healing ulceration of his right foot. The wound definitely looks improved from the last time I saw it. He has been doing a good job at not bearing weight upon his right foot.

At this point, I think it would be appropriate to place him in some extra-depth shoes or boots with accommodative insoles to help reduce pressure in the forefoot area. I am concerned that he has a very high potential for ulceration beneath the third metatarsal due to increased loading in this area.

I wrote a prescription and sent him to an orthotic specialist for new shoes and to have accommodative insoles constructed. I think the patient has an unrealistic outlook in regards to what type of insoles will be in his shoes. He is currently wearing a very rigid functional device. This is not the appropriate device to reduce pressure in the forefoot area. The prosthesis I am recommending should help cushion and distribute his weight evenly in the forefoot area as well as help maintain the rear foot in a better functioning position. Please feel free to contact me if you have any questions in regard to this matter.

Sincerely

Harry A. Medulla, MD

xx

Current date

Arthur Guttenberg, MD
5723 North Front Street
New York, NY 10010

Re: Martha Ultress
   Date of Birth: June 19, 1959

Dear Dr. Guttenberg

Thank you for seeing Martha for her right rotator cuff tendinitis. She has had intermittent pain of the right shoulder during the past two months. Over the past few days the pain has gotten very severe.

On examination, she could barely abduct past 30 degrees. The x-ray was notable for some calcific tendinitis. I injected the subacromial bursa with steroids, and obtained a rather dramatic improvement in her bursitis, only to have it return again one week later. I started her on a physical therapy program and would appreciate your evaluation concerning the continuing care and treatment of this patient.

Very truly yours

Harry A. Medulla, MD

xx

CHART NOTE

Patient Name: Ramirez, Jose

Date of Birth: May 23, 19xx

Examination Date: *Current date*

HISTORY OF PRESENT ILLNESS: This 15-year-old male is seen for a follow up on his acne. He has been using Clearasil Medicated Astringent and Oxy Wash for about two months with no improvement. He is on no oral medications, denies any allergies, and is in good health.

PHYSICAL EXAMINATION: Today's exam reveals inflammatory cystic lesions along the jaw line and upper back. Some deep cysts are palpable on the chin and over the right shoulder area.

PLAN: He is to start E-Mycin 250 mg b.i.d. and 10% Benzac topically h.s. after washing. He is to continue washing with Oxy Wash × 3 a day as tolerated. He has been cautioned not to pick at the lesions. We discussed the need to keep his hands away from his face as much as possible and to stop leaning on his elbow with his chin in his hand. It is a bad habit that only promotes the spread of bacteria and should be discontinued. He will be seen again in 4-6 weeks.

Allan Pore, MD/xx

CHART NOTE

Patient Name: Smithers, Linda

Date of Birth: August 13, 19xx

Examination Date: *Current date*

CHIEF COMPLAINT: Itching and a rash.

SUBJECTIVE: The patient is a pleasant, 26-year-old female, who is quite cooperative and in no acute distress. She complains of a rash that began about two weeks ago. She is taking Benadryl at bedtime with no relief. Upon questioning, she admits to using a new, perfumed body lotion after her shower.

OBJECTIVE: Vital Signs: Temperature 98.6, BP 136/72, weight 165 lb, height 5 ft 3 in, pulse 74, respirations 22/min. Smooth, erythematous rash over neck extending over trunk and back. On the upper extremities, she has an erythematous rash extending to her wrists.

ASSESSMENT: Contact dermatitis, secondary to allergy to perfume.

PLAN:
1. Discontinue use of perfumed body lotion.
2. Wash all clothing and bed linen that were exposed to the perfumed lotion.
3. Take Benadryl 25 mg q.6h. × 3 days

Allan Pore, MD/xx

CHAPTER 4 / PRETEST

1. T	14. T	27. d	39. d
2. T	15. T	28. c	40. a
3. T	16. F	29. d	41. a
4. F	17. F	30. a	42. c
5. F	18. F	31. c	43. c
6. T	19. F	32. b	44. c
7. T	20. F	33. a	45. a
8. T	21. F	34. c	46. b
9. F	22. F	35. a	47. c
10. T	23. T	36. d	48. a
11. T	24. F	37. a	49. a
12. F	25. T	38. c	50. c
13. T	26. a		

CHAPTER 4 / ACTIVITY 1

1. a	10. d	19. d	28. b
2. d	11. d	20. c	29. c
3. d	12. a	21. d	30. a
4. d	13. c	22. a	31. b
5. a	14. d	23. b	32. c
6. d	15. a	24. a	33. d
7. b	16. c	25. b	34. a
8. a	17. c	26. c	35. c
9. c	18. a	27. a	

---

1. d	10. d	19. b	28. b
2. d	11. d	20. a	29. d
3. b	12. a	21. c	30. a
4. d	13. c	22. b	31. c
5. a	14. d	23. a	32. b
6. d	15. a	24. a	33. a
7. b	16. c	25. d	34. a
8. a	17. a	26. a	35. d
9. c	18. b	27. c	

CHAPTER 4 / ACTIVITY 3 (4T-1)

‡top margin 1″ (line 6)
CHART NOTE
‡double space
Patient Name: Felter, Michael
‡double space
Date of Birth: July 3, 1954
‡double space
Examination Date: *Current date*
‡double space
SUBJECTIVE: Patient complains of right elbow pain for past three months. He has been playing tennis once a week over the summer with gradually worsening pain.
‡double space
OBJECTIVE: Tenderness over right medial epicondyle. Pain radiates to the forearm and back of the hand with flexion and supination.
‡double space
ASSESSMENT: Epicondylitis.
‡double space
PLAN: Advised patient to stop playing tennis for three weeks and rest elbow until inflammation subsides. Prescribed Motrin 200 mg p.o. q.i.d. Urged the patient to wear an elastic strap for support, when playing tennis in the future.
‡quadruple space

Harry A. Medulla MD
Harry A. Medulla, MD/xx

CHAPTER 4 / ACTIVITY 3 (4T-2)

‡top margin 1″ (line 6)

HISTORY AND PHYSICAL EXAMINATION REPORT
‡double space
Patient Name: Rouf, Andrea
‡double space
File Number: 2348901
‡double space
Date of Birth: April 10, 19xx
‡double space
Examination Date: *Current date*
‡double space
Physician: Gwenn Maltase, MD
‡double space
HISTORY
‡double space
CHIEF COMPLAINT: Abdominal pain, right lower quadrant for three days.
‡double space

HISTORY OF PRESENT ILLNESS: The patient is a 27-year-old legal secretary, who first noted the onset of colicky lower abdominal pain situated slightly to the right of midline, below the umbilicus and above the pubic bone three days ago. The pain has been getting worse and is associated for the past 36 hours with anorexia and nausea. She has vomited 4-5 times in the past 24 hours, mostly a bile-colored, watery liquid. The pain is not affected by positional change or ingestion of food. There is no radiation of pain. She denies fever, chills, hematemesis or change in bowel habits.
‡double space
PAST HISTORY: The patient had varicella at age 2 and the mumps at age 4. She had a tonsillectomy and adenoidectomy at age 11. There is no family history of diabetes.
‡double space
REVIEW OF SYSTEMS:
‡double space
HEENT: Mild upper respiratory infection two weeks prior to present illness manifested by rhinitis and sore throat.
‡double space
GENITOURINARY: Gravida II, para II, ab 0. No frequency, hematuria, or nocturia.
‡double space
PHYSICAL EXAMINATION
‡double space
GENERAL: The patient is alert, oriented and in moderate distress. BP 120/80, pulse 106 and regular, temperature 37.2 C, respirations 14/min.
‡double space
LUNGS: Clear to P&A.
‡double space

---------------------- begin page 2 ----------------------

HEART: Normal sinus rhythm, no cardiomegaly, no murmurs, gallops, or thrills.
‡double space
ABDOMEN: Flat. Tenderness with muscle guarding in right lower quadrant. Rebound tenderness was present. Bowel sounds are normal. No organomegaly.
‡double space
PELVIC: Bartholins, urethral, and Skene's gland normal. Adnexa normal. Uterus not enlarged.
‡double space
EXTREMITIES: Within normal limits. No edema. Good range of motion.
‡double space
NEUROLOGICAL: Grossly intact.
‡double space
IMPRESSION:
1. Acute appendicitis.
2. Rule out ureteral calculus.
‡double space
PLAN:
1. Refer to John Smithson, MD for surgical consult.
2. Patient to be admitted to General Hospital.
3. WBC and IVP ordered upon admission.
‡quadruple space

Gwenn Maltase MD
Gwenn Maltase, MD/xx

FedDes Wellness Center
Diagnostic Imaging Division, Suite 157
101 Wellness Way Drive
New York, NY 10036

Current date
‡quadruple space
Charles P. Davis, MD
FedDes Wellness Center
Family Practice Division, Suite 300
101 Wellness Way Drive
New York, NY 10036
‡double space
Re: Betty McWilliams
     Date of Birth: February 2, 1949
     ‡double space
Dear Dr. Davis
‡double space
Comparison is made to the prior mammogram dated
January 25, 20xx. An 18 × 8 × 20 mm well-demarcated simple cyst
is demonstrated within the central 12 o'clock position of the right
breast corresponding to the well-demarcated density noted on
mammography in this region. The cyst exhibits posterior wall
enhancement and sound through transmission.
‡double space
A second cyst measuring 6.1 × 7.1 × 4.4 mm is present in the
approximate 10 o'clock position of the breast projecting 6-7 mm from
the nipple corresponding to the density noted on mammography in
this region.
‡double space
No additional lesions are identified.
‡double space
IMPRESSION: The two densities noted in the right breast on the recent
mammogram correspond to simple cysts as described.
‡double space
Thank you for the opportunity to participate in the care of this
patient.
‡double space
Sincerely yours
‡quadruple space

Peter T. Bucky MD
Peter T. Bucky, MD
‡double space
xx

CHAPTER 4 / CHECK YOUR PROGRESS

1. F	14. F	27. a	39. a
2. T	15. T	28. a	40. a
3. T	16. T	29. a	41. c
4. T	17. F	30. c	42. a
5. T	18. T	31. d	43. c
6. T	19. F	32. a	44. a
7. T	20. F	33. c	45. b
8. F	21. T	34. a	46. a
9. F	22. F	35. a	47. c
10. F	23. T	36. c	48. a
11. T	24. T	37. a	49. d
12. F	25. F	38. d	50. b
13. T	26. d		

CHAPTER 5 / PART I PRETEST

1. a	24. c	47. d	69. d
2. c	25. a	48. a	70. a
3. a	26. b	49. c	71. a
4. b	27. c	50. b	72. c
5. d	28. a	51. a	73. b
6. c	29. a	52. c	74. c
7. a	30. c	53. b	75. b
8. b	31. c	54. a	76. a
9. c	32. a	55. a	77. b
10. d	33. a	56. c	78. b
11. a	34. a	57. c	79. c
12. a	35. d	58. a	80. a
13. b	36. c	59. b	81. d
14. c	37. a	60. b	82. b
15. a	38. c	61. c	83. a
16. b	39. c	62. a	84. c
17. c	40. c	63. b	85. c
18. a	41. d	64. c	86. d
19. d	42. a	65. d	87. b
20. b	43. a	66. c	88. c
21. b	44. b	67. a	89. a
22. d	45. a	68. c	90. a
23. c	46. b		

CHAPTER 5 / PART I ACTIVITY 3 (5T-1)

1. Adenoma is a benign tumor in which cells are derived from
   glandular epithelium.
   The patient had an adenomatous polyp.
2. Adenopathy is the enlargement of the glands, especially the
   lymph nodes.
   She has no cervical adenopathy.
3. Adnexa are the tissues or body parts that are near or next to one
   another.
   The adnexa are without masses or tenderness.
4. Aeration is the exchange of carbon dioxide for oxygen by the
   blood in the lungs.
   The lungs are clear to aeration.
5. Amenorrhea is the absence of the menses.
   She is 12 weeks amenorrhea with complaints of vaginal spotting.
6. Auscultation is the act of listening for sounds produced within
   the body with the unaided ear or with a stethoscope.
   The chest is clear to auscultation.
7. Bimanual is the use of both hands.
   Bimanual palpation was ineffective.
8. Blepharospasm is a spasm of the orbicular muscle of the eyelid.
   Renee has a history of blepharospasm.
9. Bleb is a bulla or blister.
   Using sterile procedure and raising a small bleb of lidocaine, a
   #22 gauge needle was introduced.
10. Bruit is a sound or murmur heard on auscultation.
    No abdominal bruits were heard.
11. Buccal pertains to the cheek.
    Buccal mucosa is moist.
12. Chlamydia is a widespread genus of gram-negative, nonmotile
    bacteria.
    DNA probe for chlamydia was obtained.
13. Cyanosis is the bluish discoloration of the skin and mucous
    membranes due to excessive concentration of reduced
    hemoglobin in the blood.
    The patient's extremities were without clubbing, cyanosis, or
    pedal edema.
14. Decubitus is the state of lying down.
    The patient was placed in the left lateral decubitus position, and
    a digital rectal exam was performed.

15. Distal is the farthest from any point of reference, remote.
Distal pulses are intact.
16. Doxycycline is a generic name for a broad-spectrum antibiotic that is active against a wide range of gram-positive and gram-negative organisms.
I will begin treatment with doxycycline.
17. Dysmenorrhea is painful menstruation.
She presents with a one-year history of dysmenorrhea that has worsened over the past three months.
18. Dyspnea is labored or difficult breathing.
No chest pain, leg cramps or exertional dyspnea was noted.
19. Dysuria is painful or difficult urination.
She denies any dysuria.
20. Edema is the accumulation of excess fluid in the tissues of the body.
Extremities show no edema.
21. Effusion is the escape of fluid from blood vessels because of rupture or seepage, usually into a body cavity.
There is no evidence of effusion.
22. Erythema is redness of the skin.
We are concerned about the erythema and associated warmth that is occurring after only minimal amounts of time on her feet.
23. Evert is to turn inside out.
The eyelid was everted and examined.
24. Exacerbation is the increase in the severity of a disease or its symptoms.
Mr. Franklin has had further exacerbation of multiple sclerosis.
25. Exudate is an accumulation of fluid in the tissues.
The pharynx appears injected with some possible left anterior tonsillar exudates.
26. Flank is the side of the body between the ribs and ilium.
The patient had no organomegaly or flank discomfort.
27. Fundus is the bottom or base of an organ.
Fundi of the eyes were benign.
28. Gallop is an abnormal rhythm of the heart.
The cardiac exam revealed heart regular in rate and rhythm without murmurs, rubs, or gallops appreciated.
29. Ganglion is a knot or knotlike mass.
She has a history of a previous carpal tunnel release and ganglion cyst excision.
30. Granuloma is a small nodular, tumor, or growth.
Calcified granuloma is noted in the right lung, laterally.
31. Guarding is a body defense method to prevent movement of an injured part.
Normal bowel sounds with no masses or guarding.
32. Hemoptysis is the coughing and spitting of blood.
No cough, hemoptysis, or SOB was noted.
33. Hepatosplenomegaly is the enlargement of the liver and spleen.
No hepatosplenomegaly or masses were noted.
34. Hyperlipidemia is the elevated concentrations of any or all lipids in the plasma.
Her history is also notable for hyperlipidemia.
35. Labyrinthitis is the inflammation of the internal ear, otitis interna.
The patient was assessed with probable acute labyrinthitis.
36. Lamina is a thin, flat layer.
Mild lamina propria edema was noted of the mucosa.
37. Laparoscope is an endoscope for examining the peritoneal cavity.
In 1988 she underwent a laparoscopy at Community Hospital that showed pelvic adhesions.
38. Lingula is a small tongue-shaped anatomic structure.
There is a questionable early lingular infiltrate on the left.
39. Meclizine is a generic name for an antiemetic especially effective for control of nausea and vomiting for motion sickness.
The patient will be treated with 25 mg of meclizine p.r.n.
40. Mucosa is the mucous membrane.
Nasal mucosa is clear.
41. Myalgia is muscular pain.
A 32-year-old white male presents with sore throat, nonproductive cough, nasal congestion, and myalgia for the past 4 days.
42. Myringotomy is a incision of the tympanic membrane.
She has had a myringotomy as a child.

43. Nystagmus is an involuntary rapid rhythmic movement of the eyeball.
No nystagmus was noted.
44. Orthopnea is the ability to breathe easily only in an upright position.
No chest pain, edema, orthopnea, leg cramps or exertional dyspnea was noted.
45. Os is an opening, mouth, or bone.
Examination reveals small amount of blood from the cervical os.
46. Palpitation is an unusually rapid, strong, or irregular heartbeat.
No chest pain, edema, palpitations, orthopnea, leg cramps or exertional dyspnea was noted.
47. Penicillin is a generic name for any of a large group of natural or semisynthetic antibacterial antibiotics.
He is allergic to penicillin.
48. Perirectal is around the rectum.
Her perirectal area appeared normal.
49. Polypoid resembles a polyp.
A small polypoid lesion was identified in the sigmoid colon.
50. Pruritus ani is the intense chronic itching in the anal region.
I am referring Ms. Biscuit to you for pruritus ani.
51. Rebound is a reversed response occurring upon withdrawal of a stimulus.
The abdomen was soft, nontender, without guarding or rebound.
52. Rhinitis is the inflammation of the mucous membrane of the nose.
Renee has a history of seasonal allergic rhinitis.
53. Rhonchus is an abnormal sound heard on chest auscultation due to an obstructed airway.
The lungs are clear to aeration, but positive to transient rhonchi in the mid and upper lung fields.
54. Sigmoidoscopy is the examination of the interior of the sigmoid colon.
Ms. Biscuit has had persistent rectal itching and was advised to have a sigmoidoscopy.
55. Sputum is the mucous secretion from the lungs, bronchi, and trachea that is ejected through the mouth.
No cough, sputum production, hemoptysis or SOB was noted.
56. Sulfacetamide is a generic name for an ophthalmic antibiotic.
Two drops of sulfacetamide were placed in the eye.
57. Terpin is used as an expectorant.
We will treat the patient with terpin hydrate with codeine, 1-2 tsp. at h.s.
58. Thyromegaly is an enlargement of the thyroid gland.
There is no thyromegaly or mass.
59. Uvula is a small soft structure hanging from the free edge of the soft palate.
Tongue and uvula are midline.
60. Vulva is the external genital organs in the female.
She also had noticed some itching in the vulva area.
61. Amoxil is the trade name for a preparation of amoxicillin, an antibiotic.
The patient was placed on Amoxil 500 mg p.o. t.i.d. × 10 days.
62. Augmentin is the trade name for a preparation of amoxicillin, an antibiotic.
The patient was placed on Augmentin 500 mg p.o. t.i.d. × 2 weeks.
63. Biaxin is the trade name for an antibiotic.
He was treated with Biaxin 500 mg b.i.d.
64. Botox is the trade name for a powder for extraocular muscle injection.
Renee has a history of blepharospasm, for which she receives Botox injections, as well as seasonal allergic rhinitis.
65. Claritin is the trade name for a nonsedating antihistamine.
Claritin is controlling her allergy symptoms.
66. Copolymer is the trade name for one of the immune modulating drugs.
The disease has progressed to the point that it would be beneficial to place him on Copolymer.
67. Cytotec is the trade name for a drug used for the prevention of NSAID-induced gastric ulcers.
I have placed him on Cytotec 100 mg q.i.d.

68. Darvocet is the trade name for a fixed combination preparation analgesic and an antipyretic.
The patient occasionally used Darvocet for pain.

69. Ditropan is the trade name for an urinary antispasmodic.
She states the Ditropan has worked wonders for her bladder.

70. E.E.S. is the trade name for an antibiotic.
We will treat the patient with E.E.S. 400 mg 1 q.i.d. and terpin hydrate with codeine 1-2 teaspoons at h.s. only.

71. Evista is the trade name for a selective estrogen receptor modulator (SERM) for the prevention of postmenopausal osteoporosis.
Her current medications include Evista 60 mg p.o. q.d.

72. Indocin is the trade name for a nonsteroidal anti-inflammatory drug, NSAID.
I have placed him on Indocin 50 mg p.o. t.i.d.

73. Klonopin is the trade name for an anticonvulsant.
She attributes her improvement, in part, to her B-12 injections, and Klonopin.

74. Lipitor is the trade name for an antihyperlipidemic that reduces cholesterol synthesis.
She is also taking Lipitor 10 mg p.o. q.h.s.

75. Lo-Ovral is the trade name for an oral contraceptive.
She was on the Lo-Ovral for about two weeks but continued to have bleeding.

76. Melatonex is the trade name for a sleep aid.
Melatonex did not help her sleep; in fact, it made her insomnia worse.

77. Naprosyn is the trade name for a nonsteroidal anti-inflammatory drug, NSAID.
I have discontinued his Naprosyn and placed him on Indocin 50 mg p.o. t.i.d., which is in addition to his Cytotec 100 mg q.i.d.

78. Neosporin is the trade name for a topical antibiotic.
She is intolerant to Neosporin.

79. Norvasc is the trade name for a calcium channel blocker, antihypertensive.
I am increasing the Norvasc to 5 mg b.i.d.

80. Ophthetic is the trade name for proparacaine hydrochloride, eye drops.
The eye was instilled with some Ophthetic eye drops.

81. Ortho-Tri-Cyclen is the trade name for a triphasic oral contraceptive.
Milly has a two-month history of persistent bleeding out of cycle while taking Ortho-Tri-Cyclen.

82. Paxil is the trade name for an antidepressant.
She attributes her improvement, in part, to her B-12 injections, and the Paxil and Klonopin medications.

83. Persantine is the trade name for an antiplatelet agent.
He is allergic to penicillin and Persantine.

84. Phenergan is the trade name for an antihistamine, antiemetic.
He was given a prescription for Phenergan 25 mg p.o. b.i.d.

85. Prilosec is the trade name for a gastric acid secretion inhibitor.
He was treated with Prilosec 20 mg b.i.d.

86. Proctocream HC is the trade name for topical corticosteroidal anti-inflammatory used as anorectal cream.
Ms. Biscuit has tried Proctocream HC several months prior to this appointment with no improvement noted.

87. Skelaxin is the trade name for a skeletal muscle relaxant.
I have prescribed Skelaxin 400 mg t.i.d. p.r.n.

88. Triamcinolone is the trade name for a corticosteroid.
She did have a vulvar dermatitis, which responded well to treatment with Triamcinolone.

89. Vancenase is the trade name for a corticosteroid for bronchial asthma; pocket inhaler.
The patient was prescribed Vancenase AQ inhaler 1 puff each nostril t.i.d.

90. Xylocaine is the trade name for preparations of lidocaine and is classified as an antiarrhythmic, anesthetic.
There is marked trigger point tenderness in the left rhomboid area, which had been treated with a 1% Xylocaine injection.

CHAPTER 5 / PART I CHECK YOUR PROGRESS

1. a	24. d	47. b	69. a
2. b	25. b	48. c	70. a
3. a	26. c	49. b	71. a
4. d	27. c	50. a	72. a
5. c	28. a	51. c	73. c
6. c	29. d	52. a	74. b
7. b	30. c	53. a	75. b
8. c	31. a	54. a	76. b
9. a	32. a	55. c	77. b
10. a	33. a	56. b	78. c
11. a	34. d	57. a	79. c
12. b	35. b	58. b	80. b
13. d	36. a	59. c	81. d
14. a	37. a	60. b	82. b
15. b	38. c	61. a	83. a
16. c	39. c	62. b	84. c
17. c	40. c	63. c	85. c
18. d	41. a	64. d	86. d
19. a	42. a	65. c	87. b
20. b	43. c	66. c	88. c
21. a	44. a	67. c	89. a
22. c	45. b	68. d	90. a
23. b	46. d		

Current date

Barry Cortex, MD
Southside Urological Associates
767 Lithiasis Drive
New York, NY 10001

Re: Thomas Gier
     Date of Birth: December 9, 19xx

Dear Dr. Cortex

I am referring this 76-year-old white male to you for evaluation of an abnormal urine analysis discovered during a physical examination performed (current date). He has a long history of vascular disease, diabetes, and hypertension. He has undergone CABG surgery as well as bilateral carotid endarterectomies. He has no pulses in his lower extremities and is, therefore, not a candidate for vascular surgery. He is allergic to penicillin and Persantine. He cannot receive ACE inhibitors because of right renal atrophy. His latest multiphasic screen of two weeks ago revealed blood sugar of 137, creatinine of 1.6, BUN of 33, and uric acid of 8.8. His urinalysis revealed 4+ occult blood, 2+ protein, and his PSA was 0.5. He is on chronic anticoagulation, and his prothrombin time was 26.4 with an INR of 5.4. This has since been corrected. His sedimentation rate is 42. He also had three negative urine cytology evaluations. A retroperitoneal ultrasound showed significant renal size asymmetry, with evidence of right renal atrophy, but no hydronephrosis.

Although the abnormal urine findings are consistent with his abnormal kidney, I would appreciate your opinion as to whether a cystoscopy is indicated. If you have any questions regarding this patient, please call me at your pleasure.

Sincerely

P.H. Waters, MD

xx

Errors are indicated in bold and italics. Margins are formatted at 1 inch.
CHART NOTE

Patient Name: Harris, Donna

Date of Birth: *October 21, 1950*

Examination Date: *Current date*

SUBJECTIVE: Donna comes in today for *a follow up.* Her weight *has,* fortunately, stayed the same. She still feels weak. Her blood *work* looks good. X-ray demonstrates prominent markings in the *right* middle lobe and a questionable nodular density in the *right* apex. Her appetite remains about the same. Her living situation is unchanged*;* and despite our best efforts, we have really not been able to help her significantly with this.

OBJECTIVE: Weight 92 *lb,* BP 120/68. She has no cervical *adenopathy.* Lungs show decreased *breath* sounds. Cardiac exam *regular in rate and rhythm* without murmurs, rubs, or gallops appreciated. She has normal chest *wall* excursion. Abdomen is soft. She has some tenderness in the right rib cage.

ASSESSMENT:
1. *Chronic obstructive pulmonary disease.*
2. Weight loss which, at this point, has stabilized.

PLAN: I am planning to check apical lordotic views of this abnormality in her lung and have them compared to previous films. I will continue to follow her weight loss. I doubt that she has lung cancer*;* but just to make sure, I will *re-evaluate the* right upper lobe a little better. At this point, I plan to follow her rib pain as well. I really *was not* able to elicit much information today.

Charles P. Davis, MD/xx

CHAPTER 5 / PART II ACTIVITY 5

Current date

J. Thomas Geiger, MD
Family Practice Division, Suite 300
101 Wellness Way Drive
New York, NY 10036

Re: Charlotte Mekola
     Date of Birth: October 19, 1958
     Examination: CHEST

Dear Dr. Geiger

There is a substantial area of alveolar infiltrate that involves the superior segment of the right lower lobe. I do not identify a mass or any definite hilar adenopathy. The lungs are otherwise clear. There is probably an element of COPD. The heart is mildly enlarged, but the pulmonary vessels do not appear prominent. There is no effusion. The visualized bony thorax and soft tissues are remarkable for an accentuated kyphosis and probable osteoporosis.

IMPRESSION: Alveolar infiltrate in the superior segment of the right lower lobe. Simple pneumonia is the most likely diagnosis. A follow up until clearing is recommended.

Thank you for referring this patient to us.

Yours truly

Potter Bucky, MD

xx

CHAPTER 5 / PART II ACTIVITY 6 (5T-3)

CHART NOTE

Patient Name: Synder, Patty

Date of Birth: May 10, 1958

Examination Date: *Current date*

CHIEF COMPLAINT: Right shoulder pain.

SUBJECTIVE: She presents today with intermittent pain of the right shoulder for the past two months. The pain has become increasingly more severe over the past two days. One week ago, I injected the subacromial bursa with steroids, resulting in a rather dramatic improvement in her bursitis. Unfortunately this was short lived as she returns today with complaints of right shoulder pain.

OBJECTIVE: Upon examination, the patient could barely abduct past 30 degrees. An x-ray in AP internal and external rotation was obtained that showed notable calcific tendinitis.

ASSESSMENT: Right rotator cuff tendinitis.

PLAN: I have placed her on a physical therapy program. We have discussed her referral to an orthopedic specialist if no improvement is seen.

_____

Izzy Sertoli, MD/xx

CHAPTER 5 / PART II ACTIVITY 7 (5T-4)

Current date

FedDes Wellness Center
Gastroenterology Division, Suite 279
101 Wellness Way Drive
New York, NY 10036

Re: George Jenum
     Date of Birth: April 30, 19xx

Dear Dr. Cobalamin

I am referring Mr. George Jenum to you for further evaluation of a mild anemia. George is a 59-year-old gentleman who presented with a viral syndrome at the end of October 20xx. He had symptoms consistent with a viral gastrointestinal infection, but because of persistent epigastric discomfort, an H. pylori titer was obtained. It was positive for H. pylori antibodies, and he was treated with Prilosec 20 mg b.i.d., Biaxin 500 mg b.i.d., and Amoxicillin 1 gm b.i.d. × 10 days. Mr. Jenum's gastritis and abdominal pain has resolved, but he has persistent leukopenia, monocytosis, and a borderline anemia.

Despite serial monitoring, he continued with mild, yet persistent abnormalities in his CBC. A manual differential count shows increasing anemia. Other recent anemia studies, including iron studies, failed to suggest an etiology for his anemia. CEA and PSA tests also came back normal.

I believe you have already received the results of all of Mr. Jenum's laboratory studies. I hope this information is helpful. I look forward to hearing from you regarding suggestions toward the evaluation and care of Mr. Jenum.

Sincerely

Izzy Sertoli, MD

xx

CHAPTER 5 / PART II CHECK YOUR PROGRESS

See Pretest (5T-2).

CHART NOTE

Patient Name: Lang, Stewart

Date of Birth: September 9, 1968

Examination Date: *Current date*

SUBJECTIVE: Patient presents today with an eight-day course of flu symptoms. He complains of head congestion and a persistent cough. He also reports intermittent vomiting and diarrhea for three days. The last time he vomited was 4-5 hours ago. The diarrhea has been less frequent over the last 12 hours. He has been eating saltine crackers, dry toast, and Jell-O. He is not using any over-the-counter medications for self-treatment.

OBJECTIVE: Weight 178 lb, temperature 97.6, BP 136/86, pulse 76. Stewart appears in no acute distress. TMs are normal bilaterally. Nasopharynx is clear. Neck is supple without adenopathy. Lungs are clear to A&P. Heart is regular in rate and rhythm. The abdomen is soft and nontender. Normal bowel sounds with no masses or guarding.

ASSESSMENT: Flu syndrome and viral gastroenteritis.

PLAN:
1. He was given a prescription for Phenergan 25 mg. He may take 1 q.4-6h. as needed for the nausea and vomiting over the next 48 hours.
2. He is to continue with the bland diet and increase fluids.
3. I will recheck if symptoms persist.

J. Thomas Geiger, MD/xx

HISTORY AND PHYSICAL EXAMINATION REPORT

Patient Name: Miers, Tamara

File Number: 245689

Date of Birth: July 1, 19xx

Examination Date: *Current date*

Physician: Charles P. Davis, MD

HISTORY

CHIEF COMPLAINT: Right knee pain.

HISTORY OF PRESENT ILLNESS: The patient is a 68-year-old female with a past medical history significant for aortic valve replacement.

PAST MEDICAL HISTORY: The patient has a long history of DJD of both knees. She recalls no specific injury to the right knee, but has noticed increasing pain over the past several months. An MRI of the right knee revealed a tear of the medial meniscus.

Her past medical history is also significant for aortic valve replacement that was performed in August of 1999 at University Hospital. She has a St. Jude-type valve in place. Her history is also notable for hyperlipidemia. She is postmenopausal.

ALLERGIES: The patient has experienced hives with pencillin. She is intolerant to Neosporin.

MEDICATIONS: Her current medications include Evista 60 mg p.o. q.d. and Lipitor 10 mg p.o. q.h.s.

FAMILY HISTORY: Remarkable for coronary artery disease and lung cancer.

SOCIAL HISTORY: The patient smokes one pack of cigarettes per day. She rarely drinks alcohol. She does not exercise regularly. She wears her seat belt. She is a retired engineer. She is widowed, but resides with one of her three children.

REVIEW OF SYSTEMS

HEENT: No complaints.

CARDIOVASCULAR: No chest pain, edema, palpitations, orthopnea, leg cramps or exertional dyspnea.

------------------------ begin page 2 ------------------------

RESPIRATORY: No cough, sputum production, hemoptysis or SOB.

GASTROINTESTINAL: No nausea, vomiting, diarrhea, or constipation.

GENITOURINARY: No problems.

MUSCULOSKELETAL: See HPI.

SKIN: No problems.

NEUROPSYCHIATRIC: No problems.

PHYSICAL EXAMINATION

GENERAL: Widowed, white female in no active distress. Weight 176 lb, BP 120/60, pulse 76 and regular.

EYES: Conjunctivae clear, PERRLA, EOMs intact. Fundi benign.

EARS, NOSE, THROAT: Ears and nose normal, externally. EACs and TMs normal. Oropharynx is clear.

NECK: Supple. There is no thyromegaly or mass.

LUNGS: Clear to auscultation.

HEART: Regular sinus rhythm. Carotid upstrokes were 2+. No bruits.

ABDOMEN: Soft, nontender, normal abdominal bowel sounds. No hepatosplenomegaly or masses. No abdominal bruits.

EXTREMITIES: Distal pulses are intact.

NEUROLOGICAL: Exam is unremarkable.

------------------------ begin page 3 ------------------------

IMPRESSION: The patient is an 68-year-old female with a past medical history significant for aortic valve replacement.

PLAN: She will be referred to an orthopedist for possible arthroscopic surgery of the right knee.

Charles P. Davis, MD/xx

CHAPTER 5 / 5T-7

CHART NOTE

Patient Name: Clark, Bertram

Date of Birth: November 20, 1926

Examination Date: *Current date*

SUBJECTIVE: He was grinding stones and got some metal in his left eye even though he was wearing protective glasses at the time of the injury. He presents with pain and a feeling that something is in his eye. This happened late this afternoon.

OBJECTIVE: His eye is slightly injected. There also appears to be a fine piece of steel in the lower eyelid. He also has a small speck of metal embedded into the cornea at approximately the 3 o'clock position.

ASSESSMENT: Foreign body, left eye.

PLAN: The eye was instilled with some Ophthetic eye drops. The eye was irrigated with sterile saline solution. A small metallic-looking speck was removed from the lower eyelid. The eyelid was everted and examined. No other abnormalities or foreign bodies were found. The eye was stained. I did not see any other ulcerations other than where the speck of what appeared to be a piece of metal was in the 3 o'clock position. However, this did not have any rust ring around it. The eye again was irrigated. The small piece of metal was gingerly removed from the 3 o'clock position with a #25 gauge needle. The entire foreign body was removed. There did not appear to be any rust ring associated with it. There was a small area of scratching noted where the foreign body was embedded and also from the needle. Again the eye was irrigated. At that point two drops of sulfacetamide were placed in the eye. He is to place in eye 2 drops q.2h. He will return tomorrow for a follow up.

_____

Charles P. Davis, MD/xx

CHAPTER 5 / 5T-8

CHART NOTE

Patient Name: Meckonni, James

Date of Birth: November 3, 1978

Examination Date: *Current date*

CHIEF COMPLAINT: Nasal congestion and facial pain.

SUBJECTIVE: His symptoms have been ongoing for approximately two weeks. He states that his upper teeth hurt at times and experiences increasing cranial pressure upon bending.

OBJECTIVE: Temperature 98.4, weight 144 lb, BP 128/74, pulse 56. The neck is supple with no adenopathy noted. The maxillary sinuses are minimally tender. Evaluation of the throat reveals only thick postnasal discharge. The chest is clear to auscultation. The heart is regular in rate and rhythm.

ASSESSMENT: Clinical sinusitis.

PLAN:
1. Augmentin 500 mg p.o. t.i.d. × 2 weeks.
2. Vancenase AQ inhaler 1 puff each nostril t.i.d.
3. Patient to return if not improving.

_____

Charles P. Davis, MD/xx

CHAPTER 5 / 5T-9

CHART NOTE

Patient Name: Chesterfield, Fredrick

Date of Birth: February 17, 1981

Examination Date: *Current date*

SUBJECTIVE: The patient presents today with a cough and sore throat for a week and a half. He presently has a slightly productive cough. He states that he coughs essentially nonstop. He has taken over-the-counter cough medicine and NyQuil with no relief. He also complains of feeling a catch in his throat.

OBJECTIVE: Weight 137 lb, BP 110/78, pulse 68, temperature 98. The patient appears in no acute distress. TMs are within normal limits, with no erythema noted. The pharynx is mildly erythematous without swelling. The neck is supple without adenopathy. The heart is regular in rate and rhythm. The lungs are clear to auscultation, but positive to transient rhonchi in the mid and upper lung fields.

ASSESSMENT: Bronchitis.

PLAN: We will treat the patient with E.E.S. 400 mg 1 q.i.d. and terpin hydrate with codeine 1-2 tsp at h.s. only. The patient is to use plain Robitussin 4-5 times during the day. Mr. Chesterfield will return in ten days for a recheck of his lungs.

_____

Charles P. Davis, MD/xx

CHAPTER 5 / 5T-10

CHART NOTE

Patient Name: Trepidor, Rodrigues

Date of Birth: May 18, 19xx

Examination Date: *Current date*

SUBJECTIVE: A 32-year-old white male presents with sore throat, nonproductive cough, nasal congestion, and myalgia for the past four days. The patient initially has had an intermittent low grade fever of 101.

OBJECTIVE: BP 98/60, pulse 72, temperature 98.2. His general appearance is that of a pleasant, nontoxic appearing 32-year-old male. TMs appear clear. The pharynx appears injected with some possible left anterior tonsillar exudates. The neck is supple with some mildly enlarged anterior adenopathy. The lungs are clear to A&P.

ASSESSMENT: Flu with possible exudative pharyngitis.

PLAN: Patient will be placed on Amoxil 500 mg p.o. t.i.d. × 10 days. He will return if no improvement is noted.

Charles P. Davis, MD/xx

CHART NOTE

Patient Name: Aswart, Sabine

Date of Birth: September 28, 1982

Examination Date: *Current date*

SUBJECTIVE: Patient comes in with episode of dizziness. She had vertigo last evening and again today. As long as her head was still, it was not a problem. If she moved her head quickly, it was much worse. She had no other associated neurological symptoms. She has had no earache, runny nose, sore throat, or cough.

OBJECTIVE: Neurological assessment is normal. No nystagmus. Carotids are equal bilaterally. TMs are normal. Reflexes symmetrical. Coordination and Romberg's sign were all within normal limits.

ASSESSMENT: Probable acute labyrinthitis.

PLAN: The patient will be treated with 25 mg of meclizine p.r.n. She has been instructed to take 1 aspirin tablet a day for an antiplatelet effect. The patient is return to us if there are any more problems. Sabine said she is feeling better than she felt in a long time, notably prior to the onset of this vertigo. She attributes this improvement, in part, to her B-12 injections, and the Paxil and Klonopin medications.

Charles P. Davis, MD/xx

PROCEDURE REPORT

Patient Name: Inshetski, Ann

File Number: 199022000

Date of Birth: July 3, 19xx

Examination Date: *Current date*

Procedure: FLEXIBLE SIGMOIDOSCOPY WITH BIOPSY.

ANESTHESIA: None.

PROCEDURE: After obtaining appropriate informed consent, the patient was placed in the left lateral decubitus position and a digital rectal exam was performed. A flexible sigmoidoscope was inserted in the usual fashion and passed approximately 55 cm, freely through the colon. A small polypoid lesion was identified in the sigmoid colon. Biopsies were taken and the scope was retracted and removed. No other abnormalities were noted.

I have informed the patient that if this is an adenomatous polyp, a colonoscopy is indicated. If this is a benign polyp, no other invasive procedures will be recommended.

IMPRESSION: Sigmoid polyp, diminutive, approximately 5 mm.

PLAN: Rule out adenoma.

Charles P. Davis, MD/xx

HISTORY AND PHYSICAL EXAMINATION REPORT

Patient Name: Stephano, Jennifer

File Number: 78901

Date of Birth: October 18, 1979

Examination Date: *Current date*

HISTORY

CHIEF COMPLAINT: Jenny comes in today for a sports physical examination.

HISTORY OF PRESENT ILLNESS: She has no complaints or concerns. She does wear contact lenses or glasses. No chest pain or SOB. Her bowels move regularly. No urinary symptoms.

PAST HISTORY: She has had no major medical problems or recent hospitalizations. She attained menarche about age 12. Her periods are regular, moderate in intensity, and last about seven days. She has had a myringotomy as a child.

ALLERGIES: No known allergies.

MEDICATIONS: None.

PHYSICAL EXAMINATION

GENERAL: Weight 148 lb, height 67 in., BP 122/60. Visual acuity is 20/30 both in the left and right eye, but corrected 20/25.

HEENT: TMs within normal limits, bilaterally.

EYES: PERRLA, EOMs intact. Fundi benign.

EARS: Oropharynx, normal.

NOSE, MOUTH, THROAT, TEETH: Tongue and uvula are midline. Buccal mucosa is moist. Dentition is in good repair.

NECK: Supple, no adenopathy. No thyroid masses palpated.

HEART: Regular.

----------------------- begin page 2 -----------------------

LUNGS: Clear to P&A.

ABDOMEN: Soft, nontender. No organomegaly or flank discomfort.

EXTREMITIES: No edema. No laxity of the knees or ankles. Good ROM is noted. Good strength. Good grips, bilaterally. DTRs intact.

NEUROLOGICAL: Intact.

ASSESSMENT: Well-child sports physical examination.

PLAN: May play soccer. No restriction. Patient to follow up as needed.

_____

Charles P. Davis, MD/xx

CHAPTER 5 / 5T-14

CHART NOTE

Patient Name: Smythers, Jane

Date of Birth: March 15, 1973

Examination Date: *Current date*

CHIEF COMPLAINT: Cold symptoms.

HISTORY OF PRESENT ILLNESS: Cold symptoms since Friday. Patient complains of sore throat, congestion and fever. No change in appetite. Cough is sometimes minimally productive. There is some SOB, but no wheezing or tightness in the chest. No history of asthma. No nausea, vomiting, diarrhea, or constipation. She has had some abdominal cramps.

PHYSICAL EXAMINATION

GENERAL: Weight 154 lb, temperature 98.

EYES: Conjunctivae clear.

HEENT: Ears and nose normal externally. TMs normal. EACs clear. Nasal mucosa is clear. Oropharynx is injected.

NECK: Supple. There is no thyromegaly, mass, or adenopathy.

LUNGS: Clear to P&A.

HEART: Regular sinus rhythm.

LABORATORY: Rapid Strep test is negative.

ASSESSMENT: Viral upper respiratory infection.

PLAN: Advised patient to increase fluids and rest. Over-the-counter cold medications p.r.n. Patient is to return for a follow-up visit if there is no improvement.

_____

P. H. Waters, MD/xx

CHART NOTE

Patient Name: Mermain, Devon

Date of Birth: March 25, 19xx

Examination Date: *Current date*

CHIEF COMPLAINT: Patient presents for a yearly check up.

HISTORY OF PRESENT ILLNESS. He is a third grader and is doing well. He does have allergies. Immunizations are up to date.

PHYSICAL EXAMINATION

GENERAL: He weighs 85 lb and is 55 in tall. He is a rather pleasant youngster in no active distress.

HEENT: Negative. No nodes.

CHEST: Clear to P&A.

HEART: The heart is regular in rhythm with no murmur.

ABDOMEN: Negative.

GENITOURINARY: Testes descended bilaterally.

BACK: No scoliosis. Gait normal.

NEUROLOGICAL: Intact.

ASSESSMENT: Normal 9-year-old exam.

PLAN: We should see him again in 2-3 years at his school physical assessment or yearly as the mother wishes.

_____

Izzy Sertoli, MD/xx

X-RAY REPORT

Patient Name: Holtzworth, Max

File Number: 498321

Date of Birth: August 28, 1962

Examination Date: *Current date*

Examination: PA AND LATERAL CHEST X-RAY

HISTORY: Cough, shortness of breath. History of colon cancer.

FINDINGS: PA and lateral views of the chest are compared to a previous study dated (1 month ago). There is hyperexpansion, compatible with COPD. There is no evidence of effusion. The bones are intact. Calcified granuloma is noted in the right lung, laterally. Chronic changes are noted in the right base. There is a questionable early lingular infiltrate on the left. A repeat chest x-ray is recommended to document clearing. The cardiac silhouette is not enlarged. The hilum, mediastinum, and trachea are unremarkable.

IMPRESSION:
1. Marked hyperexpansion, compatible with COPD.
2. Questionable early lingular infiltrate.
3. Chronic changes, bilaterally.

P. H. Waters, MD/xx

CHART NOTE

Patient Name: Margolis, Davy

Date of Birth: September 5, 1973

Examination Date: *Current date*

CHIEF COMPLAINT: Patient returns today for a recheck of his left ankle pain.

HISTORY OF PRESENT ILLNESS: He has had some improvement, but not much. Radiologist review of his x-ray is consistent with an ankle effusion. Recent blood work is notable for a negative ASO. Sedimentation rate is slightly elevated at 17. There remains some swelling about the left ankle. The effusion seems to be less prominent. There is normal ROM. No pain with ROM.

PROCEDURE: Using sterile procedure and raising a small bleb of lidocaine, a #22 gauge needle was introduced just medial to the medial malleolus and 3 cc of yellow serous fluid was removed. The synovial fluid will be sent for analysis.

ASSESSMENT: Right ankle arthritis with effusion.

PLAN: I have discontinued his Naprosyn and placed him on Indocin 50 mg p.o. t.i.d., which is in addition to his Cytotec 100 mg q.i.d. I have ordered additional blood work to include an ANA, CBC, uric acid and lipid analysis. He is to return for a recheck in one week.

P. H. Waters, MD/xx

CHART NOTE

Patient Name: Duke, Marge

Date of Birth: October 15, 1983

Examination Date: *Current date*

CHIEF COMPLAINT: Nasal congestion with maxillary and frontal sinus pain.

HISTORY OF PRESENT ILLNESS: Patient presents with nasal congestion and maxillary and frontal sinus discomfort. Thick yellow nasal discharge with low grade x 2 weeks. There is some dyspnea, but no wheezing or tightness in the chest.

PHYSICAL EXAMINATION: Weight 124 lb, temperature 102. Eyes: Conjunctivae are clear. Frontal and maxillary sinuses are sensitive to palpation. Thick yellow discharge noted. TMs normal. Oropharynx is injected. Neck is supple. The lungs are clear to auscultation. Heart is in regular sinus rhythm.

ASSESSMENT: Sinusitis.

PLAN: The patient will use over-the-counter decongestants and ibuprofen for fever and pain. Erythromycin 250 mg t.i.d. x 10 days. She will return for a follow-up visit if there is no improvement.

Gwenn Maltase, MD/xx

CHART NOTE

Patient Name: Levy, Susan

Date of Birth: December 20, 1977

Examination Date: *Current date*

CHIEF COMPLAINT: Patient complains since Thursday of being achy with a sore throat and a slight stiff neck.

HISTORY OF PRESENT ILLNESS: She denies fever, chills, or rash. She has a slight headache. Some loss of appetite, but no nausea, vomiting, or diarrhea. No sinus symptoms. No other family members are currently ill. No history of recent travel.

PHYSICAL EXAMINATION: Weight is 169, BP 122/85, pulse 64 and regular, temperature 98.2. HEENT: Ears appear normal. Sinuses are nontender. Throat shows mild erythema; no exudate. Neck: Supple, with no lymphadenopathy. Some tenderness experienced in the posterior cervical muscles. Lungs are clear. Heart is regular in rate and rhythm. Abdomen is negative. Rapid Strep test negative.

ASSESSMENT: Probable viral illness.

PLAN: Will just treat with ibuprofen, rest and fluids. She will call if not improving over the next 24-48 hours, or if new symptoms develop.

_____

Gwenn Maltase, MD/xx

CHAPTER 5 / 5T-20

Current date

Mr. Ben Over
Customer Services
Simon Seez Managed Care, Inc.
911 Dividend Drive
Cashflow, NY 10039

Re: Samuel Franklin
    Date of Birth: January 1, 1986

Dear Mr. Over

Mr. Franklin has had further exacerbation of multiple sclerosis. His legs became weak a couple of months ago, but his strength has gradually returned. Today he complains of leg cramps, along with stiffness in the left leg and deterioration of ambulation.

On exam, he walks without help but does have a limp. The strength in his legs is normal, but coordination is definitely affected. Reflexes are symmetrical. He is also having bladder and bowel difficulties.

The disease has progressed to the point that it would be beneficial to place him on one of the immune modulating drugs, preferably, Copolymer. He is very willing to undergo treatment with this drug. Since he is an HMO patient, I am requesting that approval be granted for placing him on this treatment regimen. If approved, I will need to see him every couple of months for the first six months. Follow-up visits will be adjusted according to his response to the medication.

Thank you for your timely assistance in Mr. Franklin's treatment plan.

Sincerely

J. Thomas Geiger, MD

xx

CHAPTER 5 / 5T-21

Current date

David Treppe, MD
Orthopedic Division, Suite 133
FedDes Wellness Center
New York, NY 10036

Re: Betty Ross
    Date of Birth: September 15, 19xx

Dear Dr. Treppe

Thank you for the physical therapy referral of your patient.

The patient is a 44-year-old female presenting today with a diagnosis of cervical myalgia and a trapezius muscle spasm of the left shoulder. Mrs. Ross reports onset of symptoms related to 22 hours of nearly continuous sewing of a 30-foot flag for a high school production. She has been placed on anti-inflammatory medication, a muscle relaxant, and pain medication. She reports loss of strength affecting the left upper extremity as a pre-existing condition. She has a history of a previous carpal tunnel release and ganglion cyst excision. She has a history of asthma and is a smoker.

PHYSICAL THERAPY EVALUATION: Her left glenohumeral mobility is essentially within normal limits, with slight end range pain in internal rotation. There is tenderness to palpation of the anterior glenohumeral capsule. Cervical range of motion is restricted at 75% of normal rotation to the left side. Flexion, extension, and right-side bending are essentially within normal limits. There is left-sided point tenderness over the C5-C6 paraspinal areas. There is marked trigger point tenderness in the left rhomboid area, which had been treated with a 1% Xylocaine injection.

I started her on a treatment program today of applying moist heat to the neck and left shoulder. This was followed by massage and ultrasound therapy. My plan is to have Mrs. Ross returning here for three additional sessions as you prescribed. Goals of the physical therapy will be to restore normal, pain-free cervical and left shoulder biomechanics. Mrs. Ross is currently off work at both her regular

---------------------- begin page 2 ----------------------

part-time secretarial job Enterprise Catering Services and additionally from her self-employed status as a seamstress. My long-term objective will be to have her be able to return to unrestricted employment.

Thank you again for this referral.

Sincerely

Melissa A. Anconeus, MS, PT

xx

CHAPTER 5 / 5T-22

CHART NOTE

Patient Name: Lee, My

Date of Birth: May 26, 1959

Examination Date: *Current date*

SUBJECTIVE: Patient presents today for a Pap smear and physical examination. She has also been having some problems with neck discomfort for the last six months. She has noticed that the discomfort is worse when she is under stress or has worked more than eight hours.

OBJECTIVE: Weight 128 lb, height 5 ft 5 in, BP 120/78, pulse 71 and regular. The patient is gravida I, para I. She had a cyst removed from the right breast in 1998.

ASSESSMENT: The physical examination is normal except for the previously mentioned cervical spine pain. Cervical spine x-rays are within normal limits, although they did reveal some cervical spasm.

PLAN: Recommended that the patient begin cervical neck exercises. I have prescribed Skelaxin 400 t.i.d. p.r.n. She is to return to the office for a fasting Astra IV, a TSH, and an erythrocyte sedimentation rate laboratory test. Education for the prevention of sexually transmitted diseases and birth control measures was reinforced.

_____

Izzy Sertoli, MD/xx

CHAPTER 5 / 5T-23

HISTORY AND PHYSICAL EXAMINATION REPORT

Patient Name: Feiffer, Madeline

File Number: 59011

Date of Birth: April 27, 19xx

Examination Date: *Current date*

HISTORY

HISTORY OF PRESENT ILLNESS: Madeline is a 25-year-old white female, gravida II, para II whose last menstrual period was two months ago. She is 12-weeks amenorrheic with complaints of vaginal spotting for the past 3 days. Her symptoms have progressed to increased bleeding, cramping, and passing vaginal clots. No shortness of breath or chest pain is noted. No change in bowel or bladder habits.

PAST MEDICAL HISTORY: No history of tubal infections or other gynecologic problems.

ALLERGIES: No known drug allergies.

FAMILY HISTORY: Noncontributory.

SOCIAL HISTORY: Noncontributory.

REVIEW OF SYSTEMS: See HPI. No other complaints.

PHYSICAL EXAMINATION

GENERAL: The patient is well-nourished, well-developed and alert. The skin is warm, dry, and without rashes. BP 128/84, temperature 99, pulse 92.

NECK: Supple. No thyroid enlargement.

BREASTS: Nontender without masses or discharge.

HEART: Regular rate and rhythm without murmurs or gallops.

LUNGS: Clear.

ABDOMEN: Soft, nontender, without guarding or rebound. No organomegaly.

----------------------- begin page 2 -----------------------

EXTERNAL GENITALIA: The vagina is without lesions. Vaginal bleeding and clots are present. The cervix is open 1-2 cm, with clots at the cervix and also bleeding. The uterus itself is anterior. It is soft, mobile and of a 12-week size. The adnexa are without masses or tenderness.

EXTREMITIES: Without clubbing, cyanosis, or pedal edema.

NEUROLOGICAL: Grossly intact.

IMPRESSION: Intrauterine pregnancy at 12 weeks with inevitable abortion.

PLAN: The patient will be sent for an obstetrics and gynecology consultation with a probable dilation and curettage.

_____

Matthew Sponch, MD/xx

CHAPTER 5 / PART III CHECK YOUR PROGRESS

See Pretests (5T-5) and (5T-6).

1. a: digit
2. b: Colles fracture
3. c: Smith fracture
4. c: rotator cuff tendinitis
5. d: synovia
6. a: avulsion
7. a: impingement
8. d: exostosis
9. b: lipoma
10. c: bilateral
11. a: Valsalva maneuver
12. c: osteophyte
13. a: apophysis
14. d: interarticular
15. a: genu varum
16. a: contusion
17. c: purulence
18. c: AP x-ray
19. b: posteromedial
20. a: ecchymosis
21. d: aspirate
22. a: lymphedema
23. c: effusion
24. a: arthroscopy
25. c: phalanx
26. a: crepitus
27. b: hypertrophy
28. a: tendinitis
29. a: greater trochanter
30. c: flexion
31. c: abduction
32. d: adduction
33. b: callus
34. a: turgor
35. c: peripheral
36. b: gluteus medius
37. a: pisiform
38. c: Fabre test
39. c: acromion

40. c: volar
41. c: arthroplasty
42. a: plantar
43. d: debridement
44. b: interosseous
45. a: fusiform
46. a: weightbearing
47. d: meniscectomy
48. b: symptomatology
49. b: trigger finger
50. c: radiation
51. b: work hardening
52. a: dorsiflexion
53. d: fasciculations
54. d: asymptomatic
55. b: trapezius
56. a: lymphadenopathy
57. a: meniscus
58. c: ulna
59. a: metatarsus
60. a: malleolus
61. b: calcaneus
62. a: radiculitis
63. d: paronychia
64. a: Lopressor
65. d: tetracycline
66. b: Percocet
67. b: Lipitor
68. c: Lanoxin
69. b: cortisone
70. a: codeine
71. a: Xylocaine
72. b: spironolactone
73. b: Biaxin
74. c: Vicoprofen
75. a: Keflex
76. b: Dolobid
77. c: Vicodin
78. d: penicillin

CHAPTER 6 / PART I ACTIVITY 3 (6T-1)

1. Abduction is the movement of an extremity away from midline.
   Her strength is mildly diminished in external rotation, good in internal and abduction.
2. Acromion is a spinous projection off the scapula.
   A Magnetic Resonance Imaging scan showed acromial spur, but no sign of a rotator cuff tear.
3. Adduction is the movement of an extremity toward the midline.
   She has pain with cross-chest adduction.
4. Apophysis is any outgrowth or swelling; a process or projection of a bone.
   X-rays show a fracture at the apophysis of the proximal fifth metatarsal that is displaced somewhat.
5. Arthroplasty is the reconstruction surgery to repair or reshape a diseased joint.
   As you know, she underwent hip arthroplasty in 1995 with an excellent result.
6. Arthroscopy is the examination of the interior of a joint with an arthroscope.
   We are going to proceed with arthroscopic subacromial decompression.
7. Aspirate is to draw in or out by suction.
   Her right knee was aspirated, and cortisone was injected today.
8. Asymptomatic is without symptoms.
   She, at this point, is asymptomatic.

9. Avulsion is the tearing away forcibly of a part or structure.
   He is a 39-year-old, right-hand dominant male who injured his left third finger yesterday at work and had an avulsion of the tip.
10. Bilateral is affecting or relating to two sides.
    She has well-healed carpal tunnel incisions bilaterally.
11. Calcaneus is the heel bone or os calcis.
    There are moderately sized posterior and plantar calcaneal spurs.
12. Callus is the new growth of bony tissue surrounding the bone ends in a fracture; part of the repair process of a fractured bone.
    X-ray examination shows no remarkable change in the position of the fragments, but I also do not see any remarkable callus formation yet.
13. Codeine is the generic name for an opioid analgesic.
    The patient is allergic to codeine.
14. Contusion is commonly called a *bruise*, where there is trauma to the body part but there is no break in the skin surface.
    There is some increased signal in the rotator cuff, but I think this more contusion.
15. Cortisone is the generic name for a corticosteroid, used to treat inflammations.
    The patient received cortisone injection to relieve the inflammation.
16. Crepitus is the grating sound of bone fragments rubbing together.
    He has had about a three-month history of pain and crepitus around the shoulder.
17. Debridement is the removal of dead or damaged tissue.
    It was stated to him that if it does not show improvement over the next 2-3 months, wrist arthroscopy could be entertained with debridement of his TFCC.
18. Digit is a finger or toe.
    On my exam today, she is no longer painful with resisted wrist or digit extension.
19. Dorsiflexion is to bend the joint toward the posterior aspect of the body.
    Dorsiflexion is 10 to 15 degrees with plantar flexion to 25 degrees.
20. Ecchymosis is the black and blue appearance of the skin.
    There is considerable ecchymosis and a little bit of deformity of the wrist.
21. Effusion is the escape of fluid from blood vessels because of rupture or seepage, usually into a body cavity.
    He has no effusion and good motion.
22. Exostosis is an abnormal, benign growth on the surface of a bone, also called *hyperostosis*.
    Tom returns with a chief complaint that his right lower leg is still painful in the area where the exostosis was removed.
23. Fasciculations are the uncontrolled twitching of a group of muscle fibers.
    No paraspinal spasm nor fasciculations were noted.
24. Flexion is the movement by a joint that decreases the angle between the two adjoining bones; the bending of a joint.
    Flexion was severely limited.
25. Fusiform is a spindle-shaped structure that is tapered at both ends.
    On examination today, she had 45 degrees of active flexion, fusiform swelling on the ulnar side of the PIP joint and tenderness of the synovium.
26. Genu varum is the Latin term for *bowleg*.
    Patient's gait is genu varum.
27. Gluteus medius is one of the three muscles that form the buttocks; acts to abduct and rotate the thigh.
    I have reviewed with her what was done in therapy; unfortunately, they did not initiate a gluteus medius stretching and strengthening program as I had ordered.
28. Greater trochanter is the large projection at the proximal end of the femur.
    The patient continues to demonstrate significant weakness with pain over the greater trochanter.
29. Hypertrophy is an increase in the size of an organ or structure.
    She has a large hypertrophic callus over the PIP joint, with an ingrown corn.

30. Interarticular is between two joints.
With his ulnar-sided wrist pain, recommendations today are interarticular cortisone injection to help with his discomfort and a removable Futura wrist splint to wear intermittently when doing activities.

31. Interosseous is situated or occurring between bone.
On examination, she had a deep, soft cystic mass in the area of the first dorsal interosseous, which was slightly tender to touch.

32. Lipoma is a benign tumor composed mostly of fat cells.
I ordered an MRI of the hand to determine if it was indeed a cystic or lipomatous lesion.

33. Lymphadenopathy is the disease of the lymph nodes.
He does have good sensation and good peripheral circulation with no edema or lymphadenopathy.

34. Lymphedema is edema due to obstruction of lymph vessels.
There is no lymphedema.

35. Malleolus is either of the two rounded projections on either side of the ankle joint.
Soft tissue swelling is present over both malleoli, particularly over the lateral malleolus.

36. Meniscectomy is the surgical removal of a meniscus.
Tom returns one week status post arthroscopy and partial medial meniscectomy, right knee.

37. Meniscus is the crescent-shaped fibrocartilage in the knee joint.
The lateral meniscus appears intact.

38. Metatarsus is any of the five long bones of the foot between the ankle and the toes.
X-rays show a fracture at the apophysis of the proximal fifth metatarsal that is displaced somewhat.

39. Osteophyte is an outgrowth of bone that is usually found around a joint.
His lumbar spine x-rays show only anterior osteophytes without disc space narrowing at the thoracolumbar junction, L2 and L4.

40. Paronychia is the inflammation involving the folds of tissue surrounding the nail.
The nail bed on the right great toe is healing well following removal of the nail for paronychia infection.

41. Penicillin is the generic name of any of a large group of antibacterial antibiotics derived from strains of fungi of the genus *Penicillium*.
The patient is allergic to penicillin.

42. Peripheral is occurring away from the center.
She can move her fingers okay and has good peripheral circulation and sensation.

43. Phalanx is the general term for any bone of a finger or toe.
On physical exam of his left third finger, there is a tip avulsion of soft tissue with bare bony exposure of his distal phalanx.

44. Pisiform is a pea-shaped, smallest carpal bone.
The pisiform is nontender to palpation and compression.

45. Plantar relates to the sole of the foot.
Dorsiflexion is 10 to 15 degrees with plantar flexion to 25 degrees.

46. Purulence means containing pus.
The right great toe has significant nail bed infection, erythema, purulence, and tenderness, particularly on the lateral nail fold area.

47. Radiculitis is the inflammation of a spinal nerve root.
He does get some aches around the upper back and neck area, but no true radiculitis symptoms.

48. Spironolactone is the generic name for a diuretic.
His medications included spironolactone, Lopressor, and aspirin.

49. Symptomatology is the symptoms of a specific disease.
She has shown improvement within her left trochanteric symptomatology, but incomplete resolution of her problems.

50. Synovia is the lubricating fluid of joints.
On examination today, she had 45 degrees of active flexion, fusiform swelling on the ulnar side of the PIP joint, and tenderness of the synovium.

51. Tendinitis is the inflammation of a tendon.
He appears to have a chronic cuff tendinitis with a mild impingement syndrome.

52. Tetracycline is the generic name for an antibiotic.
The patient was given tetracycline for the infection.

53. Trapezius is the muscles of the back of the neck and shoulder.
He has tenderness of the lower cervical spine and over the left trapezius, but he has full range of motion of his C-spine.

54. Turgor is the normal resiliency of the skin.
His skin turgor is normal.

55. Ulna is the inner and larger bone of the forearm, on the side opposite the thumb.
She noted both pain and swelling primarily on the ulnar side of the PIP joint.

56. Volar pertains to the palm of the hand or sole of the foot.
Left third fingertip amputation with exposed distal phalanx and loss of volar skin.

57. Biaxin is the trade name for an antibiotic.
The patient is allergic to Biaxin.

58. Dolobid is the trade name for an analgesic, anti-inflammatory.
I have changed his prescription to Dolobid 500 mg to be taken on a b.i.d. basis.

59. Keflex is the trade name for an antibiotic.
I have started him on Keflex 250 mg q.i.d. and soaks three times a day.

60. Lanoxin is the trade name for an antiarrhythmic, cardiotonic.
She is currently taking Lanoxin.

61. Lipitor is the trade name for an antihyperlipidemic.
Her medications included Lipitor, baby aspirin, and vitamin supplements.

62. Lopressor is the trade name for a beta-adrenergic blocker.
Her medications included Lopressor, Lipitor, Lanoxin, and baby aspirin.

63. Percocet is the trade name for an opioid analgesic.
I did renew a prescription for Percocet just to take at night as needed.

64. Vicodin is the trade name for a narcotic analgesic.
He is taking Vicodin as needed.

65. Vicoprofen is the trade name for a narcotic analgesic.
The patient was treated in February by Dr. Enrique Hernandez who has had the patient on Vicoprofen.

66. Xylocaine is the trade name for an antiarrhythmic, anesthetic.
I have proceeded with reduction of the fracture with 1% Xylocaine local anesthesia.

1. a: digit
2. d: synovia
3. a: avulsion
4. d: exostosis
5. b: lipoma
6. c: bilateral
7. c: osteophyte
8. a: apophysis
9. d: interarticular
10. a: genu varum
11. c: contusion
12. c: purulence
13. a: ecchymosis
14. d: aspirate
15. a: lymphedema
16. c: effusion
17. a: arthroscopy
18. c: phalanx
19. a: crepitus
20. b: hypertrophy
21. a: greater trochanter
22. c: flexion
23. c: abduction
24. d: adduction
25. b: callus
26. a: turgor
27. b: gluteus medius
28. a: pisiform
29. c: acromion
30. c: volar
31. c: arthroplasty
32. a: plantar
33. b: interosseous
34. a: fusiform
35. d: meniscectomy
36. b: symptomatology
37. a: dorsiflexion
38. d: fasciculations
39. d: asymptomatic
40. b: trapezius
41. a: lymphadenopathy
42. a: meniscus
43. c: ulna
44. a: metatarsus
45. d: malleolus
46. b: calcaneus
47. d: paronychia
48. a: Lopressor
49. d: tetracycline
50. b: Percocet
51. b: Lipitor
52. c: Lanoxin
53. b: cortisone
54. a: codeine
55. a: Xylocaine
56. b: spironolactone
57. b: Biaxin
58. c: Vicoprofen
59. a: Reflex
60. b: Dolobid
61. c: Vicodin
62. d: penicillin

CHAPTER 6 / PART II PRETEST (6T-2)

CHART NOTE

Patient Name: Book, Sally

Date of Birth: January 16, 1982

Examination Date: *Current date*

HISTORY OF PRESENT ILLNESS: Sally continues to play varsity basketball and sustained an injury to her left index finger in early December of 1998. She noted both pain and swelling, primarily on the ulnar side of the PIP joint. She continued to play and experienced pain, particularly when the finger was struck and after competitions. She has been unable to flex the finger completely.

PHYSICAL EXAMINATION: On examination today, she had 45 degrees of active flexion, fusiform swelling on the ulnar side of the PIP joint and tenderness of the synovium.

X-RAY: X-rays of the joint showed only a very tiny avulsion fracture. Flexion was severely limited.

PLAN: I asked her to start using passive flexion techniques with a rubber band and active range of motion exercises, protecting the finger during competition if at all possible. A return visit was scheduled in three weeks to reassess finger motion.

James P. Osseous, MD/xx

Errors are indicated in bold and italics. Margins are formatted at 1 inch.

HISTORY AND PHYSICAL EXAMINATION

Patient Name: Winster, Penny

File Number: 41390

Date of ***B***irth: March 16, 19xx

Examination Date: *Current date*

Physician: James P. Osseous, MD

HISTORY

HISTORY OF PRESENT ILLNESS: I had the pleasure of seeing Penny in the office today. This is a ***43-year-old right-hand*** dominant woman who saw ***Dr. Zart*** for left rotator cuff tendinitis. She has ***impingement. An*** MRI ***showed*** acromial spur, no sign of a rotator cuff tear. ***She*** has an early ***cyst*** formation. She has undergone two injections. The first did not help. The second seemed to help her for a few days. She has had physical therapy for three months.
Double space
PAST MEDICAL HISTORY: Significant for cardiac ***arrhythmia.***
Double space
MEDICATIONS: She is intermittently on ***Lopressor.*** She ***has not*** always been real compliant with that if she is not having any problems.
Double space
ALLERGIES: ***Codeine***
Double space
REVIEW OF SYMPTOMS: She denies liver or kidney disease. She has had an ulcer in the remote past. She has not had any problems with it recently.
Double space
SOCIAL HISTORY: ***One-half*** pack per day smoker for ***15*** years.
Double space
PHYSICAL EXAMINATION: On examination, this is a ***well-developed*** woman in no ***acute*** distress. She has full, ***painless*** range of motion of her neck. Has ***had*** pain in the Neer and Hawkins ***impingements*** tests. Active ***abduction*** is 135 degrees. Forward flexion is 125 degrees. Passively, I could take her the rest of the way. Her strength is mildly diminished in external rotation, good in internal and abduction. She has a negative lift-off test. She is missing about two levels internal rotation up her back. She has pain with ***cross-chest*** adduction. There is no pain at the SC or AC joint. No clavicular tenderness is noted. Neurovascularly, she is intact.

DIAGNOSTIC TESTS: I reviewed the MRI as above. We got an AP and outlet x-ray which shows a type III ***acromion.***

------------------------- begin page 2 -------------------------

PLAN: Penny has chronic ***impingement.*** We discussed the options. We are going to ***proceed*** with ***arthroscopic*** subacromial ***decompression.*** We discussed the surgery and the risks involved which she understands. All questions were answered and an ***instructional*** booklet given. We will schedule this in a timely fashion after appropriate ***preoperative*** testing.
Quadruple space

James P. Osseous, MD/xx

CHAPTER 6 / PART II ACTIVITY 5

CHART NOTE

Patient Name: Smith, Lucy

Date of Birth: February 28, 19xx

Examination Date: *Current date*

SUBJECTIVE: Lucy is an 84-year-old female who fell directly onto her right hand yesterday.

OBJECTIVE: She suffered a wrist fracture. She is right-hand dominant. She can move her fingers okay and has good peripheral circulation and sensation. There is considerable ecchymosis and a little bit of deformity of the wrist. X-rays show a reversed Colles or Smith fracture.

ASSESSMENT: Reversed Colles fracture, right wrist.

PLAN: I have proceeded with reduction of the fracture with 1% Xylocaine local anesthesia and have placed her in a sugar tong splint. Post reduction x-rays show essentially an anatomic reduction. I am going to plan to keep her immobilized for six weeks. I will have her return to the office in one week for a x-ray through the cast.

_____

James P. Osseous, MD/xx

CHAPTER 6 / PART II ACTIVITY 6 (6T-3)

CHART NOTE

Patient Name: Juanez, Paula

Date of Birth: March 29, 1943

Examination Date: *Current date*

HISTORY OF PRESENT ILLNESS: Paula is seen for a follow-up evaluation in the office today. She has shown improvement within her left trochanteric symptomatology, but some problems persist.

PAST MEDICAL HISTORY: I have reviewed with her what was done in therapy, and unfortunately they did not initiate a gluteus medius stretching and strengthening program as I had ordered.

PHYSICAL EXAMINATION: The patient continues to demonstrate significant weakness with pain over the greater trochanter.

PLAN: I have reinjected this area today and have ordered therapy through an alternative provider. I feel that unless Paula strengthens the muscle significantly, she will continue to have symptoms. I have asked her to follow up with me in eight weeks if she is still having problems after completion of her therapy program.

_____

David Treppe, MD/xx

CHAPTER 6 / PART II ACTIVITY 7 (6T-4)

CHART NOTE

Patient Name: Pentzler, Sandra

Date of Birth: October 21, 1956

Examination Date: *Current date*

HISTORY OF PRESENT ILLNESS: I saw Sandra in the office today for a follow-up evaluation. She is having less pain in her ankle.

PHYSICAL EXAMINATION: Today, on exam, the cast is in satisfactory condition. Her neurovascular status is intact.

ASSESSMENT: Follow up x-ray shows anatomic reduction of her mortise.

PLAN: Our plan is to keep her in a short leg cast for four weeks, still nonweightbearing. We will see her back at that time, get an x-ray in the cast, and probably put her in a short leg walking cast for 2-3 weeks at that time. I did renew a prescription for Percocet just to take at night as needed.

_____

Harry A. Medulla, MD/xx

CHAPTER 6 / PART II CHECK YOUR PROGRESS

See *Pretest (6T-2).*

CHAPTER 6 / PART III PRETEST (6T-5)

CHART NOTE

Patient Name: Memmler, Thomas

Date of Birth: August 18, 1941

Examination Date: *Current date*

SUBJECTIVE: Tom returns one week status post arthroscopy and partial medial meniscectomy, right knee.

OBJECTIVE: The knee looks good with very minimal effusion. The incisions are clean. He has nearly full range of motion at this point.

ASSESSMENT: Status post arthroscopy and partial medial meniscectomy, right knee.

PLAN: We will keep him off work as the knee is still somewhat irritable when he is on his feet all day. I will see him again in four weeks. He will work on some squat sets and range of motion exercises. He will call if there are any problems.

_____

Harry A. Medulla, MD/xx

CHART NOTE

Patient Name: Harris, Tim

Date of Birth: July 16, 1975

Examination Date: *Current date*

CHIEF COMPLAINT: Right great toe infection.

PAST MEDICAL HISTORY: This patient persists with pain, redness, and tenderness in the right great toe. He underwent removal of the nail plate from the left great toe several months ago.

PHYSICAL EXAMINATION: The left toe is healed well. The toenail has grown back without evidence of paronychia infection. The right great toe has significant nail bed infection, erythema, purulence, and tenderness, particularly on the lateral nail fold area.

TREATMENT: I have started him on Keflex 250 mg q.i.d. and soaks three times a day. I will recheck his progress in about 4-5 days. If he is not improved, he will require removal of the nail, and we will likely give him some preprocedure analgesic medication in preparation for this.

PLAN: He will be rechecked in one week. The patient will defer removing the nail until after the weekend, since he is apparently competing in a karate tournament this weekend.

Harry A. Medulla/xx

X-RAY REPORT

Patient Name: Dubroy, Mary Ann

File Number: 3457

Date of Birth: September 2, 19xx

Examination Date: *Current date*

Ordering Physician: Izzy Sertoli, MD

Examination: LEFT HAND X-RAY

HISTORY: This is a 21-year-old female gymnast who fell off the uneven parallel bars during practice. Patient complains of swelling and tenderness at the base of the fifth metacarpal.

FINDINGS: There is a slightly offset oblique fracture through the fifth metacarpal. The fragments are maintained in good alignment. No additional fractures are identified. Hand is otherwise normal.

IMPRESSION: Left hand fracture.

Harry A. Medulla, MD/xx

CHART NOTE

Patient Name: Hammer, Peter

Date of Birth: May 28, 1980

Examination Date: *Current date*

HISTORY OF PRESENT ILLNESS: Peter returned for follow up today. He is approximately five weeks status post his lateral ligamentous repair. He started weightbearing approximately nine days ago and felt his cast was very loose. He was brought in for a cast change.

TREATMENT: The cast was removed. His wound is clean and dry. Steri-strips were removed. He was placed back into a new short leg walking cast.

PLAN: We will plan to see the patient again in three weeks for re-evaluation.

James P. Osseous, MD/xx

X-RAY REPORT

Patient Name: Winterman, Rachel

File Number: 100456

Date of Birth: May 1, 19xx

Examination Date: *Current date*

Ordering Physician: Charles P. Davis, MD

Examination: LEFT ANKLE X-RAY

HISTORY: This is a 54-year-old female who slipped on an ice patch in front of her home.

FINDINGS: Soft tissue swelling is present over both malleoli, particularly over the lateral malleolus. There is a small ankle joint effusion. The ankle is otherwise normal. There are moderately sized posterior and plantar calcaneal spurs. There are no fractures noted.

IMPRESSION: Rule out fibular fracture

David Treppe, MD/xx

X-RAY REPORT

Patient Name: Newhouse, Lance

File Number: 8903
Date of Birth: January 14, 19xx

Examination Date: *Current date*

Ordering Physician: P. H. Waters, MD

Examination: LEFT FOURTH FINGER X-RAY

HISTORY: This is a 10-year-old male who got his finger caught in the door.

FINDINGS: Some soft tissue is present at the PIP joint. There is minimal irregularity along the dorsolateral margin of the base of the fourth middle phalanx. This could represent a small, nondisplaced avulsion fracture, but no definite fracture line is visible. The finger is otherwise normal.

Harry A. Medulla, MD/xx

CHART NOTE

Patient Name: Butger, Tommy

Date of Birth: February 22, 19xx

Examination Date: *Current date*

HISTORY OF PRESENT ILLNESS: I had the pleasure of seeing Tommy in the office today. This is a 13-year-old male who was fooling around with his brother, per his report. Apparently, he kicked a chair suffering an injury to the base of the fifth metatarsal of the right foot. This was about three weeks ago, and he continues to have pain and swelling in the area.

PAST MEDICAL HISTORY: No history of other injury is noted.

PHYSICAL EXAMINATION: On exam, his ankle is nontender. He has pain and swelling about the proximal fifth metatarsal. Point tenderness is noted. Neurovascularly, he is intact.

IMPRESSION: X-rays show a fracture at the apophysis of the proximal fifth metatarsal that is displaced somewhat. We repeated the x-rays today. There is some healing noted. He has been in a hard sole shoe.

PLAN: We are going to put him in a weightbearing cast. I will see him back in three weeks for removal and examination.

David Treppe, MD/xx

CHART NOTE

Patient Name: Harris, James

Date of Birth: April 10, 1977

Examination Date: *Current date*

HISTORY OF PRESENT ILLNESS: I had the pleasure of seeing Jim back in the office today for eight-week follow up of right tibia and fibular fracture. He tells me he has been putting a little bit more weight on the leg the last couple of days because of the ice and he has been feeling some pain.

PHYSICAL EXAMINATION: On examination, he has minimal swelling at the distal tibia with no swelling in the foot. All incisions are healing nicely, and there is no evidence of infection at this point. Subtalar motion is good. Dorsiflexion is 10-15 degrees with plantar flexion to 25 degrees.

X-RAY: X-ray examination shows no remarkable change in the position of the fragments, but I also do not see any remarkable callus formation yet.

TREATMENT: I have cautioned Jim to continue with his current weightbearing precautions and to continue using his cast brace. We will see the patient back in the office in six weeks for repeat x-rays.

David Treppe, MD/xx

CHART NOTE

Willis, Patricia

Date of Birth: August 12, 19xx

Examination Date: *Current date*

HISTORY OF PRESENT ILLNESS: Pat is a self-referred, 31-year-old woman who came to the office complaining of a mass on the radial side of her second metacarpal on the right. This has been present for several months.

PAST MEDICAL HISTORY: She normally works as a housewife, and complained of increasing weakness, intermittent swelling of the mass, and a poorly defined loss of feeling. She denied, however, any sensory change on the palmar side of the hand, and had no significant night pain.

PHYSICAL EXAMINATION: On examination, she had a deep, soft cystic mass in the area of the first dorsal interosseous, which was slightly tender to touch. It was oblong and its size, location, and depth were difficult to assess.

PLAN: I ordered an MRI of the hand to determine if it was indeed cystic or a lipomatous lesion. The study was scheduled for next Monday.

James P. Osseous, MD/xx

Current date

John Mastersetti, MD
Pleasantville Family Health
792 West Walnut Street
Westerville, OH 78910

Re: Juan Rodriquez
   Date of Birth: February 14, 19xx

Dear Dr. Mastersetti:

HISTORY OF PRESENT ILLNESS: I had the pleasure of seeing Juan in the office today. He is a 39-year-old, right-hand dominant male who injured his left third finger yesterday at work and had an avulsion of the tip. He was seen in the County Hospital Emergency Room where he had an I&D. He received a tetanus shot, was placed on p.o. antibiotics and referred here for treatment. He is an otherwise healthy male and works for Alpha Printing.

ALLERGIES: No known allergies.

MEDICATIONS: None other than what was prescribed at the emergency room yesterday.

PHYSICAL EXAMINATION: On physical exam of his left third finger, there is a tip avulsion of soft tissue with bare bony exposure of his distal phalanx. His DIP joint is not involved. He only has a few millimeters left of nail bed.

PLAN: Left third finger tip amputation with exposed distal phalanx and loss of volar skin. The plan now is for a revision amputation of the left third finger with shortening of the distal phalanx and flap coverage with some distal skin to cover the tip. Due to the exposed bone, I would not recommend he undergo healing by secondary intention and skin grafting will not work because there is exposed bone. Surgery will be scheduled in the next couple of days.

Best wishes to you and your family. With warmest regards,

Harry A. Medulla, MD

xx

CHART NOTE

Patient Name: Grant, William

Date of Birth: July 15, 1960

Examination Date: *Current date*

HISTORY OF PRESENT ILLNESS: Bill returns two months status post tibial plateau fracture and medial collateral ligament sprain, right knee. He is doing reasonably well. He still walks with a limp and is complaining of a lot of pain, especially with the cold weather.

PHYSICAL EXAMINATION: On today's examination, he has intact MCL and tenderness on the medial and posteromedial tibial plateau. He has no effusion and good motion.

PLAN: At this point, I would like to keep him using his cane, and we will start him on some physical therapy. We will see him again back in three weeks for re-evaluation. He would be capable of sedentary work, but not much more than that.

Harry A. Medulla, MD/xx

CHART NOTE

Patient Name: Phillips, John

Date of Birth: November 5, 19xx

Examination Date: *Current date*

CHIEF COMPLAINT: John is a 45-year-old, right-hand dominant gentleman who fell on the ice Saturday sustaining an injury to his right shoulder. He complains of persistent pain.

DIAGNOSIS: His MRI scan shows an essentially nondisplaced greater tuberosity fracture. There is some increased signal in the rotator cuff, but I think this is more contusion. Neurovascularly, he is intact.

TREATMENT: At this point, we will keep him in a shoulder immobilizer full time. He is taking Vicodin as needed. He will ice the area. We will see him next week for an x-ray of his shoulder, an AP in external rotation. We will let the fracture heal and monitor his progress for a potential rotator cuff tear. We will see him again in one month for re-evaluation.

Harry A. Medulla, MD/xx

HISTORY AND PHYSICAL EXAMINATION

Patient Name: Evertson, Sam

File Number: 79022

Date of Birth: July 2, 19xx

Examination Date: *Current date*

Physician: Harry A. Medulla, MD

HISTORY

HISTORY OF PRESENT ILLNESS: I saw Sam Evertson in the office today. He is a pleasant, 61-year-old gentleman who comes in for evaluation of right shoulder pain. He has had about a three-month history of pain and crepitus around the shoulder. He does not know of any injury to the shoulder. The pain stays primarily around the shoulder girdle with no radiation. He does get some aches around his upper back and neck area, but not true radiculitis symptoms.

PAST MEDICAL HISTORY: He has been in good health otherwise.

ALLERGIES: Penicillin

PHYSICAL EXAMINATION

GENERAL: BP 112/74, pulse 64 and regular, respirations 16/min. On physical examination, he is a 61-year-old gentleman appearing to be his stated age.

EXTREMITIES: His pulses are intact in the upper extremity. There is no lymphedema. He has full active range of motion of the shoulder. He is not tender over the AC joint, nor over the rotator cuff. He does have some mild subdeltoid crepitus. He has positive rotator cuff signs and impingement signs.

X-RAY: A two-view x-ray of the shoulder in AP and outlet view reveals degenerative changes of the AC joint.

IMPRESSION: He appears to have a chronic cuff tendinitis with a mild impingement syndrome.

PLAN: I am going to inject the subdeltoid space today and have him see a physical therapist. I will see him back if he continues to have difficulty.

Harry A. Medulla, MD/xx

HISTORY AND PHYSICAL EXAMINATION

Patient Name: Madison, Jerry

File Number: 90234

Date of Birth: June 17, 19xx

Examination Date: *Current date*

Physician: James P. Osseous, MD

HISTORY

CHIEF COMPLAINT: Back pain.

HISTORY OF PRESENT ILLNESS: Jerry is a 42-year-old gentleman with an initial injury that he sustained on December 12, 2000, when he was pulling an 80 lb drum at work and noted pain the following day. He was seen for evaluation by a local physician, who recommended he remain off work. Additional evaluation was requested from the University Hospital Emergency Room. They started the patient on oral medication and light-duty activity. Within a two-week period of time, his back pain had resolved. He was able to continue with his normal activity until approximately four months later when he pulled an air conditioner out of a window and noted recurrent symptoms. He again treated this with oral medication with good response. Intermittently, the patient has been aware of pain in his back with twisting. He did reasonably well until this past July when he was aware of pain and aches along the medial aspect of the thigh and lateral aspect of the thigh radiating to the level of the knee. He is not aware of any specific injury but felt that his overall symptoms were attributed to the December 2000 injury when he first injured his back. The patient was treated in February by Dr. Enrique Hernandez who has had the patient on Vicoprofen. Jerry has been able to participate in normal activity. He has no bowel or bladder problems. He has no pain with coughing or sneezing other than when his symptoms seem to be more severe at which time he does note pain with Valsalva. He has not had any tendency to trip or fall. He does not have discomfort with awakening but notes increased symptoms as the day progresses, and as he is called upon to participate in heavy bending and lifting activities.

GENERAL: The patient is a healthy gentleman. He is 6 ft tall and weighs 165 lb. BP 110/58, pulse 64.

SOCIAL HISTORY: The patient smokes 2 packs per day and has done so for 24 years. He does not drink.

PRIOR SURGERY: Removal of a bone from beneath his eye as well as wisdom teeth extraction.

------------------------ begin page 2 ------------------------

ALLERGIES: None.

REVIEW OF SYSTEMS: Negative.

PHYSICAL EXAMINATION: Jerry was a cooperative gentleman. He stood erect. He was able to flex forward touching his fingers within four inches to the ground. He extended normally. No evidence of involuntary spasm was noted. No paraspinal spasm nor fasciculations were noted.

The patient did note that he had increased symptomatology with right and left lateral bending which he described as a tightness within the back. In the sitting position, there was no pain with straight leg raising and no pain with femoral stretch. Internal and external rotation of the hip did not cause significant pain. The patient had normal sensation to pin prick. He had 2+ and symmetric patella as well as Achilles reflexes. Motor evaluation revealed evidence of slightly diminished strength on hip flexion testing on the right.

IMPRESSION: I reviewed the patient's x-rays. There is evidence of discogenic abnormality at L4-5, a small degenerative disc with bulges noted L4-5.

PLAN: I have changed his prescription to Dolobid 500 mg to be taken on a b.i.d. basis. I have given him a prescription for 30 tablets with two refills. The patient's symptoms are predominately L4. I have recommended that we proceed with a flexion back exercise program. In addition, I would like the patient to start with epidural steroids to see if we cannot decrease the symptoms with cortisone. We will plan to see the patient back for follow-up evaluation in six weeks to see how he is coming along.

James P. Osseous, MD/xx

c: The Pain Center

CHAPTER 6 / 6T-19

Current date

Peter R. Desman, MD
Orange Hill Family Practice
214 Orchard Road
Brooklyn, NY 11245

Re: Clara B. Jackson
    Date of Birth: March 17, 1952

Dear Dr. Desman

HISTORY OF PRESENT ILLNESS: I had the pleasure of seeing Clara in the office today. She is doing much better status post epicondylar injection on the left elbow. She, at this point, is asymptomatic.

PHYSICAL EXAMINATION: On my exam today, she is no longer painful with resisted wrist or digit extension. She still has some sensitivity around both the lateral and medial epicondyles. Her elbow motion is full. There is no crepitus or instability. She is currently undergoing a work-up for some scarring in her lungs, which the Pulmonary Care Center is handling. She also tells me a lupus test was done which she has not had the results of yet. She has evidence of osteoarthritis.

IMPRESSION: Clinically, I do not see any signs of other significant inflammatory arthritis.

PLAN: At this point, only p.r.n. follow-up care is needed.

It was a pleasure caring for her.

Sincerely

James P. Osseous, MD

xx

CHAPTER 6 / PART II Check Your Progress

See Pretests (6T-5) and (6T-6).

CHAPTER 7 / PART I PRETEST

1. a	22. a	43. a	63. a
2. c	23. c	44. a	64. b
3. d	24. b	45. b	65. a
4. a	25. a	46. a	66. d
5. b	26. c	47. c	67. a
6. c	27. a	48. c	68. c
7. d	28. c	49. d	69. b
8. a	29. b	50. c	70. b
9. a	30. d	51. b	71. d
10. b	31. b	52. a	72. a
11. c	32. d	53. a	73. a
12. c	33. c	54. d	74. b
13. d	34. a	55. a	75. c
14. c	35. a	56. b	76. b
15. a	36. c	57. a	77. c
16. d	37. b	58. d	78. c
17. c	38. a	59. a	79. d
18. a	39. a	60. a	80. a
19. a	40. b	61. c	81. b
20. b	41. d	62. b	82. c
21. c	42. a		

CHAPTER 7 / PART I ACTIVITY 3 (7T-1)

1. Amoxicillin is a generic name for an antibiotic.
   At this point in time, we will use amoxicillin.
2. Arteriogram is a radiograph of an artery.
   The patient is admitted at this time for further evaluation that includes an arteriogram of the right collecting system.
3. Atrioventricular pertains to an atrium and the ventricle of the heart.
   Rule out atrioventricular malformation.
4. Bacitracin is a generic name for a bactericidal antibiotic.
   The wound was cleaned with bacitracin ointment, sterile fluff dressing, and a supporter.
5. Bradycardia is the slowness of the heart beat.
   The patient's EKGs have been remarkable for the presence of left ventricular sinus bradycardia.
6. Calculus is an abnormal concretion, stone.
   The patient had a history of ureteral calculus.
7. Captopril is a generic name for an angiotensin-converting enzyme inhibitor.
   He is maintained on captopril 25 mg t.i.d.
8. Cholecystectomy is the removal of the gallbladder.
   She had a cholecystectomy.
9. Cholecystitis is the inflammation of the gallbladder.
   The etiology of the pain remains unclear, although possibilities would include a calculus cholecystitis or another ovarian cyst.
10. Coapt is to bring together, as suturing a laceration.
    With the Valsalva maneuver, the bladder neck was not well coapted.
11. Colporrhaphy is the suture of the vagina.
    The patient was scheduled for a vaginal hysterectomy, anterior colporrhaphy, and endoscopic urethral suspension.
12. Concomitant takes place at the same time.
    The patient was diagnosed with possible concomitant urinary tract infection.
13. Coude' is bent or elbowed.
    The existing catheter was removed and a #24 French coude' catheter was passed with little difficulty.
14. Creatinine is a normal alkaline constituent of urine and blood.
    Her creatinine is normal.
15. Cystitis is the inflammation of the urinary bladder.
    There is no history of cystitis.

16. Cystocele is the herniation of the urinary bladder into the vagina.
Examination at that time demonstrated a marked cystocele and a positive Marshall test.
17. Cystometrography is the graphic record of the pressure in the bladder at varying stages of filling.
Cystometrogram in my office revealed normal bladder compliance.
18. Cystoscope is an endoscope especially designed for passing through the urethra into the bladder to permit visual inspection of its interior.
Subsequently, the rigid cystoscope was inserted and the cystoscopy was performed.
19. Cystourethroscope is an instrument for examining the posterior urethra and bladder.
The 23.5 cystourethroscope was assembled, lubricated, and advanced through the urethra and into the bladder.
20. Diuresis is an increased excretion of urine.
A diuresis renogram was performed and this study was normal, with no evidence of obstruction of either collecting system.
21. Diverticulum is a sac or pouch in the walls of a canal or organ.
The patient had a history of hypertension and Crohn's disease and diverticulitis.
22. Dyspneic is labored or difficult breathing.
He currently presents in an acute anxiety state and is dyspneic.
23. Ecchymosis is a skin discoloration caused by a hemorrhage.
No hematoma or ecchymosis is noted.
24. Extravasation is a discharge or escape of fluid from a vessel into the tissues.
There is no sign of any extravasation.
25. Flank is the side of the body between the ribs and ilium.
The patient is a 38-year-old male in mild distress secondary to right-sided flank discomfort.
26. Fossa is a hollow or depressed area.
The prostatic fossa demonstrates grade II/IV obstruction as viewed from the veru.
27. Fulguration is the destruction of living tissue by electric sparks generated by a high-frequency current.
Fulguration of the lumens of both the cut ends was performed with electrocautery.
28. Genitourinary pertains to the genitalia and urinary organs.
There is no previous history of urinary tract infections, stones, or genitourinary surgery.
29. Hematuria is the discharge of blood in the urine.
An examination revealed microscopic hematuria.
30. Heme is the nonprotein, insoluble, iron constituent of hemoglobin.
Urinalysis shows 3+ heme which is greater than 30 per high-power field.
31. Hydrocele is an accumulation of fluid in a sac-like cavity.
The right testicle is noteworthy for a moderate-sized hydrocele.
32. Hydrochlorothiazide is a generic name for a diuretic, antihypertensive agent.
The patient was given hydrochlorothiazide 25 mg daily for hypertension.
33. Hydronephrosis is the distention of the renal pelvis and calices with urine.
This newborn has very mild, yet persistent hydronephrosis, with no evidence of progression.
34. Incontinence is the inability to control excretory functions.
The patient's chief complaint was urinary incontinence.
35. Laminectomy is the surgical excision of the lamina.
He is hypertensive, with a previous history of a laminectomy for a herniated disc.
36. Leukocytes are colorless blood corpuscles.
Urinalysis shows 2+ leukocytes which were greater than 10 per high-power field and 3+ heme which is greater than 30 per high-power field.
37. Lithotomy is an incision of a duct or organ for the removal of calculi.
The patient was brought to the cytoscopy suite and placed in the dorsal lithotomy position.

38. Meatus is an opening.
The penis is circumcised and the meatus adequate.
39. Meclizine is a generic name for an antiemetic, antihistamine, motion sickness relief.
The patient was given meclizine on a p.r.n basis for dizziness.
40. Nephrectomy is the surgical removal of the kidney.
The patient was admitted to University Hospital for a right nephrectomy.
41. Occlude is to close tight.
Two clips were placed in opposing directions on both cut ends to further occlude the lumen.
42. Oophorectomy is the excision of one or both ovaries.
She has had an oophorectomy but has her uterus.
43. Panendoscope is a cystoscope that gives a wide-angle view of the bladder.
The panendoscopy was performed with a #16 French flexible panendoscope.
44. Parenchyma are the essential elements of an organ.
No deformity to the parenchyma or fluid loss is noted.
45. Periumbilical is around the umbilicus.
The pain appeared to start in the periumbilical area and then improved.
46. Pessary is an instrument placed in the vagina to support the uterus or rectum.
Because of her age, I convinced her to try therapy with a pessary, and a 2-inch Gellhorn pessary was inserted.
47. Phallus is the penis.
The phallus is uncircumcised, with normal full foreskin.
48. Pyelogram is a x-ray study of the renal pelvis and uterus.
An intravenous pyelogram and voiding cystourethrogram were normal as well as urine cytology and urine culture.
49. Pyelonephritis is the inflammation of the kidney and renal pelvis.
The negative urinalysis would also mitigate against a pyelonephritis and the pain is clearly abdominal rather than in the CVA region.
50. Pyuria is pus in the urine.
She has a three-month history of persistent pyuria.
51. Raphe is a seam or ridge noting the line of junction of halves of a part.
The left vas was regrasped and brought into the median raphe.
52. Rectocele is a hernia protrusion of part of the rectum into the vagina.
Upon removal of the pessary, there is a large cystocele and a small rectocele.
53. Resect is to cut off or cut out a portion of a tissue or organ.
The patient underwent prostatic resection and hernia repair in 1998.
54. Staghorn is the calculus of the renal pelvis usually extending into multiple calices.
X-rays reveal a large, staghorn calculus with minimal obstruction.
55. Suprapubic is above the pubis.
The abdomen is soft and tender in the suprapubic region.
56. Syncope is the temporary suspension of consciousness; fainting.
The patient is free of any dizziness, lightheadedness, syncope, or near syncope.
57. Trabeculation is a small beam or supporting structure.
The mucosa was examined in full circumferential fashion and was without tumors, trabeculation, or diverticula.
58. Trigone is a triangular area.
The bladder showed a normal trigone with normal orifices bilaterally.
59. Urethrocele is the prolapse of the female urethra through the urinary meatus.
GENITALIA: Moderate urethrocele.
60. Urethrotrigonitis is the inflammation of the urethra and trigone of the bladder.
Cystoscopy revealed some mild changes of urethrotrigonitis, and stress incontinence was demonstrated.
61. Urogram is a diagnostic x-ray study of kidneys, ureter, and bladder.
A recent urogram showed a filling defect of the left kidney.

62. Urosepsis is the poisoning from retained and absorbed urinary substances.
The patient was seen and evaluated several years ago for a suspected urosepsis with an associated high fever, secondary to a staghorn calculus and chronic urinary infection.

63. Vas deferens is the excretory duct of the testis.
The vas deferens was grasped and brought into the median raphe and anesthesia infiltrated.

64. Vasculature is the supply of vessels to a specific region.
The patient is scheduled for an arteriogram later today to further define the vasculature of the left kidney and hopefully identify the bleeding site.

65. Verumontanum is the elevation on the floor of the prostatic portion of the urethra where the seminal ducts enter.
The flexible cystourethroscope was advanced through the urethra to the level of the verumontanum.

66. Aldactone is the trade name for a diuretic.
The patient's medication included Aldactone.

67. Bactrim is the trade name for an antibiotic.
Medications include a recent course of Bactrim, which has caused nausea and headache.

68. Betadine is the trade name for a topical antibacterial, antiseptic.
The genitalia were prepped with a Betadine scrub and draped in a sterile fashion.

69. Calan is the trade name for an antianginal, antiarrhythmic, antihypertensive.
His only medication was Calan SR 240 mg 1 p.o. daily.

70. Cardura is the trade name for an antihypertensive, antiadrenergic.
His only medication includes Cardura 3 mg at bedtime.

71. Cipro is the trade name for a fluoroquinolone antiobiotic, antibacterial drug.
Antibiotics in the form of Cipro were given.

72. Imodium is the trade name for an antidiarrheal.
Her medication included Imodium.

73. Lopressor is the trade name for an antianginal, antihypertensive.
Her medications included Aldactone, Imodium, and Lopressor.

74. Maxaquin is the trade name for a fluoroquinolone antibiotic, antibacterial.
The patient was started on Maxaquin 400 mg p.o. q.d. for a 7-day course.

75. Neptazane is the trade name for a diuretic, antiglaucoma agent.
He takes one aspirin a day and is maintained on Neptazane 1 b.i.d.

76. Noroxin is the trade name for an antibacterial, urinary tract anti-infective.
I have placed her on Noroxin, 400 mg p.o. b.i.d. for 5 days.

77. Propine is the trade name for an antiglaucoma agent, eyedrops.
He also uses Propine eye drops.

78. Timoptic is the trade name for a topical antiglaucoma agent.
He also uses Propine and Timoptic eye drops.

79. Tolinase is the trade name for an antidiabetic agent.
He is maintained on Tolinase 250 mg p.o. q.d., as well as captopril 25 mg t.i.d.

80. Toradol is the trade name for a nonsteroidal anti-inflammatory drug; analgesic for acute, moderately severe pain.
His pain is quite severe, but was relieved with intravenous Toradol.

81. Trimpex is the trade name for an antibacterial, antibiotic.
After he finishes the Bactrim, I will place him on Trimpex 100 mg daily.

82. Xylocaine (zi-lo-kan) is the trade name for an anesthetic, antiarrhythmic.
Xylocaine jelly was injected into the urethra.

CHAPTER 7 / PART I CHECK YOUR PROGRESS

See *Part I Pretest*.

CHAPTER 7 / PART II PRETEST (7T-2)

HISTORY AND PHYSICAL EXAMINATION REPORT

Patient Name: Mead, Jay

File Number: 001256

Date of Birth: January 2, 1948

Examination Date: *Current date*

Physician: Benjamin Keytone, MD

HISTORY

CHIEF COMPLAINT: Left flank pain.

HISTORY OF PRESENT ILLNESS: A patient with a known chronic obstructive lung presents in the Emergency Care Unit this evening with left flank pain. An examination revealed microscopic hematuria. His pain is quite severe, but was relieved with intravenous Toradol. He has a history of kidney stones. He was previously evaluated by Dr. Keytone in the past for a prostatic nodule. Previous biopsies for a prostatic nodule by Dr. Keytone proved to be negative. He currently presents in an acute anxiety state and is dyspneic. Because of his pronounced anxiety, he is unable to provide a complete history. He does state that he has had no significant urinary distress.

PAST HISTORY: The patient was admitted two weeks ago. The patient has COPD and chronic anxiety, as noted above. He is hypertensive, with a previous history of a laminectomy for herniated disc. He has a history of asbestos exposure as well as a TB exposure.

FAMILY HISTORY: His father had emphysema. His mother suffered from Alzheimer's disease. One brother had an MI.

REVIEW OF SYSTEMS: Noncontributory, except for shortness of breath and anxiety.

PHYSICAL EXAMINATION

GENERAL: Well-nourished, well-developed male in acute distress with anxiety and dyspnea.

HEENT: Normal.

NECK: Supple, no masses.

HEART: Normal sinus rhythm. No murmurs or enlargement.

----------------------- begin page 2 -----------------------

LUNGS: Increased AP diameter, with diminished breath sounds and poor expansion bilaterally.

ABDOMEN: Soft, no palpable mass or organ enlargement. No CVA tenderness.

GENITALIA: Normal male.

RECTAL: The prostate is benign in consistency but enlarged 1+.

EXTREMITIES: No edema or deformity.

PLAN:
1. Possible ureteral calculus. The patient has a history of renal calculi.
2. Chronic obstructive pulmonary disease.
3. Anxiety state

_____

Benjamin Keytone, MD/xx

Errors are indicated in bold and italics. Margins are formatted at 1 inch.

CONSULTATION REPORT

Patient Name: Barnes, Franklyn

File Number: 003416

Date of Birth: February 13, 19xx

Examination Date: *Current date*

Requesting Physician: Izzy Sertoli, MD

HISTORY OF PRESENT ILLNESS: This ***22-year-old*** gentleman fell approximately ***27 feet*** off a scaffold. He landed on a large screw top object and sustained an abrasion of his right flank. The patient informs me that he did not have much pain immediately after the fall and***, therefore,*** did not come to see you for evaluation until later in the day. A urine ***analysis*** performed in your office showed 20-50 ***RBCs.*** Due to your concern about ***right*** flank trauma, I was asked to evaluate the patient.

The patient is ***alert*** and oriented. There is no tenderness over the abdomen. There is a ***right*** flank abrasion measuring about 4 ***cm.*** No ***hematoma*** or ***ecchymosis is*** noted. The left flank area is smooth and unremarkable. There is no tenderness in the lower abdomen. The testicles are normal. The prostate is 1+, smooth and nontender. His hemoglobin is ***14.***
Double space
An IVP was performed that showed a large ***gas*** pattern over the entire ***abdomen.*** The left kidney functions promptly and is smooth. The right kidney shows good function in both the upper and lower poles. There is some decreased ***filling*** of the renal ***pelvis,*** but there is good ***excretion*** of ***contrast.*** The renal pelvis does not really fill out ***well*** in the entire ***midline*** area***,*** which I think is consistent with a renal ***contusion.*** There is no sign of any ***extravasation.***
Double space
A renal ***sonogram*** also shows the kidney to be totally ***intact.*** No deformity to the ***parenchyma*** or fluid loss is noted. It is essentially a normal appearing kidney.
Double space
IMPRESSION: Right renal contusion. No signs of any ***extravasation.***
Double space
PLAN: The patient will be admitted to ***University Hospital*** and placed on ***bed rest*** with observation. I will order a urine culture and sensitivity test. He will be started on IV antibiotics, and I will follow along with you in his care. Thank you for ***referring*** this patient to us.
Quadruple space

_____

Benjamin Keytone, MD/xx

OPERATIVE REPORT

Patient Name: Cruise, Jason

File Number: 0045612

Date of Birth: March 16, 1967

Examination Date: *Current date*

Preoperative Diagnosis: Carcinoma of the prostate.

Postoperative Diagnosis: Carcinoma of the prostate.

Operation: FLEXIBLE CYSTOSCOPY

PROCEDURE: Flexible cystoscopy

The patient was identified by me, prepped and draped in the usual fashion. The panendoscopy was performed with a #16 French flexible panendoscope. The anterior urethra was unremarkable. The membranous urethra is intact. There is no evidence of any stricture.

The prostatic fossa demonstrates grade II/IV obstruction as viewed from the veru. This probably represents 15-20 gm of resectable adenoma. There is no evidence of tumor within the prostatic fossa. The bladder neck anatomy is unremarkable. The bladder mucosa is healthy throughout. There were no stones, tumors, or diverticula identified.

Right and left ureteral orifices were in normal position and normal configuration. Clear efflux is seen bilaterally. The bladder neck anatomy is unremarkable as noted from a retroflex position. There is no evidence of any tumor invasion into the bladder base.

The scope was withdrawn. The patient tolerated the procedure well.

PLAN:
1. Trimpex 100 mg b.i.d.
2. Schedule a follow-up appointment in two weeks to discuss treatment options for carcinoma of the prostate.

_____

Theodore Trigone, MD/xx

CONSULTATION REPORT

Patient Name: Delado, Lucille

File Number: 004218

Date of Birth: February 23, 19xx

Examination Date: *Current date*

Requesting Physician: J. Thomas Geiger, MD

HISTORY OF PRESENT ILLNESS: This 59-year-old lady admitted to University Hospital by Dr. Geiger for acute bronchopneumonia. I was asked to see the patient because of persistent, significant microscopic hematuria.

On admission, she had urine that showed greater than 100 red cells per high-powered field. Urinalysis further revealed 3-5 white cells, small bacterial, and small yeast. Her creatinine is normal.

The patient states she has had absolutely no urinary symptoms. She denies burning, frequency, or urgency. There is no family history of kidney stones, bladder tumors, or kidney tumors. She has had an oophorectomy but has her uterus. She had a cholecystectomy. She does not smoke.

On examination, she is a very pleasant, well-developed, slightly obese lady in no acute distress. Her abdomen is slightly obese, but it is soft. I cannot palpate an enlarged liver or spleen. I cannot palpate any flank or bladder masses.

IMPRESSION: Significant microscopic hematuria.

PLAN: Repeat urinalysis, culture and sensitivity and cytology studies. I will schedule her for an IVP and cystoscopy to rule out any other significant problems. I will follow along with you. Thank you for your kind referral.

_____

Helen Loop, MD/xx

Current date

J. Thomas Geiger, MD
FedDes Wellness Center
Family Practice Division, Suite 300
101 Wellness Way Drive
New York, NY 10036

Re: Janice Rapaport
    Date of Birth: November 2, 1953

Dear Dr. Geiger

The patient was seen and evaluated several years ago for a suspected urosepsis with an associated high fever, secondary to a staghorn calculus and chronic urinary infection. The patient elected not to pursue surgical intervention at the time the initial diagnosis was made.

On this admission to the hospital, x-rays reveal a large, staghorn calculus with minimal obstruction. A renal scan shows differential function to be only slightly diminished on the right side. The right kidney is working reasonably well. After discussing the situation and potential options with Miss Rapaport and with Adam Valence, MD from the Cardiology Division, it was decided that surgical intervention would be risky. We will try to manage this conservatively with long term antibiotic therapy and frequent follow-up visits.

The patient was transferred from the acute center to the transitional unit where she has been for five days during which time she has recovered. Antibiotics in the form of Cipro were given. She is now ready for discharge.

I have discussed the situation again with Miss Rapaport. She will continue with her Cipro 500 mg daily. I will see her back in the office in one month for a follow up. Thank you for allowing us to assist in the care of this patient.

Sincerely

Helen Loop, MD

xx

CHAPTER 7 / PART II CHECK YOUR PROGRESS

See Pretest (7T-2).

HISTORY AND PHYSICAL EXAMINATION

Patient Name: Shapiro, Adam

File Number: 00134

Date of Birth: April 8, 19xx

Examination Date: *Current date*

Physician: Benjamin Keytone, MD

HISTORY

CHIEF COMPLAINT: Gross hematuria.

HISTORY OF PRESENT ILLNESS: This 29-year-old man presented with an episode of gross hematuria that occurred about five weeks ago and spontaneously resolved itself. The patient took a course of Cipro, with a resultant clearing of the blood. He denies any associated voiding symptoms at that time. The bleeding has returned over the past 48 hours often heavy with clots. He was again started on an antibiotic, but the bleeding continued. The cystoscopy performed as an outpatient procedure today demonstrated blood emanating from the right ureteral orifice. The bladder was otherwise normal with no blood seen from left side. The patient is admitted at this time for further evaluation that includes an arteriogram of the right collecting system.

PAST MEDICAL HISTORY: Negative for serious illness. Past surgery includes a tonsillectomy. Medications include a recent course of Bactrim, which has caused nausea and headache.

ALLERGIES: None known, although the patient has had recent nausea and headache after taking Bactrim.

FAMILY HISTORY: Positive for heart disease and lung cancer.

SOCIAL HISTORY: Positive for one pack of cigarettes a day for more than nine years.

REVIEW OF SYSTEMS: Negative for chest pain, dyspnea on exertion or change in weight or bowel habit.

PHYSICAL EXAMINATION

GENERAL: The patient is a healthy appearing 29-year-old male in no acute distress.

HEENT: Clear.

- begin page 2 -

NECK: Supple without masses.

HEART: Regular rhythm with no murmur or gallop.

ABDOMEN: Thin, soft, nontender, no active bowel sounds and no masses.

BREAST: Without CVA tenderness.

EXTREMITIES: Without pretibial edema.

NEUROLOGICAL: Grossly intact.

IMPRESSION: Gross hematuria originating from the right kidney and/or collecting system.

PLAN: The patient is scheduled for an arteriogram later today to further define the vasculature of the right kidney and hopefully identify the bleeding site. Rule out atrioventricular malformation. Rule out carcinoma.

Benjamin Keytone, MD/xx

CHAPTER 7 / PART III PRETEST (7T-6)

OPERATIVE REPORT

Patient Name: Shroder, Sally

File Number: 005689

Date of Birth: June 19, 19xx

Examination Date: *Current date*

Preoperative Diagnosis: Urinary incontinence.

Postoperative Diagnosis: Urinary incontinence with stress and urge incontinence.

Operation: VIDEO CYSTOURETHROSCOPE

CHIEF COMPLAINT: This is a 76-year-old female who presented with the complaint of severe urinary incontinence. She had recently undergone a vaginal hysterectomy. An intravenous pyelogram and voiding cystourethrogram were normal as well as urine cytology and urine culture. Cytoscopy was suggested and agreed upon by the patient as a way to investigate the cause of her incontinence.

PROCEDURE: The patient was brought to the cytoscopy suite and placed in the dorsal lithotomy position. The genitalia were prepped with a Betadine scrub and draped in a sterile fashion.

The 23.5 cystourethroscope was assembled, lubricated, and advanced through the urethra and into the bladder. The mucosa was examined in full circumferential fashion and was without tumors, trabeculation, or diverticula. No calculus was seen. The right and left urethral orifices were identified in their usual anatomic position and found normal. The scope was advanced to the mid-urethra and the bladder neck was visualized. With the Valsalva maneuver, the bladder neck was not well coapted. The scope was removed. The patient was asked to cough and during so, marked urinary leakage from the urethra was noted. This event was stopped via a finger in the vagina to the right of the urethra at the level of the bladder neck, which is consistent with a positive Marshall test. The scope was removed. The patient tolerated the procedure well and there were no complications.

IMPRESSION: Urinary incontinence with stress and urge incontinence.

Helen Loop, MD/xx

CHAPTER 7 / 7T-7

CONSULTATION REPORT

Patient Name: Stewartson, Jason

File Number: 18790

Date of Birth: January 1, 19xx

Examination Date: *Current date*

Requesting Physician: Charles P. Davis, MD

REASON FOR REFERRAL: Prenatal hydronephrosis.

HISTORY: Newborn baby boy, 40 weeks gestation born to a 24-year-old mother. An older sibling had prenatal hydronephrosis and is currently under the care of this practice. This newborn has very mild, yet persistent hydronephrosis, with no evidence of progression.

The baby boy is unremarkable. The abdomen is soft, nontender, with no palpable masses. The bladder is not distended. The phallus is uncircumcised, with normal full foreskin. The testes are descended bilaterally with no masses noted.

IMPRESSION: Bilateral, prenatal hydronephrosis.

PLAN:
1. Prophylactic antibiotics. At this point in time, we will use amoxicillin.
2. Repeat renal ultrasound in 48 hours.
3. Recommend a voiding cystourethrogram if hydronephrosis is present.

Benjamin Keytone, MD/xx

CHAPTER 7 / 7T-8

OPERATIVE REPORT

Patient Name: Yonie, Soshia

File Number: 000236

Date of Birth: March 31, 19xx

Examination Date: *Current date*

Preoperative Diagnosis: Sterile pyuria.

Postoperative Diagnosis: Negative exam.

Operation: CYSTOSCOPY

This 65-year-old white female, recently involved in a motor vehicle accident, was noted to have sterile pyuria. She has a three-month history of persistent pyuria and has been through multiple courses of antimicrobial pharmaceuticals. Preoperative studies did include a urine culture that showed no growth. An intravenous pyelogram showed the upper tracts to be normal.

The patient was counseled in the risks and benefits of this procedure and gave informed consent for further evaluation of her condition via cystoscopy.

PROCEDURE: The patient was taken to the urology suite and placed in the lithotomy position. The perineum was prepped with Betadine and draped in a sterile manner. Xylocaine jelly was injected into the urethra. Subsequently, the rigid cystoscope was inserted and the cystoscopy was performed. The urethra appeared normal. The bladder showed a normal trigone with normal orifices bilaterally. There was clear urine effluxing from both orifices. The mucosal pattern of the bladder was normal. No foreign bodies or stones in the bladder were seen. The bladder was drained and the cystoscope was removed.

IMPRESSION: Normal examination.

Helen Loop, MD/xx

CHAPTER 7 / 7T-9

HISTORY AND PHYSICAL EXAMINATION

Patient Name: Diaz, Roal

File Number: 8023

Date of Birth: July 3, 19xx

Examination Date: *Current date*

Physician: Benjamin Keytone, MD

HISTORY

CHIEF COMPLAINT: Urinary distress.

HISTORY OF PRESENT ILLNESS: The patient has been followed for one year with intermittent frequency, urgency, incontinence, and weakness in the voiding stream. He had a previous TURP in 1989. A recent cystoscopic evaluation revealed recurrent benign prostatic hyperplasia. The patient was reluctant to undergo surgery again and has been treated with conservative measures over the past several months. His symptoms have become worse and now present for further direction.

PAST MEDICAL HISTORY: The patient underwent prostatic resection and hernia repair in 1998. He has a history of questionable coronary artery disease but takes no medication. He has no stated allergies.

FAMILY HISTORY: Noncontributory.

SOCIAL HISTORY: Negative for chest pain or shortness of breath. Occasional problems with constipation.

PHYSICAL EXAMINATION

GENERAL: The patient is a well-developed male in no acute distress.

HEENT: Normal.

NECK: Supple. No masses.

·HEART: Heart sounds are of good quality. No murmurs or cardiomegaly noted.

LUNGS: Lungs are free and equal in expansion, bilaterally. No rales.

----------------------- begin page 2 -----------------------

ABDOMEN: Soft. Liver, spleen, and kidneys not palpable. The bladder is not distended.

EXTREMITIES: No edema.

NEUROLOGICAL: Negative.

IMPRESSION: Benign prostatic hypertrophy with recurrent outlet obstruction.

PLAN: Transurethral resection of the prostate.

Benjamin Keytone, MD/xx

CHART NOTE

Patient Name: Jackson-Jones, Betty Ann

Date of Birth: November 2, 19xx

Examination Date: *Current date*

HISTORY OF PRESENT ILLNESS: This a 49-year-old black female who is status post Marshall-Marchetti-Krantz bladder neck suspension in (*current month and year*). She was in retention while in the hospital, but was discharged voiding spontaneously. She called today complaining of suprapubic discomfort, urinary frequency, with small volume voids. She complained of feeling warm, although her temperature was not taken at home. No chills or sweats. She is complaining of malaise.

PHYSICAL EXAMINATION

VITAL SIGNS: Temperature 97.8, pulse 79, respirations 22/min. BP 157/86.

LUNGS: Clear to auscultation.

HEART: Regular rhythm and rate. No murmurs. CVA regions are without tenderness.

ABDOMEN: The abdomen is soft and tender in the suprapubic region, right more so than left. The bladder is nonpalpable. No rebound or masses. Her midline infraumbilical wound is healing nicely.

PELVIC: Pelvic exam reveals an exquisitely tender bladder base and trigone area. No other abnormalities noted.

LABORATORY DATA: Her WBC is 6.8. Urinalysis reveals 3-5 white cells and 3-5 red cells per high-powered field.

IMPRESSION: Probable cystitis.

PLAN: I have placed her on Noroxin, 400 mg p.o. b.i.d. for 5 days. She is instructed to drink plenty of fluids. She is to return in one week for a follow-up visit.

_____
Helen Loop, MD/xx

HISTORY AND PHYSICAL EXAMINATION

Patient Name: Pierre, Julia

File Number: 814790

Date of Birth: September 6, 19xx

Examination Date: *Current date*

Physician: Helen Loop, MD

HISTORY

HISTORY OF PRESENT ILLNESS: This 73-year-old female presents with episodes of intermittent gross hematuria. A recent urogram showed a filling defect of the left kidney. A subsequent CT renal scan revealed a 6 mm mass involving the upper pole of the left kidney.

PAST MEDICAL HISTORY: History of hypertension and Crohn's disease and diverticulitis. The patient had a laparotomy for a perforated bowel in October of 1995. The patient continues with the colostomy that was performed at that time. A hysterectomy was performed in 1974.

MEDICATIONS:
1. Lopressor
2. Aldactone
3. Imodium

ALLERGIES: None known.

FAMILY HISTORY: Noncontributory.

SOCIAL HISTORY: Positive for tobacco until the past year.

REVIEW OF SYSTEMS: Negative for chest pain or dyspnea on exertion. No change in weight or bowel habits. The patient has trouble with arthritis of the left hip.

PHYSICAL EXAMINATION

GENERAL: Julia is a healthy appearing 73-year-old female in no acute distress.

HEENT: Clear.

NECK: Supple, without masses.

------------------------ begin page 2 ------------------------

HEART: Regular rhythm. No murmurs or gallops.

ABDOMEN: Soft, nontender, with active bowel sounds and no masses. The left lower quadrant colostomy is noted.

GENITALIA: External genitalia is normal.

EXTREMITIES: No pretibial edema.

NEUROLOGIC: Grossly intact.

IMPRESSION:
1. Large mass of left kidney with a filling defect of the left renal pelvis. Carcinoma is suspected, although cell type (transitional cell versus clear cell) remains unclear.
2. History of Crohn's disease.
3. Status post colostomy and bowel resection of October 1995.
4. Hypertension.

PLAN: Admit patient to University Hospital for a right nephrectomy. If the cell type is identified as transitional cell carcinoma, the ureter will also be resected.

_____
Helen Loop, MD/xx

HISTORY AND PHYSICAL EXAMINATION

Patient Name: Dawson, Thomas

File Number: 08081

Date of Birth: March 25, 1948

Examination Date: *Current date*

Physician: Theodore Trigone, MD

HISTORY

CHIEF COMPLAINT: Dysuria

HISTORY OF PRESENT ILLNESS: Patient presents today complaining of some discomfort with urination. He states that he felt fine while he was taking the Bactrim. He did not have any problems with urination. Now he is complaining of some discomfort prior to and after voiding. He denies chest pain. No respiratory problems. He denies any fever or chills with these symptoms. His appetite is good. He does have joint aches and pains which have been a common occurrence for him. He tolerated the journey to his daughter's wedding very well.

PHYSICAL EXAMINATION

GENERAL: Weight 187, up 2 lb. BP 132/58, pulse 60. The heart is regular and without murmur.

CHEST: Lungs are clear. No rales, rhonchi or wheezing.

ABDOMEN: Soft. No suprapubic tenderness or CVA tenderness.

EXTREMITIES: Some persistent edema noted. He has deformity of the knees and hands secondary to arthritis.

LABORATORY TESTS: Urinalysis shows 2+ leukocytes which were greater than 10 per high-powered field and 3+ heme which is greater than 30 per high-powered field.

ASSESSMENT:
1. Urinary tract infection.
2. Probable chronic cystitis.
3. Degenerative joint disease.
4. History of Parkinson's disease.

---------------------- begin page 2 ----------------------

5. History of prostate cancer.
6. Status post radiation therapy.

PLAN: The patient will resume a regimen of Bactrim DS 1 b.i.d. × 10 days. Repeat UA and C&S in two weeks. After he finishes the Bactrim, I will place him on Trimpex 100 mg daily. This can be taken at nighttime. We will see if it keeps him from experiencing further urinary symptoms. He is to schedule a follow-up appointment in three months or p.r.n. basis.

Theodore Trigone, MD/xx

Current date

J. Thomas Geiger, MD
FedDes Wellness Center
Family Practice Division, Suite 300
101 Wellness Way Drive
New York, NY 10036

Re: Mary Ross
    Date of Birth: June 11, 19xx

Dear Dr. Geiger

This 43-year-old female noticed the onset of vague abdominal pain 3-4 days ago. The pain appeared to start in the periumbilical area and then improved. Shortly thereafter, the pain returned to the lower abdomen, particularly on the left side. She presented to the University Hospital Emergency Department yesterday evening, at which time the pain was described as subcostal. She also reported episodes of gross hematuria. She experienced some nausea with vomiting. She denied fever, chills, dysuria, frequency, or other voiding symptoms. There is no previous history of urinary tract infections, stones, or genitourinary surgery.

The past medical history is remarkable for an appendectomy. The patient also has had a tubal ligation and surgery for an ovarian cyst.

On physical examination, the abdomen appears relatively soft, but diffuses tender, particularly on the left upper and left lower quadrants. Some guarding was noted, with no clearly elicited rebound. There were no abdominal masses. The patient has no CVA masses or tenderness. A rectal examination was performed which shows no evidence of masses or pain. The stool was guaiac negative.

The laboratory studies showed a white blood count of 8.8 on the evening of *(yesterday's date)* and 10.6 earlier today. The urinalysis on *(yesterday's date)* was described as "turbid yellow" with greater than 100 red cells per high-powered field. Urinalysis today shows 6-10 red cells. There is no suggestion of infection with white cells or bacteria.

A renal ultrasound was performed, showing no evidence of hydronephrosis or renal masses. A KUB showed no evidence of stone overlying the urinary tract. A diuresis renogram was performed and this study was normal, with no evidence of obstruction of either collecting system.

---------------------- begin page 2 ----------------------

The etiology of the pain remains unclear, although possibilities would include a calculus cholecystitis or another ovarian cyst. With the absence of obstruction on the renogram, the cause of pain is not suggestive of a stone or other cause of renal colic. The negative urinalysis would also mitigate against a pyelonephritis and the pain is clearly abdominal rather than in the CVA region. The etiology of the reported gross hematuria remains unclear.

RECOMMENDATION: A surgical consultation is advised to further evaluate the abdomen. At some future time, a steroid prep urogram and cystoscopy would be prudent to further evaluate the cause of the reported hematuria.

Thank you for allowing us to see this very pleasant patient in consultation. I will follow along with you.

Sincerely

Helen Loop, MD

xx

CHAPTER 7 / 7T-14

HISTORY AND PHYSICAL EXAMINATION

Patient Name: Resch, Gladys

File Number: 60954

Date of Birth: August 28, 19xx

Examination Date: *Current date*

Physician: Helen Loop, MD

HISTORY

CHIEF COMPLAINT: Incontinence of urine.

HISTORY OF PRESENT ILLNESS: This 93-year-old white female saw me for the first time on July 21, 1996, with complaints of urinary incontinence of about one month duration. Examination at that time demonstrated a marked cystocele and a positive Marshall test. Because of her age, I convinced her to try therapy with a pessary, and a 2-inch Gellhorn pessary was inserted. She is now able to empty the bladder with her pessary, but is constantly dribbling. She has become constipated with a pessary and does not like it. She desires surgical correction of her problem.

PAST MEDICAL HISTORY: Unremarkable for a 93-year-old female. Her only surgical procedures include laparotomy for ectopic pregnancy almost 72 years ago. No known allergies.

MEDICATIONS: Hydrochlorothiazide 25 mg daily for hypertension. Meclizine on a p.r.n basis for dizziness.

PHYSICAL EXAMINATION

GENERAL: Mrs. Resch is a well-developed, well-nourished, alert, white female appearing much younger than her stated age. Blood pressure is 134/66. Her weight is 143 pounds.

HEENT: Pupils are equal and reactive to light and accommodation. Extraocular muscles intact.

NECK: Supple. No masses or adenopathy. Thyroid not enlarged. Oropharynx is clear.

CHEST: Clear to percussion and auscultation.

HEART: Regular rate and rhythm. No murmurs or gallops.

- begin page 2 -

BREASTS: No masses.

ABDOMEN: Flat, soft, nontender. Scars appropriate to noted previous surgeries.

PELVIC: Remarkable for a 2-inch Gellhorn pessary in place. She desires that it be left in place until the surgery. Upon removal of the pessary, there is a large cystocele and a small rectocele, which is currently asymptomatic. The cervix and uterus are unremarkable. No unusual adnexal masses are noted. The remainder of the exam is normal.

IMPRESSION: Stress urinary incontinence and genital prolapse that is unresponsive to a pessary.

PLAN: Vaginal hysterectomy, anterior colporrhaphy, and endoscopic urethral suspension. Depending upon my findings at surgery, a posterior repair may be performed. The procedures, its complications, particularly related to urinary retention, recurrence of stress incontinence, and discharge with a suprapubic tube have been discussed. She understands and desires to proceed.

Helen Loop, MD/xx

CHAPTER 7 / 7T-15

CONSULTATION REPORT

Patient Name: Sever, Jed

File Number: 90258

Date of Birth: November 18, 19xx

Examination Date: *Current date*

Requesting Physician: Izzy Sertoli, MD

I was asked by Dr. Izzy Sertoli to evaluate Mr. Sever for urinary retention.

SUBJECTIVE: Jed Sever is a 75-year-old gentleman who was recently admitted to University Hospital for urinary retention. He had a #18 French Foley catheter inserted upon admission. He subsequently developed gross hematuria with clotting and a nondraining catheter.

OBJECTIVE: His temperature is 98.9. His blood pressure is 120/71. His abdomen is soft and nontender with a noted midline scar from a previous exploratory procedure. The bladder is not distended. The #18 French Foley catheter is draining blood-tinged urine. There are several worm-like clots in the drainage bag. The left testicle and adnexa are normal. The right testicle is noteworthy for a moderate-sized hydrocele.

The existing catheter was removed and a #24 French coude' catheter was passed with little difficulty. The catheter irrigates well. The balloon was inflated with 10 cc of saline. Several small clots were recovered. Currently, the urine is clear. The catheter was connected to closed drainage.

ASSESSMENT: Urinary retention and hematuria.

PLAN: The patient was started on Maxaquin 400 mg p.o. q.d. for a 7-day course. The patient will be discharged tomorrow. In two weeks, he is scheduled for a renal ultrasound and cystourethroscope.

Benjamin Keytone, MD/xx

See Pretests (7T-5) and (7T-6).

CHAPTER 8 / PART I PRETEST

1. a	26. a	51. a	75. c
2. a	27. a	52. c	76. a
3. a	28. d	53. b	77. a
4. b	29. a	54. b	78. c
5. b	30. c	55. d	79. c
6. c	31. a	56. d	80. b
7. a	32. d	57. c	81. b
8. d	33. c	58. a	82. c
9. b	34. a	59. d	83. a
10. d	35. d	60. b	84. b
11. c	36. a	61. b	85. d
12. b	37. b	62. a	86. a
13. b	38. b	63. d	87. c
14. d	39. c	64. b	88. a
15. c	40. d	65. c	89. b
16. b	41. a	66. a	90. c
17. c	42. b	67. c	91. a
18. c	43. c	68. a	92. c
19. c	44. c	69. c	93. d
20. a	45. b	70. a	94. a
21. a	46. b	71. a	95. b
22. a	47. d	72. a	96. a
23. c	48. a	73. b	97. d
24. b	49. d	74. a	98. c
25. b	50. b		

CHAPTER 8 / ACTIVITY 3 (8T-1)

1. Adenocarcinoma is a malignant tumor of the glands.
   She is status postabdominal surgery for adenocarcinoma of uterus in 1990.
2. Adenopathy is the enlargement of the glands, especially the lymph nodes.
   The neck was bull-like without adenopathy or venous distention.
3. Afebrile is without fever.
   The patient has been afebrile.
4. Amoxicillin is the generic name for an aminopenicillin antibiotic.
   She was also started on another antibiotic, which may have been amoxicillin.
5. Aneurysm is a localized dilitation of the wall of a blood vessel.
   He is six weeks status post aortic aneurysm repair.
6. Arteriogram is the radiographic visualization of an artery after injection of a contrast medium.
   Previous assessment includes a carotid arteriogram.
7. Ascites is the accumulation of fluid in the peritoneal cavity.
   The abdomen is distended, and there may be ascites.
8. Atelectasis is the collapse of a portion of the lung.
   Chest x-ray showed atelectasis in the right upper lobe.
9. Auscultation is the act of listening for sounds produced within the body with an unaided ear or with a stethoscope.
   The chest is clear to auscultation.
10. Bilateral is affecting both sides.
    He had a bilateral hernia repair three years ago.
11. Bronchodilator is any drug that has the capacity of increasing the capacity of the pulmonary air passages and improve ventilation to the lungs.
    After his hospital course we will try to get him to stop smoking and start him on an inhaled bronchodilator program for his obstructive lung disease.

12. Bruit is a sound or murmur heard on auscultation.
    There is a short right carotid bruit.
13. Caries is the condition of decay and destruction of a tooth.
    Periodontal disease and caries were noted in various stages.
14. Cephalosporin is a generic name for any of the large group of broad-spectrum antibiotics.
    A first generation cephalosporin would cover his staph aureus.
15. Claudication is cramping pains of the calves caused by poor circulation to the leg muscles.
    He does not have symptoms of claudication.
16. Continent is the ability to control urination and defecation urges.
    He does have bladder spasms and remains partially continent.
17. Cor pulmonale is an abnormal heart condition characterized by the increased size of the right ventricle.
    The patient exhibited cor pulmonale, severe emphysema, and hypertension.
18. Cyanosis is the bluish-purple discoloration of the skin due to lack of oxygenated blood.
    No clubbing or cyanosis was noted in the extremities.
19. Dentition refers to the position and condition of the teeth.
    There was poor dentition with some periodontal disease noted and caries in various stages.
20. Diuresis is the increased excretion of urine.
    We will have an answer if the next chest x-ray results show improvement with diuresis.
21. Diuretic is a substance that promotes the excretion of urine.
    Diuretics have already been ordered.
22. Doxepin is the generic name for an antidepressant.
    Her current medication included doxepin 1 tablet t.i.d.
23. Dyspnea is the labored or difficult breathing.
    The dyspnea is worse on exertion, especially when climbing stairs and doing his job as a janitor.
24. Dysrhythmia is a disordered rhythm.
    Heather Williams is a 78-year-old lady with a long history of hypertension and recurrent supraventricular dysrhythmia.
25. Echocardiogram is a diagnostic procedure using ultrasound to study heart structure and motion.
    Previous assessment includes a carotid arteriogram and an echocardiogram for left ventricular function that was normal.
26. Edema is the accumulation of excess fluid in the tissues of the body.
    There was no edema noted in the extremities.
27. Effusion is the escape of fluid into a body cavity.
    The patient's past history was remarkable for a hospital admission two months ago for a large pleural effusion and mass.
28. Embolus is a mass that is brought by the blood from another vessel that obstructs blood circulation.
    I suspect there is a substantial chance this may yet be a pulmonary embolus.
29. Emesis is to vomit.
    She was starting to spike fevers of 102 and felt toxic with coughing and emesis.
30. Empiric is treating a disease based upon observation and experience rather than reasoning alone.
    I would empirically proceed with pulmonary angiography.
31. Erythema is redness of the skin.
    Over the past 2-3 months, she has noticed increasing pedal edema although there has been no erythema, inflammation, or calf tenderness.
32. Erythromycin is a generic name for a broad-spectrum antibiotic.
    The patient was seen a couple of weeks ago and was started on erythromycin.
33. Fibrillation is the uncoordinated twitching of muscle fibers.
    This is a 49-year-old white male admitted with new onset of atrial fibrillation.
34. Flora are normally occurring microorganisms that live within the body that provide natural immunity against certain organisms.
    A first generation cephalosporin would cover both his normal flora and staph aureus.
35. Gallop is an abnormal heart rhythm.
    The heartbeat was regular without murmur, gallop, or rub.

36. Hemoptysis is the coughing or spitting up blood from the respiratory tract.
    She has had some mild pleuritic pain, but no hemoptysis.
37. Heparin is the generic name for an anticoagulant.
    He was treated initially with intravenous nitroglycerin and intravenous heparin.
38. Homans' sign is a calf pain with dorsiflexion of foot.
    No clubbing, cyanosis, edema or Homans' sign was noted in the extremities.
39. Hydrate is a compound containing water molecules.
    We will also gently hydrate her over the next 24 hours and get a follow-up chest x-ray.
40. Infiltrate is when fluid, cells, or other substances pass into tissue spaces.
    Chest x-ray shows left lower lobe infiltrate.
41. Intrauterine means within the uterus.
    Her last normal menstrual period was approximately one month ago, but she denies the possibility of intrauterine pregnancy.
42. Ischemia is a decreased supply of oxygenated blood to a body part.
    Perhaps a dobutamine MUGA scan will also be required at some point to exclude myocardial ischemia.
43. Isosorbide is the generic name for a nitrate based antianginal agent.
    Her medications included isosorbide 10 mg p.o. q.i.d.
44. Lorazepam is a generic antianxiety drug.
    She is taking lorazepam 1 mg t.i.d. p.r.n.
45. Metastasis is the transfer of disease from one organ or part to another not directly connected with it.
    My impression is that we are dealing with a man with a known mass in his right lung with probable metastasis to his brain.
46. Nebulization is a treatment by a spray.
    The patient was placed on nebulization p.r.n.
47. Nifedipine is a generic calcium channel blocker drug.
    He is taking nifedipine 1 tablet t.i.d.
48. Nitroglycerin is a generic name for a coronary vasodilator, antianginal.
    The patient's medications include nitroglycerin spray, p.r.n.
49. Nocturnal is something that occurs at night.
    We will arrange a nocturnal oxygen saturation test along with a chest x-ray, pulmonary function tests, and a room air arterial blood gas.
50. Nystagmus is the involuntary, rapid, rhythmic movement of the eyeball.
    Extraocular movements were intact without nystagmus.
51. Occlusion is the act of closure or state of being closed.
    Previous assessment includes a carotid arteriogram that showed a right carotid occlusion and an echocardiogram for left ventricular function that was normal.
52. Pedal is a term relating to the foot.
    Over the past 2-3 months, she has noticed increasing pedal edema although there has been no erythema, inflammation, or calf tenderness.
53. Pneumonectomy is the surgical removal of all or a segment of the lung.
    A pneumonectomy was recommended because of evidence of cancer.
54. Pneumothorax is the presence of air or gas in the pleural cavity.
    Chest x-ray showed no evidence of pneumothorax with some hyperinflation and chronic obstructive pulmonary disease changes.
55. Prednisone is a generic corticosteroid drug.
    We will admit, treat with IV antibiotics, oral prednisone, and aerosol bronchodilators.
56. Pulmonary toilet is the cleansing of the trachea and bronchial tree.
    The patient was admitted to the hospital and placed on intravenous antibiotic therapy with pulmonary toilet.
57. Purulent means containing pus.
    She denies fever, sweats, chills, purulent sputum, hemoptysis, or chest pain.
58. Rale is an abnormal crackle sound heard on chest auscultation.
    Chest exam showed decreased breath sound and wheezes without local rales.
59. Rhonchus is an abnormal sound heard on chest auscultation due to an obstructed airway.
    Lung exam demonstrated scattered expiratory wheezes and rhonchi, but fair air excursion.
60. Rub is a sound caused by the rubbing together of two surfaces.
    There was no cardiac rub.
61. Saphenous pertains to the two main superficial veins of the lower leg.
    He has no history of ankle edema or deep vein thrombosis, although he has had coronary artery bypass grafting and a saphenous vein harvest on the left side.
62. Sequela is any abnormal condition that follows and is the result of a disease, treatment or injury.
    He also has a history of a right hip fracture, with residual pain, an appendectomy, a myocardial infarction, and a small CVA with no sequelae.
63. Somnolence is drowsiness.
    He denies any significant daytime somnolence.
64. Sputum is the material coughed up from the lungs and ejected through the mouth.
    She has had some mild pleuritic pain, scant sputum production, but no hemoptysis.
65. Stasis is an abnormal slowing or stopping of fluid flowing through a vessel.
    Extremity evaluation reveals some stasis changes of the lower extremities, with almost absent pulses at the dorsalis pedis and posterior tibialis.
66. Supraventricular refers to situated or occurring above the ventricles.
    Susan is a 65-year-old lady with a history of hypertension and recurrent supraventricular dysrhythmia.
67. Syncope is the act of fainting.
    There has been no syncope.
68. Tachycardia is an abnormally fast heartbeat.
    She had a sinus tachycardia of 110.
69. Theophylline is a generic name for a bronchodilator.
    She was complaining of staggering gait and overall weakness which was thought to be in part secondary to her theophylline level.
70. Thoracentesis is the aspiration of fluid from the chest cavity.
    She underwent thoracentesis, closed needle biopsy, and bronchoscopy under general anesthesia, which resulted in no definitive diagnosis.
71. Thyromegaly is the enlargement of the thyroid gland.
    No neck mass or thyromegaly was noted.
72. Ancef IV is the trade name for an cephalosporin antibiotic.
    We will also place him on Ancef IV and erythromycin orally.
73. Ascriptin is the trade name for a preparation of aspirin with Maalox, an analgesic and anti-inflammatory.
    Her medications included insulin NPH 30 units, regular 6 units in the morning and Ascriptin 1 tablet a day.
74. Atrovent is the trade name for a nasal spray, bronchodilator.
    Her current medications include Atrovent, 2 puffs, q.i.d.
75. Azmacort is the trade name for a corticosteroid for the prevention or treatment of bronchial asthma.
    His current medications include Azmacort 4 puffs, b.i.d.
76. Bumex is the trade name for a loop diuretic.
    The physician prescribed Bumex 2 mg q. a.m.
77. Cardizem is the trade name for a calcium channel blocker for atrial fibrillation.
    Her medications included insulin NPH 30 units, regular 6 units in the morning, Cardizem 30 b.i.d., and Ascriptin 1 tablet a day.
78. Colace is the trade name for a stool softener.
    Her medications included Cardizem 30 b.i.d., Ascriptin 1 tablet a day, and Colace.
79. Compazine is the trade name for a tranquilizer and antiemetic.
    We will place him on Compazine for nausea.
80. Darvon is the trade name for a narcotic analgesic.
    The patient was taking Darvon, 1 p.o. q.6h. p.r.n.

81. Dilantin is the trade name for an anticonvulsant used in the treatment of epilepsy.
Her epilepsy was controlled with Dilantin 100 mg q.i.d.
82. Fibercon is the trade name for a bulk-forming laxative.
Her medications included insulin NPH 30 units, regular 6 units in the morning, Cardizem 30 b.i.d., Ascriptin 1 tablet a day, FiberCon, and Colace.
83. Lopressor is the trade name for an antihypertensive.
The patient's current medications include
Lopressor 50 mg q. a.m., Bumex 2 mg q. a.m., and isosorbide 10 mg p.o. q.i.d.
84. Mevacor is the trade name for an antihyperlipidemic.
The patient's current medications include
Lopressor 50 mg q. a.m., Bumex 2 mg q. a.m.,
isosorbide 10 mg p.o. q.i.d., and Mevacor 20 mg p.o. q.d.
85. NPH (neutral protamine Hagedorn) insulin is trade name for an insulin that decreases blood sugar.
He has added additional doses of regular insulin to his usual regimen of 30 units of NPH and 6 units of regular insulin in the morning.
86. Paxil is the trade name for an antidepressant.
The physician prescribed prednisone and Paxil.
87. Pepcid is the trade name for an acid controller for heartburn and acid indigestion.
The physician prescribed Pepcid, prednisone, and Paxil.
88. Procardia is the trade name for a coronary vasodilator.
The patient is taking Dilantin 100 mg q.i.d.,
Procardia 30 mg q. a.m. and Lopressor 50 mg q. a.m.
89. Proventil MDI is a trade name for a bronchodilator, metered dose inhaler.
We will provide Proventil MDI on a p.r.n. basis.
90. Restoril is the trade name for a sedative-hypnotic.
The physician prescribed Pepcid, prednisone, Restoril, and Paxil.
91. Serevent is the trade name for an aerosol bronchodilator.
The patient was using several bronchodilators including
Serevent 2 puffs b.i.d. and Azmacort 4 puffs b.i.d.
92. Slo-bid is the trade name for an extended-release bronchodilator.
Her current medications are Slo-bid 300 mg p.o. b.i.d.,
Lorazepam 1 mg t.i.d. p.r.n., nitro-derm patch 0.2 mg daily p.r.n., and oxygen 2 liters by nasal cannula 24 hours a day.
93. Theo-Dur is the trade name for a bronchodilator.
His current medications are potassium 2 tablets t.i.d.,
doxepin 1 tablet t.i.d., nifedipine 1 tablet t.i.d.,
Xanax 1/2 tablet q.4h. as needed, and Theo-Dur b.i.d.
94. Vanceril is the trade name for a corticosteroid.
The patient's current medications are Proventil, metered dose inhaler, 2 puffs t.i.d. and Vanceril, 2 puffs, q.i.d.
95. Vasotec is the trade name for an antihypertensive.
The patient's current medications include
Lopressor 50 mg q. a.m., Bumex 2 mg q. a.m.,
Zantac 150 mg b.i.d., Vasotec 10 mg p.o. b.i.d.,
isosorbide 10 mg p.o. q.i.d., and Mevacor 20 mg p.o. q.d.
96. Ventolin is the trade name for a bronchodilator.
The patient was using several bronchodilators including
Ventolin 2 puffs q.i.d., Serevent 2 puffs b.i.d., and
Azmacort 4 puffs b.i.d.
97. Xanax is the trade name for an antianxiety agent.
She was taking Xanax 1/2 tablet q.4h. as needed and
Theo-Dur b.i.d.
98. Zantac is the trade name for an acid controller for heartburn and acid indigestion.
The patient's current medications include
Lopressor 50 mg q. a.m., Bumex 2 mg q. a.m.,
Zantac 150 mg b.i.d., Vasotec 10 mg p.o. b.i.d.,
isosorbide 10 mg p.o. q.i.d., and Mevacor 20 mg p.o. q.d.

CHAPTER 8 / PART I CHECK YOUR PROGRESS

1. b	26. c	51. c	75. a
2. b	27. a	52. d	76. a
3. d	28. d	53. b	77. c
4. a	29. b	54. b	78. c
5. d	30. d	55. a	79. b
6. c	31. c	56. d	80. b
7. b	32. a	57. b	81. c
8. b	33. a	58. c	82. a
9. c	34. b	59. a	83. b
10. b	35. a	60. c	84. d
11. b	36. c	61. d	85. a
12. a	37. b	62. c	86. c
13. b	38. b	63. a	87. a
14. d	39. a	64. d	88. b
15. c	40. d	65. c	89. c
16. a	41. a	66. d	90. a
17. b	42. c	67. a	91. c
18. b	43. a	68. b	92. d
19. a	44. a	69. b	93. a
20. a	45. a	70. c	94. b
21. c	46. a	71. a	95. a
22. a	47. a	72. b	96. d
23. d	48. d	73. a	97. c
24. b	49. a	74. c	98. c
25. a	50. b		

CHAPTER 8 / PART II PRETEST (8T-2)

HISTORY AND PHYSICAL EXAMINATION

Patient Name: Horner, Judith

File Number: 09237

Date of Birth: January 3, 19xx

Examination Date: *Current date*

Physician: Douglas Sputum, MD

HISTORY

HISTORY OF PRESENT ILLNESS: The patient is a 25-year-old white female who presents today following a three-week illness and progressive shortness of breath and cough. She has seen two different doctors in last five days regarding this problem. She got tired of the situation and self-referred herself to our office. Apparently the patient was seen a couple of weeks ago and was started on erythromycin. She was on that for a few days until she was taken off of it. She was also started on another antibiotic, which may have been amoxicillin. Nonetheless, she was not getting much better. She was starting to spike fevers of 102 and felt toxic with coughing and emesis. She has had some mild pleuritic pain, scant sputum production, but no hemoptysis.

PAST MEDICAL HISTORY: Noncontributory.

FAMILY HISTORY: Not obtained.

SOCIAL HISTORY: She works as a receptionist and smokes about a pack of cigarettes a day.

REVIEW OF SYSTEMS: Negative other than the above discussion.

PHYSICAL EXAMINATION

GENERAL: She is a well-developed, well-nourished white female.

HEENT: Reveals multiple earrings in the right ear and one in the left eyebrow. Otherwise the exam is negative.

NECK: Trachea is midline. There are no nodes.

HEART: Normal.

CHEST: Mild rub posteriorly.

------------------------- begin page 2 -------------------------

ABDOMEN: Soft.

EXTREMITIES: No clubbing, cyanosis or edema.

LABORATORY DATA: Elevated white count. Chest x-ray shows right lower lobe pneumonitis.

IMPRESSION: Right lower lobe pneumonia, unresponsive to outpatient therapy.

PLAN: Admit to hospital and place her on intravenous antibiotic therapy with pulmonary toilet. We will then convert to oral medications and stabilization, then discharge.

_____

Douglas Sputum, MD/xx

CHAPTER 8 / PART II ACTIVITY 4

Errors are indicated in bold and italics. Margins are formatted at 1 inch.

CONSULTATION REPORT

Patient Name: Calabretta, Gregory

File Number: 09451

Date of Birth: January 15, 19xx

Examination Date: *Current date*

Requesting Physician: Izzy Sertoli, MD

HISTORY OF PRESENT ILLNESS: The patient is a *42-year-old* white male who presented to the hospital with some vague chest pain as well as a history of shortness of *breath.* The patient states to me that he has had shortness of *breath* for approximately a year and *a half.* The *dyspnea* is worse on *exertion,* especially when climbing stairs and doing his job as a janitor. He has had a dry cough**,** which on occasion was productive of clear *sputum* but has not been productive of blood or *pus.* He complains of vague**,** substernal**,** *left-sided* chest pain. The pain is worse with movement or *palpation* of the area.

PAST HISTORY: His past history is significant for asthma. He had a bilateral hernia repair *three* years ago.

REVIEW OF SYSTEMS: *Negative.*

PHYSICAL EXAMINATION

GENERAL: His blood pressure is *120/70,* pulse *70,* respirations *12/min.*

HEENT: Negative. Neck veins are not *distended.* Trachea is *midline.* There are no *nodes* in the *supraclavicular* or cervical chain.

CHEST: Breath sounds reveal some *crackles* at the *bases* but are otherwise negative.

HEART: Heart sounds are normal, but distant.

EXTREMITIES: No *clubbing,* cyanosis, or edema noted.

LABORATORY DATA: Room air *ABG* shows a *PO2* of *59* without *CO2* retention. Chest x-ray reveals a diffuse *interstitial* process with no hilar *nodes.*

------------------------- begin page 2 -------------------------

IMPRESSION: I suspect that we are dealing with an inflammatory *process* in his lungs. *An* illness such as sarcoid is a *distinct* possibility as we discussed on the phone last night. Additionally, this could be *CHF,* although clinically it does not look like it. We will have an answer if the next chest x-*ray* results show improvement with *diuresis.* If it does not**, then** a more *extensive work-up* shall take place. Clinically, I doubt an infection. I suspect we end up doing a *bronchoscopy* with a biopsy.

PLAN: If there is no improvement on *tomorrow's* x-ray, we will proceed with a more *aggressive work-up.* The patient states *he* has no previous chest x-rays for comparison. *Quadruple space*

_____

Allan Bolus, MD/*xx*

FedDes Wellness Center
Pulmonary Medicine Division, Suite 451
101 Wellness Way Drive
New York, NY 10036

Current date

Charles P. Davis, MD
FedDes Wellness Center
Family Practice Division, Suite 300
101 Wellness Way Drive
New York, NY 10036

Re: Lawrence A. Rabia
    Date of Birth: January 20, 19xx

Dear Dr. Davis

Mr. Rabia is a 62-year-old white male with a past history of smoking. He is six-weeks status postaortic aneurysm repair. Postoperatively he did well and was discharged. At home, he has been fairly homebound but not bedridden. He was in his usual state of health, without an upper respiratory illness, cough, congestion, or aches, when he developed the acute onset of left-sided pleuritic chest pain. The pleuritic component of the pain has intensified and is actually positional at this time. He denied any hemoptysis. He has some mild shortness of breath and mild dyspnea or exertion. He has no history of ankle edema or deep vein thrombosis, although he has had coronary artery bypass grafting and a saphenous vein harvest on the left side.

On physical examination, the patient's temperature was 99. His other vital signs were stable. HEENT was benign. Neck showed no mass or adenopathy. Lungs showed diminished breath sounds bilaterally, with scratchy, rub-like sounds on the left side. Cardiovascular exam shows S1, S2 within normal limits and grade I/VI systolic ejection murmur at the lower left sternal border. There was no cardiac rub. Abdomen was soft. Extremities showed no edema. Calves were benign and nontender.

Chest x-ray showed no evidence of pneumothorax with some hyperinflation and chronic obstructive pulmonary disease changes. His ventilation perfusion scan showed an abnormal perfusion study with three matched defects.

IMPRESSION: Pleuritic left-sided chest pain six-weeks postoperative and an abnormal perfusion scan. Given the indeterminate scan, I suspect there is a substantial chance this may yet be a pulmonary embolus. I would empirically heparinize at this time and proceed with pulmonary angiography. I have discussed this with the patient and he understands and agrees.

Thank you for this referral.

Sincerely

Allan Bolus, MD

xx

CHART NOTE

Patient Name: Bolton, Maggie

Date of Birth: February 5, 1987

Examination Date: *Current date*

SUBJECTIVE: Maggie came in today for a follow-up visit. She still feels weak. Her appetite remains the same. Her living situation is unchanged, despite our best efforts.

OBJECTIVE: Her weight has remained stable. Her blood work looks good. Her chest x-ray demonstrates prominent markings in the right middle lobe and a questionable nodular density in the right apex. She has no cervical adenopathy. Lungs show decreased breath sounds. Cardiac exam RRR without appreciable murmurs, rubs or gallops. She has normal chest wall excursion. The abdomen is soft. She has some tenderness in the left rib cage.

ASSESSMENT:
1. COPD.
2. Weight loss, which at this point, has stabilized.

PLAN: I doubt that she has lung cancer, but to be sure I will re-evaluate the left upper lobe a little better. I have ordered apical lordotic views of her lungs and will have them compared to previous films. I will follow along in her weight loss as well as her rib pain.

_____

Douglas Sputum, MD/xx

CONSULTATION REPORT

Patient Name: Pickman, Peter

File Number: 09734

Date of Birth: February 9, 19xx

Examination Date: *Current date*

Requesting Physician: Charles P. Davis, MD

HISTORY OF PRESENT ILLNESS: This is a 49-year-old white male admitted with new onset of atrial fibrillation. He is a nonsmoker with no previous history of pulmonary disease. There is a history of asthma and allergies in his family. His atrial fibrillation has improved with IV therapy, although he still complains of some dyspnea and chest congestion. In addition, he has loud snoring and some irregular nighttime breathing. He denies any significant daytime somnolence.

On physical examination, he is in sinus rhythm with a rate of 80-88. Respiratory rate is 12/min. HEENT showed a small posterior pharynx with a large soft palate and tongue. No neck mass or thyromegaly. Lung exam demonstrated scattered expiratory wheezes and rhonchi, but fair air excursion. Cardiovascular exam revealed crisp heart sounds without murmur or S3. The abdomen was nontender. The extremities were benign.

IMPRESSION:
1. New onset of atrial fibrillation with a questionable airway disease.
2. Possible obstructive sleep apnea.

PLAN: We will arrange a nocturnal oxygen saturation test along with a chest x-ray, pulmonary function tests, and a room air arterial blood gas. We will provide Proventil MDI on a p.r.n. basis.

_____

Neal Alveoli, MD/xx

CHAPTER 8 / PART III PRETEST (8T-5)

HISTORY AND PHYSICAL EXAMINATION

Patient Name: Nachmanson, Gussie

File Number: 00824

Date of Birth: July 5, 19xx

Examination Date: *Current date*

Physician: Allan Bolus, MD

HISTORY

CHIEF COMPLAINT: Shortness of breath.

HISTORY OF PRESENT ILLNESS: This is an 89-year-old lady who lives at Shadyside Retirement Village. She presents with several days of increasing shortness of breath. She denies fever, sweats, chills, purulent sputum, hemoptysis, or chest pain. She smokes about a pack of cigarettes a day.

PAST HISTORY: Remarkable for a hospital admission two months ago for a large pleural effusion and mass. She underwent thoracentesis, closed needle biopsy, and bronchoscopy under general anesthesia, which resulted in no definitive diagnosis. However her CT scan and clinical presentation were consistent with some kind of tumor process in the right upper lobe and/or the thyroid area. She was placed on antibiotic steroids. She was felt to be too frail to pursue a more vigorous diagnostic approach and was sent home, realizing that we had no definitive diagnosis and that problems may recur.

MEDICATIONS:
1. Pepcid.
2. Prednisone.
3. Restoril.
4. Paxil.

ALLERGIES: Penicillin.

FAMILY HISTORY: Her father died from pancreatic cancer. Her mother died from complications of pneumonia. She has one sister with lung disease.

REVIEW OF SYSTEMS: Negative, except as above.

---------------------- begin page 2 ----------------------

GENERAL: Pleasant, elderly, easily confused female who is in no acute distress now that she is placed on oxygen support.

VITAL SIGNS: BP 138/60, pulse 100 and regular, respirations 24/min., and temperature 99. Saturation is 93-94 on 3 liters of oxygen.

CHEST: Clear.

NECK: Neck veins are not distended. Trachea is midline.

LUNGS: Dullness in the right chest. Left chest reveals scattered rhonchi.

HEART: Heart is regular without gallop or rub.

ABDOMEN: The abdomen is soft, without masses. There is some guarding.

EXTREMITIES: There is no clubbing, cyanosis, or peripheral edema. All extremities move well. There is no localized neurologic deficit.

DIAGNOSTIC TESTING: Chest x-ray show a mass in the right upper lobe, recurrent densities in the right lower lung, and a moderately large pleural effusion.

IMPRESSION: The patient probably has an inoperable tumor process and for this reason we did not pursue further work-up during her last admission. However, the severe dyspnea has reoccurred, although, not unexpectedly. We need to once again address the diagnosis. If no diagnosis can be made with a closed procedure, we will either proceed with an open biopsy with the surgeons or basically treat her as if this is a tumor without confirmation and make her comfortable.

PLAN: We will admit the patient and proceed with a simple thoracentesis and closed needle biopsy. If that is negative, then we will think about a more vigorous approach.

_____

Allan Bolus, MD/xx

CONSULTATION REPORT

Patient Name: Keiffer, Randy

File Number: 09661

Date of Birth: February 10, 19xx

Examination Date: *Current date*

Requesting Physician: J. Thomas Geiger, MD

HISTORY OF PRESENT ILLNESS: Mr. Keiffer is a 65-year-old white male who is referred to us by Dr. J. Thomas Geiger. About three or four weeks ago he was in South Carolina vacationing when he had an episode of hemoptysis. Subsequent chest x-ray and CT scan showed a 5 × 5 right mid to upper lobe lung field mass. He presents to us for further evaluation. He has now developed neurologic complaints of headache, dizziness, nausea, and difficulty with his gait. He describes his gait difficulty as being as if he were drunk with wobbly gait as opposed to one who feels like he is going to faint. After walking short distances, he becomes quite nauseated and has trouble keeping down food. His episode of hemoptysis was only during one or two days. It has since stopped and has not returned. He has not coughed up any other mucus. He denies any wheeze, fever, chills, chest pain, or pleurisy.

PAST MEDICAL HISTORY: His past medical history is insignificant for medical illness, no malignancy, and no TB. He is a former smoker who quit 25 years ago. He had smoked 2 packs of cigarettes a day for 30 years.

SOCIAL HISTORY: He is a retired automobile salesman.

REVIEW OF SYSTEMS: Negative other than the above.

PHYSICAL EXAMINATION

VITAL SIGNS: BP 110/70, pulse 70, and respirations 12/min.

HEENT: Negative.

NECK: Neck veins are not distended. Trachea is midline. There are no nodes in the supraclavicular or cervical chain.

CHEST: Chest is clear.

HEART: Heart sounds are normal.

---------------------- begin page 2 ----------------------

ABDOMEN: Abdomen is soft, without organomegaly. It is noted that his pants are quite loose. He reports that he has had a 10-pound weight loss.

EXTREMITIES: Extremities are without clubbing, cyanosis, or edema. I had him walk, and it is obvious that he has difficulty with his gait, especially on his tiptoes. The more he walked, the more wobbly he got and then he became nauseated.

IMPRESSION: My impression is that we are dealing with a man with a known mass in his right lung with probable metastasis to his brain. He is to the point of dehydration and falling and injuring himself as well. He needs metastatic work-up and a bronchoscopy, but his immediate needs are hydration and care with his gait.

PLAN: We will admit him to the hospital for hydration and start a work-up on his lung and probable metastases. After we get a definitive answer to his situation, we can make suggestions for treatment.

Thank you for involving us in the care of this patient.

_____

Douglas Sputum, MD/xx

_____

HISTORY AND PHYSICAL EXAMINATION

Patient Name: Banks, Francine

File Number: 09571

Date of Birth: February 25, 19xx

Examination Date: *Current date*

Physician: Allan Bolus, MD

HISTORY

HISTORY OF PRESENT ILLNESS: This is a 28-year-old white female with a history of asthma resulting in multiple hospital admissions. She had a recent upper respiratory infection of 7-10 days duration. She has complained of cough, chest burning, and congestion with blood-tinged sputum over the past 2-3 days. She was started on oral erythromycin without improvement. She presents today with increasing shortness of breath and chest discomfort. She uses only a Proventil inhaler and erythromycin at home.

PAST MEDICAL HISTORY: Noncontributory.

ALLERGIES: She has an allergic reaction to aspirin.

FAMILY HISTORY: Unremarkable.

REVIEW OF SYSTEMS: Her last normal menstrual period was approximately one month ago, but she denies the possibility of intrauterine pregnancy.

PHYSICAL EXAMINATION

VITAL SIGNS: Temperature was 100.4. She had a sinus tachycardia of 110. BP 110/60. Respiratory rate 20-24/min.

HEENT: Sclerae were clear. Conjunctivae pink and dry. Nasopharynx and TMs were clear. Oropharynx was clear.

---------------------- begin page 2 ----------------------

NECK: No masses or adenopathy. Neck was supple, without stiffness.

LUNGS: Coarse rales and rhonchi were heard in the right upper and left lower lobe region. There were a few scattered expiratory wheezes, but fair air excursion.

HEART: Sinus tachycardia without murmur or S3.

ABDOMEN: The abdomen was soft, with mild suprapubic tenderness without rebound, rigidity or mass. Bowel sounds were active.

EXTREMITIES: Extremity exam revealed no edema. Calves were benign.

NEUROLOGICAL: Grossly intact.

DIAGNOSTIC TESTING: Chest x-ray showed infiltrate and atelectasis in the right upper lobe with right middle lobe and left lower lobe infiltrates.

IMPRESSION:
1. Trilobed pneumonia.
2. History of asthma with intermittent steroid use.

PLAN:
1. We will admit her to the hospital and place her on aerosol bronchodilator, IV steroids, IV antibiotics and oral erythromycin pending sputum gram stain C&S.
2. Obtain arterial blood gas, WBC, and hematocrit.
3. We will also gently hydrate her over the next 24 hours and get a follow-up chest x-ray.

Allan Bolus, MD/xx

CHAPTER 8 / 8T-8

CONSULTATION REPORT

Patient Name: Williams, Heather

File Number: 097256

Date of Birth: March 1, 19xx

Examination Date: *Current date*

Requesting Physician: Charles P. Davis, MD

HISTORY OF PRESENT ILLNESS: Heather Williams is a 78-year-old lady with a long history of hypertension and recurrent supraventricular dysrhythmia that has been, until recently, well controlled on a medical regimen. She has also been treated for dyspnea. Previous assessment includes a carotid arteriogram that showed a right carotid occlusion and an echocardiogram for left ventricular function that was normal. During the past several days, she has noticed increasing dyspnea and some episodes of hemoptysis. Her chest x-ray was interpreted as showing congestive heart failure resulting in her admission to University Hospital.

PHYSICAL EXAMINATION

VITAL SIGNS: A physical examination shows a blood pressure of 160/90 and a pulse of 80 and regular.

NECK: There is a short right carotid bruit.

LUNGS: Scattered rhonchi are present in both lungs, with coarse rales in both lung bases and a moderately prolonged expiratory phase.

HEART: The heart is not significantly enlarged. There is a short grade II/VI innocent-sounding aortic ejection murmur.

ABDOMEN: The abdomen is unremarkable.

EXTREMITIES: Peripheral pulses are palpable, but decreased, and there is 1+ dependent edema.

IMPRESSION: Mrs. Williams has a previously, well documented, normal left ventricular function. It is possible that the present drug regimen has resulted in fluid retention or a complicated interstitial process is occurring.

------------------------- begin page 2 -------------------------

PLAN: Reassessment of her left ventricular function through echocardiography would be appropriate. Perhaps a dobutamine MUGA scan will also be required at some point to exclude myocardial ischemia. We appreciate the opportunity to participate in her care. Diuretics have already been ordered. We will follow along with you.

Douglas Sputum, MD/xx

CHAPTER 8 / 8T-9

HISTORY AND PHYSICAL EXAMINATION

Patient Name: Nelson, Quinetta

File Number: 09843

Date of Birth: March 13, 19xx

Examination Date: *Current date*

Physician: Neal Alveoli, MD

HISTORY

CHIEF COMPLAINT: Severe dyspnea.

HISTORY OF PRESENT ILLNESS: This is a 70-year-old female with a long history of smoking. Two years ago she was admitted to the hospital with bronchopneumonia and shortness of breath. Unfortunately, her respiratory symptoms have progressed from dyspnea on exertion to shortness of breath while at rest. She is barely able to perform her daily activities at home despite home oxygen and a maximal inhaler regimen. Over the past 2-3 months, she has noticed increasing pedal edema although there has been no erythema, inflammation, or calf tenderness. She presents today with severe dyspnea.

PAST MEDICAL HISTORY: Mrs. Nelson has a history of severe emphysema, DJD, hypertension and TIAs. She is status postabdominal surgery for adenocarcinoma of uterus in 1990.

MEDICATION:
1. Proventil, metered dose inhaler, 2 puffs t.i.d.
2. Vanceril, 2 puffs, q.i.d.
3. Atrovent, 2 puffs, q.i.d.
4. Nitroglycerin spray, p.r.n.
5. Darvon, 1 p.o. q.6h. p.r.n.
6. Slo-bid 300 mg p.o. b.i.d.
7. Lorazepam 1 mg t.i.d. p.r.n.
8. Nitro-derm patch 0.2 mg daily p.r.n.
9. Oxygen 2 liters by nasal cannula 24 hours a day

SOCIAL HISTORY: Former smoker who quit two years ago.

PHYSICAL EXAMINATION

VITAL SIGNS: On physical examination, the blood pressure was 152/92, pulse was 90 and regular, respiratory rate 28-32/min.

HEENT: Sclerae were clear. Conjunctivae pink and moist. Fundi showed mild AV nicking. TMs, nasal, and oropharynx were clear.

NECK: Neck showed JVD three-quarters of the way to the angle of the jaw. No thyromegaly or masses noted.

LUNGS: Diminished breath sounds bilaterally with marked hyperinflation and a few rales in both lung bases.

HEART: Increased P2 with a mid-systolic murmur. Questionable tricuspid regurgitation.

ABDOMEN: Liver was 4-5 finger breadths below the right costal margin. The abdomen is mildly obese, nontender.

EXTREMITIES: 2+ edema to the midcalf, bilaterally.

NEUROLOGICAL: Grossly intact.

IMPRESSION:
1. COPD.
2. Cor pulmonale.
3. Severe emphysema.
4. Hypertension.

PLAN: Mrs. Nelson appeared very dyspneic with respiratory rates in the 28-32 range and admission was recommended for IV steroids, diuresis, and bronchodilators. I believe with diuretics she will improve. We will follow her clinical status, arterial blood gas, and laboratory studies throughout her hospitalization.

_____

Neal Alveoli, MD/xx

CONSULTATION REPORT

Patient Name: Waye, Marty

File Number: 09523

Date of Birth: March 8, 19xx

Examination Date: *Current date*

Requesting Physician: Izzy Sertoli, MD

HISTORY OF PRESENT ILLNESS: This is a 71-year-old male who presented approximately 3-4 days ago with left-sided chest pain and dyspnea. His chest x-ray revealed a left lower lobe infiltrate. He was admitted for IV antibiotics and further therapy.

When his pneumonia did not fully clear, a CT scan was ordered which revealed some narrowing of the left main stem bronchus, a large anterior mediastinal adenopathy and/or mass, and a left pleural effusion. An ENT evaluation showed normal vocal cord movement.

PAST MEDICAL HISTORY: His past medical history includes atrial fibrillation, ischemic heart disease, hypertension, and previous inferior MI. He quit smoking 10-12 years ago. He is status postpacer implantation in July 1999.

PHYSICAL EXAMINATION: The patient has been afebrile. Vital signs are otherwise stable. HEENT was benign. Neck showed no mass or adenopathy and no JVD. Lungs showed rales and decreased breath sounds at the left base. There were no wheezes. There was good air excursion. The heart had a regular rhythm, without murmur. The abdomen was soft and nontender. The extremities showed no edema.

IMPRESSION: Left lower lobe pneumonia and a questionable malignancy. Given his chronic anticoagulation, the simplest thing may be an ultrasound guided thoracentesis when his PT is less than 16. If this is negative for malignancy, then a bronchoscopy with brush forceps biopsies. A Wang needle biopsy of the mediastinal mass would also be reasonable. At this point, I would continue his antibiotic therapy based upon sputum analysis. A first generation cephalosporin would cover both his normal flora and staph aureus.

PLAN: We will plan to do the ultrasound thoracentesis tomorrow if his PT is less than 16.

_____

Allan Bolus, MD/xx

CONSULTATION REPORT

Patient Name: Washington, John

File Number: 90023

Date of Birth: April 2, 19xx

Examination Date: *Current date*

Requesting Physician: Adam Valence, MD

HISTORY OF PRESENT ILLNESS: The patient is a 66-year-old black male whom I am asked to see preoperatively and then follow for restrictive lung disease. He was admitted to Community Hospital last month with unstable angina. He subsequently underwent heart catheterization and was found to have a 70% distal left main occlusion. He was treated initially with intravenous nitroglycerin and intravenous heparin. He was seen in consultation by Dr. Adam Valence who agreed that bypass surgery was indicated but estimated risk at 25% to 30% mortality. The patient has been transferred to University Hospital for presumed heart surgery on Thursday, and I am asked to see the patient in consultation.

He is a former pack and a half per day smoker. He denies any history of chronic cough or sputum production and gave up cigarette smoking in 1981. He denies any symptoms of exertional dyspnea, wheezing, or shortness of breath. Remarkably, he does admit to a significant amount of exertional chest pain prior to his admission at Community Hospital. He denies any history of asthma, pleurisy, TB, or exposure to TB.

PAST MEDICAL HISTORY: His past medical history is quite extensive and remarkable for coronary artery disease that dates back to at least 1992. He has a history of congestive heart failure and transient ischemic attacks. He also has a history of colon cancer, esophageal stricture, and multiple injuries from a motorcycle accident in 1982.

ALLERGIES: He denies any allergies.

SOCIAL HISTORY: Noncontributory. He has worked as a legal clerk his entire life.

FAMILY HISTORY: Markedly positive for coronary artery disease.

REVIEW OF SYSTEMS: He denies any recent fevers, chills, night sweats, weight loss, or substernal chest pain as previously described. He denies any diarrhea or constipation.

PHYSICAL EXAMINATION: He is an obese man in no acute distress. Head, eyes, ears, nose, and throat show arcus senilis present. The pupils are equal, round, and reactive to light and accommodation.

----------------------- begin page 2 -----------------------

The oropharynx is unremarkable. The neck is supple with no carotid bruits noted. The trachea is midline. The chest reveals an increased AP diameter, with a prolonged expiratory phase with diminished breath sounds bilaterally. There are no wheezes, rales, or rhonchi. Cardiac exam reveals soft S4 gallop with no murmur. His abdomen is soft and nontender. He is markedly obese. There are scars from previous surgeries in evidence. Extremity evaluation reveals some stasis changes of the lower extremities, with almost absent pulses at the dorsalis pedis and posterior tibialis.

LABORATORY DATA: Laboratory test results from Community Hospital reveal a hemoglobin of 11.2, white count 10,800, and electrolytes unremarkable. Pulmonary function tests were remarkable for a vital capacity of 2.01 liters, 42% of predicted, an FEV1 of 1.38 liters, 37% of predicted. After administration of aerosol bronchodilators, there is a 19% improvement of the vital capacity and a 22% improvement of the FEV1.

IMPRESSION:
1. Restrictive lung disease.
2. Coronary artery disease with mid-distal left main coronary artery obstruction.
3. Renal insufficiency.
4. Peripheral vascular disease and generalized atherosclerotic cardiovascular disease.

PLAN: The patient's pulmonary function tests are adequate for cardiac surgery. He does have a bronchodilator response, and we will take advantage of this by placing him on aerosol bronchodilators. We will not place him on corticosteroids, since this is likely to raises his BUN and creatinine preoperatively. We will follow along with you.

Thank you for asking me to see your patient in consultation.

_____

Douglas Sputum, MD/xx

_____

CONSULTATION REPORT

Patient Name: McMurray, Brenda

File Number: 09671

Date of Birth: May 1, 19xx

Examination Date: *Current date*

Requesting Physician: Charles P. Davis, MD

CHIEF COMPLAINT: Shortness of breath.

HISTORY OF PRESENT ILLNESS: This is a delightful, but very deaf, 63-year-old black female, with multiple admissions and multiple problems concerning breast carcinoma. According to the patient, she has undergone chemotherapy and bilateral radiation therapy for about the past five years. She was admitted for further chemotherapy. She has been progressively dyspneic for several months.

PAST MEDICAL HISTORY: Three weeks ago, at Community Hospital, she had a thoracentesis of the right side and removal of pleural fluid with transient relief of her dyspnea. Tests on the pleural fluid were done, but the results are currently not available to me. She has not smoked or had evidence of primary lung disease. No evidence of pneumonia, TB, asthma, wheezing, cough, or recent URI.

PHYSICAL EXAMINATION

GENERAL: She is a very pleasant woman, who is very deaf, but in no acute distress. She seems to understand the reason for my visit and our plans.

VITAL SIGNS: Her pulse is 100 with respirations at 20/min. BP 110/70, temperature is normal.

HEENT: Her pharynx is clear.

NECK: Neck veins are not distended. There is no cervical adenopathy.

BREASTS: The right breast is surgically absent. The left breast is without nodules.

CHEST: There is dullness of breath sounds in both lower lung fields.

HEART: The heart is hyperdynamic with normal first and second sounds. No gallop or rubs are noted.

----------------------- begin page 2 -----------------------

ABDOMEN: The abdomen is distended. There may be ascites.

EXTREMITIES: There is 3+ edema of both lower extremities, without warmth, tenderness, or redness.

DIAGNOSTIC TESTING: The chest x-ray shows moderately large bilateral pleural effusion. I noted a normal MUGA scan resting left ventricular ejection fraction.

IMPRESSION: Bilateral pleural effusion, probably related to metastatic breast cancer.

PLAN: The patient understands the aims of a diagnostic and therapeutic thoracentesis, which will probably be done tomorrow. Pending contraindications from the coagulation tests, I will tap the side with the most fluid, which is probably the left side. Further recommendations will depend upon the evaluation of that fluid and the degree of respiratory relief obtained.

Thank you for letting me assist in her care.

_____

Neal Alveoli, MD/xx

CHAPTER 8 / PART III CHECK YOUR PROGRESS

See Pretests (8T-5) and (8T-6).

CHAPTER 9 / PART I PRETEST

1. c	27. d	52. a	77. b
2. b	28. c	53. b	78. c
3. d	29. a	54. b	79. d
4. d	30. c	55. d	80. a
5. a	31. a	56. c	81. a
6. b	32. a	57. a	82. b
7. a	33. d	58. c	83. d
8. d	34. c	59. a	84. b
9. c	35. c	60. a	85. c
10. a	36. d	61. a	86. d
11. b	37. c	62. c	87. c
12. a	38. b	63. d	88. a
13. b	39. a	64. b	89. b
14. a	40. d	65. d	90. c
15. c	41. b	66. c	91. b
16. a	42. a	67. a	92. d
17. a	43. b	68. d	93. a
18. a	44. b	69. a	94. c
19. b	45. a	70. a	95. a
20. a	46. a	71. c	96. c
21. d	47. d	72. c	97. d
22. a	48. a	73. b	98. a
23. c	49. b	74. a	99. c
24. b	50. a	75. b	100. b
25. b	51. a	76. c	101. d
26. c			

CHAPTER 9 / PART I ACTIVITY 3 (9T-1)

1. Adenomatous relates to some types of glandular hyperplasia.
   Given his history of large adenomatous polyps, a repeat colonoscopy is recommended in three years.
2. Anastomosis is an opening created by surgery, disease, or trauma between two or more organs or structures.
   A vascular anastomosis was performed to bypass an aneurysm.
3. Arteriogram is a radiographic record of an artery after injection of a contrast medium into it.
   The patient had a normal coronary arteriogram in 1994.
4. Biliary relates to bile or the biliary tract.
   The physician ruled out biliary disease such as gallstones or other cholestatic liver diseases.
5. Cecum is the cul-de-sac, about 6 cm in depth, lying below the terminal ileum forming the first part of the large intestine.
   The scope was easily advanced to the cecum, with good visualization of all areas.
6. Cholecystectomy is the surgical removal of the gallbladder.
   In addition, her history is remarkable for rectocele and cystocele repair and cholecystectomy.
7. Colitis is the inflammation of the colon.
   A biopsy was taken for microscopic colitis.
8. Colonoscope is an elongated endoscope, usually fiberoptic.
   The physician used the Olympus video colonoscope.
9. Colonoscopy is the visual examination of the inner surface of the colon by means of a colonoscope.
   The patient underwent a colonoscopy using the Olympus video colonoscope.
10. Colostomy is the establishment of an artificial opening into the colon.
    There is a colostomy in the left lower quadrant which appears healthy.
11. Creatinine is a normal component of urine.
    Pertinent laboratory tests included electrolytes and creatinine, which were normal.

12. Cystocele is a hernia of the bladder usually into the vagina and introitus.
    The patient's history is remarkable for cystocele repair and cholecystectomy.
13. Decubitus is a recumbent or horizontal position.
    The patient was placed in the left lateral decubitus position.
14. Dysphagia is the difficulty in swallowing.
    He denies any regular symptoms of dysphagia.
15. Electrolyte is any solution compound that conducts electricity.
    Pertinent laboratory tests included electrolytes and creatinine, which were normal.
16. Emesis is to vomit.
    She denies emesis.
17. Endoscopy is the examination of the interior of a canal or hollow viscus by means of endoscope.
    The gastroenterologist will perform an upper endoscopy later this morning.
18. Erythema is the redness of the skin due to capillary dilatation.
    An abdominal exam revealed that the PEG tube site is somewhat erythematous, with a fungal-appearing rash.
19. Exacerbation is an increase in the severity of a disease or symptoms.
    My impression is that this patient has classic symptoms of colitis with recent exacerbation.
20. Folate is folic acid.
    Her medications included folate 1 mg daily.
21. Formalin is a 37% aqueous solution of formaldehyde.
    The liver biopsy was sent in a formalin jar for pathological analysis.
22. Gastritis is an inflammation of the stomach, especially the mucosal.
    She was noted to have some chronic gastritis, but no evidence of ulcer disease.
23. Gastroesophageal relates to both the stomach and the esophagus.
    He denies any regular symptoms of dysphagia or gastroesophageal reflux.
24. Gastrointestinal relates to the stomach and the intestines.
    The patient's transient gastrointestinal distress has since resolved.
25. Gastroparesis is a slight degree of gastroparalysis.
    The patient's past medical history is notable for diabetes mellitus, diabetic neuropathy, diabetic gastroparesis, diabetic retinopathy, and amputation of several toes.
26. Gastrostomy is the establishment of a new opening into the stomach.
    The gastroenterologist replaced the PEG tube with a new replacement balloon gastrostomy kit.
27. Hematemesis is to vomit blood indicating upper gastrointestinal bleeding.
    The patient had no prior history of ulcer disease or hematemesis.
28. Hematochezia is the passage of bloody stools.
    He presents today with four days of increasing painless hematochezia.
29. Heme is the oxygen-carrying, color-furnishing group of hemoglobin.
    She has heme positive emesis.
30. Hemicolectomy is the removal of the right or left side of the colon.
    This 79-year-old white lady presents for a 4-year follow-up colonoscopy evaluation of a right hemicolectomy performed on November 4, 1999.
31. Heparin is a generic name for an anticoagulant.
    With the colonoscopy, she would have to stop her current medication, go on heparin, get the colonoscopy done, then go back on the medication.
32. Hepatosplenomegaly is the enlargement of the liver and spleen.
    Soft and nontender abdomen, with no hepatosplenomegaly.
33. Hydrocortisone is a generic name for a corticosteroid.
    Her current medications include hydrocortisone and aspirin.

34. Icterus is jaundice.
    There is no scleral icterus.
35. Ketone is any compound containing carbon oxide.
    Urinalysis shows trace ketones and a small amount of blood.
36. Labyrinthitis is the inflammation of the otitis interna.
    The patient's past medical history was remarkable for an episode of labyrinthis.
37. Laminectomy is the surgical excision of the lamina.
    This is a 45-year-old, black female who three weeks ago underwent a cervical laminectomy of C5 and C6.
38. Lidocaine is a generic name for a local anesthetic; used as a cardiac antiarrhythmic.
    Lidocaine 1% was used for topical anesthesia of the skin, subcutaneous tissue, and down to the intercostal space.
39. Lumen is the cavity or channel within a tube.
    There were no polyps or other lesions noted upon careful inspection of the lumen upon withdrawal of the endoscope.
40. Lymphadenopathy is the disease of the lymph nodes.
    He had no lymphadenopathy.
41. Malaise is a feeling of uneasiness.
    She also has anorexia with severely decreased oral intake, as well as malaise and severe fatigue.
42. Meclizine is a generic name for an antinauseant.
    The patient was admitted for symptomatic therapy with meclizine as well as for intravenous therapy.
43. Melena is the darkening of the feces by blood pigments.
    She denies any fever, chills, diarrhea, melena, hematemesis, hematochezia, or abdominal pain.
44. Motility is the ability to move spontaneously.
    The patient is a very pleasant 48-year-old white female who I have previously seen for constipation that was due to a motility-related disturbance as a complication of her polio.
45. Myalgia is muscular pain.
    She has had episodic fevers and chills, as well as myalgia over the last three weeks.
46. Nitroglycerin is a generic name for a vasodilator and is used to relieve certain types of pain.
    Her current medications include hydrocortisone and nitroglycerin paste.
47. Nystagmus is the involuntary, rapid, rhythmic movement of the eyeball.
    The patient's extraocular movements were intact, except for horizontal nystagmus of 3-4 beats.
48. Occult is specimen hidden from view.
    A rectal exam reveals heme-negative brown stool, which tests negative for occult blood.
49. Odynophagia is the burning, squeezing pain while swallowing.
    He denies any regular symptoms of dysphagia, odynophagia, or gastroesophageal reflux.
50. Pinna is the projecting part of the ear lying outside the head.
    Pinna is normal.
51. Polyp is any growth or mass protruding from a mucous membrane.
    The patient had a past history of multiple polyps.
52. Postprandial is after a meal.
    He has a long history of postprandial heartburn and indigestion.
53. Prednisone is a generic name for an anti-inflammatory and antiallergic agent.
    The patient was treated with prednisone and antibiotics.
54. Proctitis is the inflammation of the rectum.
    He does have occasional red blood mixed in with his stool, which has been attributed to radiation proctitis.
55. Prophylatic is an agent that tends to ward off disease.
    The patient was prescribed prophylatic treatments for her asthma.
56. Prostate is a gland in the male that surrounds the neck of the bladder and urethra.
    The patient has an enlarged prostate.
57. Pyridoxine is one of the forms of vitamin B6.
    Her medication included pyridoxine 250 mg daily.

58. Rectocele is the hernial protrusion of part of the rectum into the vagina.
The patient's history is remarkable for rectocele and cystocele repair and cholecystectomy.

59. Reflux is a backward or return flow.
He denies any regular symptoms of dysphagia, odynophagia, or gastroesophageal reflux.

60. Retroflexion is the bending of an organ so that its top is thrust backward.
There were no abnormalities noted and retroflexion in the rectum was unremarkable.

61. Sclera is the tough white outer coat of the eyeball.
There is no scleral icterus.

62. Sigmoidoscope is an endoscope for use in sigmoidoscopy.
The patient had a normal sigmoidoscope examination.

63. Sigmoidoscopy is the direct examination of the interior of the sigmoid colon.
Sigmoidoscopy was completed to 60 cm into the descending colon.

64. Stenosis is the narrowing of a body passage or opening.
She has been in excellent health until approximately one month ago when she underwent aortic valve replacement due to aortic stenosis.

65. Stent is a mold for keeping a skin graft in place.
He has a history of coronary artery disease and has had stenting in the past.

66. Thyromegaly is the enlargement of the thyroid gland.
He had no thyromegaly or lymphadenopathy.

67. Titrate is to analyze a given solution component by adding a liquid reagent.
We will then titrate his dose to the lowest possible dose required to control his reflux symptoms.

68. Turgor is the condition of fullness; the expected resiliency of the skin.
Skin color, turgor and texture are normal for her age.

69. Ativan is the trade name for an antianxiety agent.
Her medications included Ativan.

70. Axid is the trade name for an antagonist for the treatment of gastric and duodenal ulcers.
He has been on Axid.

71. Bumex is the trade name for a loop diuretic.
Her current medications include hydrocortisone, Bumex, and nitroglycerin paste.

72. Chem-7 is the trade name for a profile of seven different chemical laboratory tests.
The gastroenterologist ordered a Chem-7, RBC, WBC, and partial thromboplastin time.

73. Coumadin is the trade name for an anticoagulant.
With the colonoscopy, she would have to stop her Coumadin, go on heparin, get the colonoscopy done, then go back on the heparin and Coumadin.

74. Demerol is the trade name for a synthetic narcotic analgesic.
The anesthesia administered was Demerol 25 mg IV.

75. Dilantin is the trade name for an anticonvulsant used in the treatment of epilepsy.
Her current medications include hydrocortisone, Bumex, Dilantin, and nitroglycerin paste.

76. Elavil is the trade name for an antidepressant.
Her medications included Elavil.

77. Hemoccult is the trade name for a guaiac test for occult blood.
A rectal exam showed no stool available for Hemoccult evaluation.

78. Humulin is the trade name for an antidiabetic.
The patient is diabetic and currently being treated with Humulin 45 units daily in the morning.

79. Hytrin is the trade name for an antihypertensive used in the treatment of benign prostatic hyperplasia.
His only past medical history is that of benign prostatic hypertrophy, for which he takes Hytrin.

80. Indocin is the trade name for a nonsteroidal anti-inflammatory agent.
Her medications included Indocin daily, nitroglycerin patch 0.4 mg/hr. daily, and aspirin every other day.

81. K-Dur is the trade name for a potassium supplement.
Her current medications include hydrocortisone, K-Dur, Bumex, Dilantin, and nitroglycerin paste.

82. Lopressor is the trade name for an antihypertensive.
Her current medications include hydrocortisone, K-Dur, Bumex, Lopressor, Dilantin, and nitroglycerin paste.

83. Macrobid is the trade name for an urinary bacteriostatic.
She has been taking Macrobid for the past five days for an urinary tract infection.

84. Maxzide is the trade name for a diuretic and antihypertensive.
Her only medication has been Maxzide for hypertension.

85. Metamucil is the trade name for a bulk laxative.
Her medications included Indocin daily, nitroglycerin patch 0.4 mg/hr. daily, aspirin every other day, and Metamucil.

86. Naprosyn is the trade name for a nonsteroidal anti-inflammatory agent.
She has been taking Naprosyn on a chronic basis, and over the last 4-5 days she has been having melenic stools.

87. Norvasc is the trade name for an antianginal and antihypertensive.
Her medications included Norvasc 25 mg daily, aspirin daily, folate 1 mg daily, and pyridoxine 250 mg daily.

88. Paxil is the trade name for an antidepressant.
Her medications included Paxil for her anxiety attacks.

89. Pepcid is the trade name for an acid controller for heartburn and acid indigestion.
He had been placed originally on Pepcid 20 mg t.i.d. with initial relief.

90. Prilosec is the trade name for a gastric acid secretion inhibitor.
Her medications included Norvasc 25 mg daily, aspirin daily, folate 1 mg daily, pyridoxine 250 mg daily, and most recently, Prilosec 20 mg daily.

91. Procardia is the trade name for a coronary vasodilator.
The patient was taking Procardia 30 mg t.i.d.

92. Reglan is the trade name for a gastrointestinal stimulant, antiemetic.
He reports that this problem was treated in the past with Reglan with some improvement.

93. Ritalin is the trade name for a mild central nervous system stimulant and antidepressant.
Current medications are Ritalin, which he is taking for attention deficit disorder.

94. Synthroid is the trade name for a thyroid hormone.
Her current medications include Synthroid, hydrocortisone, K-Dur, Bumex, Lopressor, Dilantin, Prilosec, and nitroglycerin paste.

95. Tenormin is the trade name for an antihypertensive.
The patient's medications include Tenormin and Pepcid.

96. Terramycin is the trade name for an antibiotic.
The patient is allergic to penicillin and Terramycin.

97. Tigan is the trade name for an antiemetic.
The patient was admitted for symptomatic therapy with meclizine and Tigan as well as for intravenous therapy.

98. Timoptic is the trade name for a beta-blocker, antiglaucoma agent.
The patient is currently on Coumadin and Timoptic.

99. Vasotec is the trade name for an antihypertensive.
Her current medications include Synthroid, hydrocortisone, K-Dur, Bumex, Lopressor, Vasotec, Dilantin, Prilosec, and nitroglycerin paste.

100. Versed is the trade name for a short-acting benzodiazepine general anesthetic adjunct for preoperative sedation.
The anesthesia administered was Demerol 25 mg IV and Versed 2 mg IV.

101. Zocor is the trade name for a reductase inhibitor for hypercholesterolemia and coronary heart disease.
Her medications included Norvasc 25 mg daily, Zocor 20 mg at bedtime, aspirin daily, folate 1 mg daily, pyridoxine 250 mg daily, and most recently, Prilosec 20 mg daily.

1. b	27. b	52. c	77. a
2. d	28. c	53. a	78. a
3. c	29. b	54. d	79. b
4. a	30. d	55. c	80. d
5. d	31. d	56. a	81. b
6. b	32. a	57. c	82. c
7. a	33. b	58. a	83. d
8. a	34. a	59. a	84. c
9. c	35. d	60. d	85. a
10. c	36. c	61. c	86. b
11. c	37. a	62. c	87. c
12. a	38. b	63. d	88. b
13. a	39. a	64. c	89. d
14. b	40. b	65. a	90. a
15. b	41. a	66. b	91. c
16. d	42. c	67. a	92. a
17. c	43. a	68. a	93. a
18. b	44. c	69. a	94. c
19. a	45. a	70. c	95. c
20. d	46. b	71. d	96. b
21. b	47. a	72. a	97. a
22. a	48. d	73. c	98. b
23. b	49. a	74. b	99. c
24. b	50. c	75. d	100. b
25. d	51. b	76. d	101. c
26. a			

CHAPTER 9 / PART II PRETEST (9T-2)

HISTORY AND PHYSICAL EXAMINATION

Patient Name: Edwards, Mona

File Number: 89034

Date of Birth: October 9, 19xx

Examination Date: *Current date*

Physician: Gwenn Maltase, MD

CHIEF COMPLAINT: Vomiting and abdominal pain.

HISTORY OF PRESENT ILLNESS: This is a 72-year-old white female with severe nausea, abdominal pain, and vomiting for the past few hours. She has heme positive emesis. The patient states that this has happened before. She is status post Miles resection in 1997 for rectal carcinoma. She has had multiple partial small bowel obstructions since that time. She has previously been decompressed with a nasogastric tube.

ALLERGIES: She is allergic to sulfa.

MEDICATIONS: She has been taking Macrobid for the past five days for an urinary tract infection.

PAST MEDICAL HISTORY: Significant for an appendectomy, two hip replacements, and an abdominoperineal resection in 1997 for colon cancer.

SOCIAL HISTORY: She lives alone. She is a nonsmoker. She occasionally drinks alcohol.

PHYSICAL EXAMINATION

GENERAL: She is alert, quite conversant and in no acute distress.

HEENT: Her pupils are equal, round and reactive to light and accommodation. There is no scleral icterus.

NECK: Supple without adenopathy.

HEART: Regular.

LUNGS: Clear.

- - - - - - - - - - - - - - - - - begin page 2 -

ABDOMEN: The abdomen is slightly distended, quiet with minimal bowel sounds. There is a colostomy in the left lower quadrant, which appears healthy. The bag is empty and there is no discharge. There is minimal tenderness on deep palpation.

EXTREMITIES: Bilateral hip replacements. There is no edema.

NEUROLOGIC: Within normal limits.

IMPRESSION:
1. Partial small bowel obstruction likely secondary to adhesions from prior abdominoperineal resection in 1997.
2. History of rectal carcinoma.

PLAN:
1. Admit, hydrate, and observe.
2. Clear liquid diet.
3. Obtain stat obstruction series x-rays and hemoglobin.

Gwenn Maltase, MD/xx

CHAPTER 9 / PART II ACTIVITY 4

Errors are indicated in bold and italics. Margins are formatted at 1 inch.

HISTORY AND PHYSICAL EXAMINATION

Patient Name: Schupp, Lacey

File Number: 00841

Date of Birth: November 2, 19xx

Examination Date: *Current date*

Physician: Anna Bolism, MD

HISTORY:
Double space
CHIEF COMPLAINT: Melenic stools.
Double space
HISTORY OF *PRESENT* ILLNESS: The patient is a very pleasant *48-year-old* white *female* who I have previously seen for constipation that was due to a *motility-related* disturbance as a complication of her polio. She has been taking *Naprosyn* on a chronic *basis,* and over the last *4-5* days she has been having melenic stools. During the same time frame, she has *noted* progressive fatigue and weakness. A *hemoglobin* study performed in Dr. Geiger's office showed that her *hemoglobin* was in the *6.5* range, and she was admitted to University Hospital. She denies any *abdominal* pain. There is *no* prior history of ulcer disease or *hematemesis.* She has lost about *3-5 pounds* over this same time frame.

PAST MEDICAL HISTORY: She has had numerous postpolio complications, including a neurogenic bladder and constipation. She has had several back *surgeries* as well as a wrist operation. *She* does not smoke or drink.

MEDICATIONS:
1. *Naprosyn.*
2. *Paxil.*
3. *Elavil.*
4. *Ativan.*

FAMILY HISTORY: Noncontributory.
Double space
PHYSICAL EXAMINATION
Double space
GENERAL: A pale white female who is in no acute distress.

HEART: Negative.

LUNGS: Negative.

---------------------- begin page 2 ----------------------

ABDOMEN: Negative.

RECTAL: A rectal exam showed *no* stool available for *Hemoccult* evaluation.

LABORATORY DATA: Lab studies showed a BUN elevated at *33* with a *creatinine* of *0.4. Her electrolytes* were normal as were her platelet count and *coagulation* time. *Hemoglobin* was *6.9.*

IMPRESSION: GI bleed. *It is* almost certainly upper GI bleeding due to nonsteroid use.

PLAN
1. Transfuse 2 units of packed *cells.*
2. Perform an upper *endoscopy* later this morning. We will make further recommendations after the *endoscopy.*
Quadruple space

_____

Anna Bolism, *MD/xx*

OPERATIVE REPORT

Patient Name: Artemis, Jacob

File Number: 00864

Date of Birth: December 12, 1958

Examination Date: *Current date*

Preoperative Diagnosis: Hepatitis C and mildly elevated liver enzymes.

Postoperative Diagnosis: Hepatitis C and mildly elevated liver enzymes.

Operation: Percutaneous liver biopsy under ultrasound guidance.

PROCEDURE: The patient was counseled. Potential complications were explained. Consent was obtained. The patient was placed supine on the exam table. Ultrasound was used to scan in the mid-axillary line. The liver margins were identified, and the best location for the liver biopsy was selected along the mid-axillary line at approximately the 10th intercostal space. The skin was then prepped and draped in the usual sterile manner. Lidocaine 1% was used for topical anesthesia of the skin, subcutaneous tissue, and down to the intercostal space. A #22 gauge spinal needle was used to sound the depth of the liver.

Because of the patient's obesity, the liver was found to be approximately 5 cm from the skin surface. The Klatskin needle was then attached to a glass syringe filled with sterile saline. The Klatskin needle was inserted into the intercostal space and then subsequently into the liver for a quick suction biopsy. The first pass yielded only a 5 mm fragment of tissue. A second pass was therefore performed which yielded a much larger 4 cm piece of tan-appearing liver. The liver biopsy was sent in a formalin jar for pathological analysis. The skin was then dressed and taped. The patient was then observed for four hours. No immediate complications were observed. Postbiopsy vital signs were normal. The patient tolerated the procedure well, without any complications.

IMPRESSION: Hepatitis C and mildly elevated liver enzymes.

_____

Kate Cobalamin, MD/xx

OPERATIVE REPORT

Patient Name: Anderson, Timothy

File Number: 01578

Date of Birth: June 1, 1956

Examination Date: *Current date*

Preoperative Diagnosis: Flexible sigmoidoscopy

Postoperative Diagnosis: Normal sigmoidoscope examination.

Anesthesia: None.

Operation: FLEXIBLE SIGMOIDOSCOPY WITH BIOPSY.

PROCEDURE: After obtaining appropriate informed consent and a fleet enema preparation, the patient was placed in the left lateral decubitus position. A digital rectal examination was performed which was unremarkable. A flexible sigmoidoscope was inserted in the usual fashion and was advanced to 60 cm without difficulty. The prep was excellent. The scope was withdrawn and the mucosa inspected. There were no abnormalities noted and retroflexion in the rectum was unremarkable.

ASSESSMENT: Normal flexible sigmoidoscopy to 60 cm.

PLAN: Repeat the procedure in 3-5 years unless the patient presents with related symptoms.

_____

Kate Cobalamin, MD/xx

_____

CHAPTER 9 / PART II ACTIVITY 7 (9T-4)

HISTORY AND PHYSICAL EXAMINATION

Patient Name: Mossier, Anthony

File Number: 002157

Date of Birth: May 7, 19xx

Examination Date: *Current date*

Physician: Gwenn Maltase, MD

HISTORY

CHIEF COMPLAINT: Sensation of a foreign body in proximal esophagus, near the hypopharynx.

HISTORY OF PRESENT ILLNESS: Mr. Anthony Mossier is a 60-year-old patient who was referred to us for an esophagogastroduodenoscopy to exclude an esophageal foreign body. He was in usual state of health until earlier today when he was eating turkey broth soup and felt that he swallowed a turkey bone. He has a continued sensation of something lodged in his proximal esophagus/hypopharyngeal area. This has happened to him before. He denies any regular symptoms of dysphagia, odynophagia, or gastroesophageal reflux.

PAST MEDICAL HISTORY: His only past medical history is that of benign prostatic hypertrophy, for which he takes Hytrin. He is a former smoker, quitting about 13 years ago.

ALLERGIES: No known allergies.

REVIEW OF SYSTEMS: Negative.

PHYSICAL EXAMINATION: Physical examination reveals the patient in no distress. His vital signs are normal. HEENT is negative. Pulmonary and cardiac auscultation is normal. His abdomen is soft and nontender with no abnormal scars or palpable masses. The extremity evaluation is negative.

IMPRESSION: Sensation of foreign body.

PLAN: We will proceed with an esophagogastroduodenoscopy. Potential risks and complications of the procedure were explained to the patient and a consent form was signed.

_____

Gwenn Maltase, MD/xx

_____

CHAPTER 9 / PART II CHECK YOUR PROGRESS

See Pretest (9T-2).

_____

CHAPTER 9 / PART III PRETEST (9T-5)

Current date

Charles P. Davis, MD
FedDes Wellness Center
Family Practice Division, Suite 300
Wellness Way Drive
New York, NY 10036

Re: Jonathan Dewey
    Date of Birth: February 29, 19xx

Dear Dr. Davis

Mr. Dewey is a 49-year-old gentleman admitted to the hospital with epigastric and chest discomfort to rule out myocardial infarction.

He has a history of coronary artery disease and has had stenting in the past. He has a long history of postprandial heartburn and indigestion. This has been more severe recently with postprandial belching and burning. He denies vomiting. He is frequently awakened by regurgitation and heartburn. He obtains relief of his symptoms by sitting and taking Alka-Seltzer. He has been on Axid. Last week Dr. Adam Valence started him on Prilosec b.i.d. When the dose was reduced to one time daily, his symptoms recurred.

He drinks two cups of coffee daily. He smokes a cigar. He frequently consumes a bowl of cereal before going to bed. He has no dysphagia or odynophagia. He has had no weight loss. His bowel habits are normal.

PAST MEDICAL HISTORY: Notable for coronary artery disease and hyperlipidemia.

MEDICATIONS: His medications include:
1. Lopressor 25 mg t.i.d.
2. Norvasc 25 mg daily.
3. Zocor 20 mg at bedtime.
4. Aspirin daily.
5. Folate 1 mg daily.
6. Pyridoxine 250 mg daily.
7. Most recently, Prilosec 20 mg daily.

PHYSICAL EXAMINATION: He is in no acute distress. His abdomen is soft with normoactive bowel sounds. There is no organomegaly. There is mild epigastric tenderness. CBC on admission is normal.

IMPRESSION: My impression is that this patient has classic symptoms of gastroesophageal reflux disease with recent exacerbation. It is highly likely that he has some degree of esophagitis.

RECOMMENDATIONS: I would recommend that we continue to treat him with Prilosec 20 mg b.i.d. If this does not completely alleviate his symptoms, he will require endoscopy. I would recommend ongoing Prilosec therapy for at least eight weeks to allow healing of any potential esophagitis. We will then titrate his dose to the lowest possible dose required to control his reflux symptoms. I have also counseled him on antireflux measures. I will be happy to follow this patient as an outpatient after discharge.

Thank you for allowing me to see him in consultation.

Sincerely

Gwenn Maltese, MD

xx

OPERATIVE REPORT

Patient Name: Nicholson, Dick

File Number: 74201

Date of Birth: October 25, 1934

Examination Date: *Current date*

Preoperative Diagnosis: Past history of multiple polyps.

Postoperative Diagnosis: Normal colonoscopy. No evidence of recurrent polyps or cancer.

Operation: TOTAL COLONOSCOPY.

Anesthesia: Demerol 25 mg IV and Versed 2 mg IV

PROCEDURE: A rectal exam was performed. The patient has an enlarged prostate. No nodules were noted. The patient then underwent a colonoscopy using the Olympus video colonoscope.

The scope was easily advanced to the cecum, with good visualization of all areas. The scope was then withdrawn, examining the entire colon a second time. Visualization and preparation were excellent. The patient was stable throughout the procedure with no changes in oxygen saturation, which remained above 90. Stable vital signs throughout the procedure. The procedure was terminated and was well tolerated by the patient.

IMPRESSION: No abnormalities were noted anywhere in the colon. No polyps could be identified. Since the patient has a normal exam after 3 years, I think his surveillance interval can be widened to every 3-5 years.

Anna Bolism, MD/xx

Current date

Charles P. Davis, MD
FedDes Wellness Center
Family Practice Division, Suite 300
101 Wellness Way Drive
New York, NY 10036

Re: Alice Kier
    Date of Birth: May 26, 19xx

Dear Dr. Davis

We were asked to see this patient for evaluation of abdominal discomfort.

Ms. Kier is a 59-year-old woman who is scheduled to undergo coronary bypass surgery. She developed a sensation of upper abdominal discomfort and left upper quadrant discomfort yesterday. It has subsequently resolved. Her description of the discomfort is really quite vague, stating that the pain "jumps around" her abdomen. She thinks it may have only been gas. She currently denies actual pain. Her bowels have been moving fine. She rarely has nausea. She has no unexplained weight loss. She denies early satiety, dysphagia, or odynophagia. Her appetite has been good. There is no family history of cancer.

Her past medical history is significant for coronary artery disease, prior removal of a pituitary tumor, and an appendectomy. She has severe left ventricular dysfunction.

Her current medications include Synthroid, hydrocortisone, K-Dur, Bumex, Lopressor, Vasotec, Dilantin, Prilosec, Zocor, and nitroglycerin paste. She is allergic to aspirin.

Physical examination reveals a well-appearing woman in no acute distress. Her abdominal examination is unremarkable. There are no palpable masses. There are no bruits. A rectal exam reveals heme-negative brown stool, which tests negative for occult blood.

IMPRESSION: Transient gastrointestinal distress that has since resolved. There is no objective evidence for ongoing organic disease. I do not think that anything further needs to be done.

Thank you for the opportunity of sharing in Ms. Kier's care.

Sincerely

Kate Cobalamin, MD

xx

OPERATIVE REPORT

Patient Name: Dubin, Raymond

File Number: 800223

Date of Birth: December 24, 1937

Examination Date: *Current date*

Preoperative Diagnosis: History of large polyps in the sigmoid colon, now for repeat inspection.

Postoperative Diagnosis: Normal sigmoidoscopy to 60 cm.

Operation: FLEXIBLE SIGMOIDOSCOPY

PROCEDURE: The patient is an elderly white male with a history of two large polyps in the sigmoid colon last year. The patient is undergoing a repeat sigmoidoscope evaluation of these areas for evidence of any residual tissue.

The indication, risks, benefits, and alternatives to the procedure were explained. The patient had the opportunity to ask questions. Informed written consent was obtained.

The patient was placed in the left lateral decubitus position. A rectal examination was significant for external hemorrhoids. The endoscope was advanced into the rectum without difficulty. Sigmoidoscopy was completed to 60 cm into the descending colon. There were no polyps or other lesions noted upon careful inspection of the lumen upon withdrawal of the endoscope. Retroflex view of the rectum was normal. Patient vital signs, cardiac rhythm and oxygen saturation were monitored throughout the procedure. The patient tolerated the procedure well.

IMPRESSION: Given his history of large adenomatous polyps, a repeat colonoscopy is recommended in three years.

Gwenn Maltase, MD/xx

HISTORY AND PHYSICAL EXAMINATION

Patient Name: Chen, Chi

File Number: 80041

Date of Birth: March 31, 19xx

Examination Date: *Current date*

Physician: Anna Bolism, MD

HISTORY

CHIEF COMPLAINT: Gastrointestinal hemorrhage.

HISTORY OF PRESENT ILLNESS: Mr. Chen is an 89-year-old gentleman with a history of prior diverticular bleeding on his last hospital admission in 1998. He presents today with four days of increasing painless hematochezia. He has no upper GI symptoms.

PAST MEDICAL HISTORY: Notable for hypertension, appendectomy, and hernia repair.

MEDICATIONS: Procardia 30 mg t.i.d.

ALLERGIES: No known drug allergies.

SOCIAL HISTORY: He does not smoke or drink alcohol. He lives at Shadyside Retirement Village.

PHYSICAL EXAMINATION

GENERAL: The patient appears well and is in no acute distress. Vital signs are normal. Afebrile.

HEENT: Negative.

LUNGS: Normal.

HEART: Normal.

ABDOMEN: Normal.

RECTAL: Exam revealed red blood on the examining finger.

----------------------- begin page 2 -----------------------

EXTREMITIES: Without edema.

IMPRESSION: My impression is that of lower gastrointestinal bleeding. Given this patient's history of diverticular hemorrhage in the past and progressive hematochezia, I suspect recurrent diverticular hemorrhage.

PLAN: I plan to admit him to the hospital for observation, given the likelihood of ongoing bleeding. I will obtain a Chem-7, RBC, WBC, and partial thromboplastin time. When the bleeding subsides, he will require a colonoscopy.

_____
Anna Bolism, MD/xx

OPERATIVE REPORT

Patient Name: Dubinsky, Ronald

File Number: 80067

Date of Birth: June 30, 1930

Examination Date: *Current date*

Preoperative Diagnosis: Abdominal pain and diarrhea.

Postoperative Diagnosis: Normal exam.

Operation: FIBEROPTIC SIGMOIDOSCOPY.

PROCEDURE: A rectal exam was done and it was normal. A fiberoptic sigmoidoscopy was performed to 60 cm using the Olympus video sigmoidoscope. The mucosa appeared completely normal. A biopsy was taken for microscopic colitis. The procedure was well tolerated by the patient.

IMPRESSION: Normal examination. The patient's symptoms are probably related to an irritable bowel syndrome.

_____
Gwenn Maltase, MD/xx

CONSULTATION REPORT

Patient Name: Landis, Micah

File Number: 80039

Date of Birth: September 30, 1984

Examination Date: *Current date*

Requesting Physician: Matthew Sponch, MD

HISTORY OF PRESENT ILLNESS: The patient has been unable to swallow saliva or liquids since last night.

PAST MEDICAL HISTORY: She has a past medical history of peptic ulcer disease and esophageal stricture with meat impaction. She has no active cardiopulmonary problems.

REVIEW OF SYSTEMS: Review of systems at this time is negative.

PHYSICAL EXAMINATION

VITAL SIGNS: Vital signs in the emergency room were stable. Pulse is 100.

HEENT: Negative.

LUNGS: Clear bilaterally.

HEART: Exam reveals normal sinus rhythm, with no abnormalities.

ABDOMEN: Negative.

IMPRESSION: Meat impaction.

PLAN: Esophagoscopy with removal of food impaction.

Anna Bolism, MD/xx

HISTORY AND PHYSICAL EXAMINATION

Patient Name: Rodriquez, Manuelo

File Number: 80078

Date of Birth: October 31, 19xx

Examination Date: *Current date*

Physician: Gwenn Maltase, MD

HISTORY

CHIEF COMPLAINT: Dysphagia.

HISTORY OF PRESENT ILLNESS: Mr. Rodriquez is a 48-year-old male with a long history of diabetes mellitus. On questioning, the patient reports a 3-4 year history of solid food dysphagia. He has particular problems with doughy foods and red meat. Over the past several months, his symptoms have been increasing. He reports no epigastric pain or weight loss. Occasionally he will have to regurgitate retained food. He reports that this problem was treated in the past with Reglan with some improvement.

PAST MEDICAL HISTORY: Notable for diabetes mellitus, diabetic neuropathy, diabetic gastroparesis, diabetic retinopathy, and amputation of several toes.

MEDICATIONS: His only medication is insulin.

ALLERGIES: He has no known drug allergies.

PHYSICAL EXAMINATION: Mr. Rodriquez is a thin, middle-aged man, appearing older than his stated age. He is in no acute distress. His vital signs are stable. He has a low-grade temperature. He has no adenopathy. His abdomen is soft and nontender. There are no masses or organomegaly.

IMPRESSION: My impression is that of a male with severe diabetes and diabetic neuropathy presenting with dysphagia. Differential diagnosis would include motility disorder or esophagitis.

PLAN:
1. Obtain CBC, total bilirubin, BUN, SGOT, and creatinine.
2. Schedule an upper GI series. If this is negative, I recommend an upper endoscopy to thoroughly examine the esophageal mucosa.

Gwenn Maltase, MD/xx

CONSULTATION REPORT

Patient Name: Chan, Alice

File Number: 80082

Date of Birth: November 30, 19xx

Examination Date: *Current date*

Requesting Physician: Izzy Sertoli, MD

HISTORY OF PRESENT ILLNESS: This is an 84-year-old white female who is known to me from prior evaluation for PEG tube replacement. The patient is postinfarct dementia that requires persistent feeding through the PEG tube. The patient is a residence at Pleasant Acres Retirement Home. Apparently, she was found this morning with the PEG tube out of the stomach with a defective, deflated balloon. The nurse placed a #22 French Foley catheter to keep the PEG tube tract open.

On examination, the patient is alert but confused. Her blood pressure is 126/88. Her temperature is 97. Pulse is 72. Respiratory rate is 20/min. Her cardiac exam revealed regular rate and rhythm. Lungs are clear. An abdominal exam revealed that the PEG tube site is somewhat erythematous, with a fungal-appearing rash. There is no drainage from the PEG site. The Foley catheter is in place. There is no tenderness in the abdomen. Bowel sounds are active.

IMPRESSION: Defective PEG tube due to breakage of the balloon.

PLAN: Replace PEG tube with a new replacement balloon gastrostomy kit.

Kate Cobalamin, MD/xx

HISTORY AND PHYSICAL EXAMINATION

Patient Name: Admad, Ahed

File Number: 80051

Date of Birth: August 31, 19xx

Examination Date: *Current date*

Physician: Gwenn Maltase, MD

HISTORY

CHIEF COMPLAINT: Lower gastrointestinal hemorrhage.

HISTORY OF PRESENT ILLNESS: Mr. Admad is an 81-year-old gentleman who was well until today when he had profuse hematochezia on 3 occasions. He had no associated abdominal pain, nausea, or vomiting. He has had no diarrhea. He has no chronic upper GI symptoms. He has a history of diverticular disease with a hospital admission in 1994. He denies prior diverticular hemorrhage. He does have occasional red blood mixed in with his stool, which has been attributed to radiation proctitis.

PAST MEDICAL HISTORY:
1. Prostate cancer. He is status post radiation therapy in 1994.
2. Diverticulitis in 1994.
3. Coronary artery disease.
4. Deep vein thrombosis.
5. Cholecystectomy.

MEDICATIONS: His medications include:
1. Indocin daily.
2. Nitroglycerin patch 0.4 mg/hr. daily.
3. Aspirin every other day.
4. Metamucil.

ALLERGIES: He has no known drug allergies.

SOCIAL HISTORY: He is a nonsmoker and social drinker. He is a retired auto mechanic who lives with his wife.

---------------------- begin page 2 ----------------------

PHYSICAL EXAMINATION

GENERAL: On physical examination he appears well and in no acute distress. Vital signs are stable. He is afebrile.

HEENT: Negative.

LUNGS: Clear to auscultation and percussion.

HEART: Cardiac exam reveals a regular rate and rhythm with a normal S1 and S2. There is a grade II/VI systolic murmur at the apex.

ABDOMEN: His abdomen is soft and nontender, with no masses or organomegaly.

RECTAL: A rectal examination revealed no masses. There was bright red blood on the examining finger.

EXTREMITIES: The extremities are without edema.

LABORATORY DATA: ECG showed no ischemic change.

IMPRESSION: My impression is that of a lower gastrointestinal hemorrhage. Most likely this is diverticular bleeding. Although the patient does take Indocin and aspirin, there is nothing to suggest that this is an acute upper gastrointestinal hemorrhage.

PLAN
1. Admit to hospital for careful observation.
2. Obtain CBC, WBC, prothrombin time, and Chem-7.
3. Proceed with a colonoscopy when the bleeding subsides. Should the bleeding continue, he will require an upper endoscopy and possibly an arteriogram.

Gwenn Maltase, MD/xx

CONSULTATION REPORT

Patient Name: Norr, Ralph

File Number: 80042

Date of Birth: May 31, 19xx

Examination Date: *Current date*

Requesting Physician: P. H. Waters, MD

HISTORY OF PRESENT ILLNESS: We were asked to assist in the evaluation and care of this 72-year-old gentleman who was admitted to University Hospital from the emergency room this morning for complaints of a rapid heart rate. He also had some complaints of retrosternal and epigastric discomfort and burning. The patient states that over the last six months to a year he has had increasing episodes of heartburn that have required an almost continuous use of antacids. Although he has had no nocturnal component to his symptoms, he also has had an increasing dry cough. The symptoms have become worse in the past month with increasing burning and epigastric pain. He had been originally placed on Pepcid 20 mg t.i.d. with some relief. However, the medication did not relieve his most recent symptoms. He denies any concomitant symptoms of dysphagia, hematemesis, or odynophagia.

PAST MEDICAL HISTORY: The patient notes a previous history of peptic ulcer disease in his 20s. This was diagnosed with an upper GI x-ray. His ulcer was not complicated with gastrointestinal bleeding. The patient does not smoke. He does not take any aspirin products or nonsteroidal anti-inflammatory drugs on a regular basis. He does drink one glass of wine per day. The patient denied any previous gastrointestinal surgeries. He has no history of a myocardial infarction or diabetes. He does have a history of hypertension. He has been treated in the past for irritable bowel syndrome with resolution of his symptoms.

MEDICATIONS: The patient's medications include Tenormin and Pepcid.

ALLERGIES: He does note allergies to certain antibiotics, but he is unsure of the particular drug.

PHYSICAL EXAMINATION: VITAL SIGNS: Blood pressure 192/102, pulse 190/minute, respirations 20/minute, and temperature 97.9. The patient appeared comfortable at the time of the consultation. He had no scleral icterus or jaundice. He had no thyromegaly or lymphadenopathy. Pulmonary auscultation revealed clear lung fields.

Cardiac auscultations revealed a regular heart rate. There were no murmurs noted. Abdominal examination revealed a soft abdomen. There were no abnormal masses palpated. He had some epigastric discomfort to palpation. Extremity examination was negative.

------------------------- begin page 2 -------------------------

Pertinent laboratory tests included electrolytes and creatinine, which were normal. Glucose was elevated at 116 CBC was normal, as were the prothrombin time, partial thromboplastin time, creatine kinase, and lactic dehydrogenase.

IMPRESSION:
1. Gastroesophageal reflux disease. Rule out peptic ulcer disease, severe esophagitis, and Barrett's esophagus.
2. Rapid heart rate.

RECOMMENDATIONS:
1. Agree with empiric Prilosec.
2. EGD to assess severity of reflux disease and/or complications resulting from it.

Anna Bolism, MD/xx

CHAPTER 9 / PART III CHECK YOUR PROGRESS

See Pretests (9T-5) and (9T-6).

CHAPTER 10 / PART I PRETEST

1. a	24. d	47. a	70. a
2. c	25. a	48. b	71. a
3. b	26. d	49. c	72. d
4. c	27. b	50. a	73. b
5. b	28. d	51. a	74. a
6. d	29. a	52. a	75. c
7. c	30. c	53. a	76. a
8. a	31. b	54. c	77. c
9. a	32. b	55. d	78. b
10. d	33. d	56. a	79. a
11. a	34. a	57. a	80. d
12. d	35. a	58. b	81. a
13. a	36. a	59. a	82. a
14. b	37. b	60. d	83. b
15. d	38. c	61. d	84. d
16. b	39. a	62. b	85. c
17. b	40. b	63. c	86. c
18. a	41. a	64. a	87. b
19. b	42. d	65. a	88. b
20. b	43. b	66. c	89. d
21. a	44. a	67. d	90. a
22. c	45. c	68. b	91. b
23. d	46. b	69. c	92. c

CHAPTER 10 / PART I ACTIVITY 3 (10T-1)

1. Afebrile is without fever.
   He is palpably afebrile.
2. Amaurosis is the loss of sight without the apparent lesion of the eye.
   She has noted some intermittent visual symptoms in her left eye; however, I would not clearly call it amaurosis fugax.
3. Aneurysm is a localized abnormal dilatation of the wall of a blood vessel.
   The physician felt no abdominal aortic aneurysm.
4. Angiography is the radiographic visualization of a blood vessel after injecting a contrast agent.
   The patient requires a coronary angiography.
5. Arrhythmia is the variation from the normal rhythm of the heartbeat.
   She has a history of hypertension, glaucoma, and arrhythmia.
6. Arteriography is the radiography of an artery after injection of a contrast medium in the bloodstream.
   Combined coronary arteriography with cerebral angiography would be appropriate.
7. Atherosclerotic is the hardening of an artery due to deposits of plaque within the vessel.
   She has a family history of atherosclerotic disease.
8. Atrial pertains to the atrium.
   She has a history of chronic atrial fibrillation and sleep apnea.
9. Bradycardia is a slow heartbeat.
   An electrocardiogram revealed bradycardia and a junctional rhythm was documented.
10. Bruit is a sound or murmur heard in auscultation.
    The abdomen contains no masses and no bruits.
11. Cardiomyopathy is the disease process of the heart muscle.
    The patient is a 35-year-old with documented cardiomyopathy.
12. Cardioverter is a device used to administer electrical shocks to the heart.
    The patient was given intravenous diuretics and readjusted her medicines to try to medically or electrically cardiovert her.
13. Carotid relates to the principal artery of the neck.
    Carotid bruits are not heard.
14. Cholecystectomy is the surgical removal of the gallbladder.
    She is scheduled next Wednesday morning for a laparoscopic cholecystectomy and possible open cholecystectomy.
15. Claudication is the cramp-like pains in the calf; limping.
    She has a history of peripheral vascular disease and is status post left iliac angioplasty with good results and no residual claudication.
16. Collateral is a secondary or accessory blood pathway.
    This is a 68-year-old male with single vessel coronary involving the left circumflex and bridging collaterals on the right coronary artery.
17. Cyanosis is a dark bluish or purplish coloration of the skin due to deficient oxygenation of the blood.
    No cyanosis or edema noted.
18. Diaphoresis is perspiration.
    He developed chest pain suddenly two hours ago with diaphoresis and nausea.
19. Digoxin is a generic name for a cardiotonic.
    Her medications included digoxin 0.125 mg daily and a laxative.
20. Diltiazem is a generic name for a coronary vasodilator.
    She denies hypertension, although she is on diltiazem at the time of her arrival in my office.
21. Dobutamine is a generic name for a cardiotonic agent.
    He was recently hospitalized several weeks ago for intravenous dobutamine therapy.
22. Duodenal relates to the duodenum, the first division of the small intestine.
    She has a history of peptic ulcer disease and a bleeding duodenal ulcer.
23. Dysrhythmia is a defective rhythm.
    She has a history of cardiac dysrhythmia in the past.

24. Echocardiogram is a diagnostic procedure using ultrasound to study heart structure and motion.
She had an echocardiogram and Holter monitor exam at that time.
25. Endarterectomy is a surgical procedure done to clear a blocked artery.
The patient underwent coronary artery bypass grafting on August 18, 1996 with right carotid endarterectomy at the same time.
26. Epiphysis is the center for the ossification at the proximal and distal ends of a long bone.
The patient's past medical history was significant for open reduction internal fixation of the right hip for what sounds like slipped capital femoral epiphysis disease.
27. Erythema is the redness of the skin due to capillary dilatation.
There is minimal erythema.
28. Expiratory relates to exhalation.
There is a moderately slight prolonged expiratory phase.
29. Fibrillation is the exceedingly rapid contractions of muscular fibrils.
She has a history of chronic atrial fibrillation and sleep apnea.
30. Gallop is a triple cadence to the heart sounds.
There are no significant murmurs or gallops.
31. Gout is a disorder associated with an inborn error of uric acid metabolism that increases production or interferes with the excretion of uric acid.
The patient also has a history of gout.
32. Hemiblock is the failure to conduct an impulse down one division of the left bundle branch.
The electrocardiogram shows a left anterior hemiblock, normal sinus rhythm, and premature arterial contractions.
33. Hemoptysis is the coughing or spitting of blood from the respiratory tract.
Negative for cough sputum or hemoptysis.
34. Heparin is a generic name for an anticoagulant.
The patient is refusing to consider intravenous heparin or any form of IV therapy or blood work.
35. Hypercholesterolemia is the presence of an abnormally large amount of cholesterol in the cells and plasma of the blood.
The patient is a 56-year-old gentleman with a history of chest pain, with negative evaluation in the past, and hypercholesterolemia.
36. Hyperkalemia is the greater than normal concentration of potassium ions in the blood.
He has hyperkalemia with an elevated potassium at 7.7.
37. Hyperlipidemia is a condition of elevated lipid levels in the blood.
The patient also has a history of mild hyperlipidemia and gout.
38. Hypotensive is characterized by low blood pressure or causing a reduction in blood pressure.
The patient would get so weak, dehydrated, and hypotensive that her diuretics would be cut back.
39. Idiopathic is a disease of unknown cause.
The patient is a 35-year-old with documented idiopathic cardiomyopathy.
40. Iliac relates to the ilium.
She has a history of peripheral vascular disease and is status post left iliac angioplasty with good results and no residual claudication.
41. Infarction is the sudden insufficiency of arterial or venous blood supply.
He presented to the University Hospital Emergency Room and an acute inferior infarction was noted by the ECG.
42. Inferolateral pertains to a location situated below and to the side.
Testing shows anteroapical and inferolateral anemia.
43. Inotropic pertains to the force of muscular contractions.
Parenteral inotropic agents will again be employed.
44. Intimal relates to the inner coat of a vessel.
In August 1994, the patient did have a heart catheterization that demonstrated decreased left ventricular function and intimal coronary artery disease.
45. Ischemia is the decreased supply of oxygenated blood to a body part.
His 12-lead ECG shows no evidence of transmural ischemia.

46. Mediastinum is the mass of tissues and organs separating the sternum in front and the vertebral column behind.
Mediastinum looks normal size.
47. Myocardial pertains to the muscular tissue of the heart.
The patient's chest discomfort could certainly be attributed to myocardial ischemia and infarction and this should be excluded.
48. Normocephalic is the normal size of the head.
The head is normocephalic, atraumatic.
49. Nortriptyline is a generic name for an antidepressant.
The patient's medications included nortriptyline 50 q.h.s.
50. Paroxysm is the sudden recurrence or increase in intensity of symptoms.
She has a history of paroxysmal atrial fibrillation and chronic atrial fibrillation.
51. Pectoralis pertains to the chest or breast.
There has been no definite angina pectoralis nor definite symptoms related to his right carotid lesion.
52. Pedal pertains to the foot or feet.
There is 1+ pedal edema.
53. Pitting is the formation of a small depression.
She has 4+ pitting edema of her lower extremities bilaterally.
54. Pleura is the serous membrane investing the lungs and lining the walls of the thoracic cavity.
She denies shortness of breath or pleuritic chest pain.
55. Polycythemia is an increase in the total red cell mass of the blood.
The patient has a history of polycythemia secondary to her COPD.
56. Quinidine is a generic name for an antiarrhythmic agent used in the treatment of atrial flutter, atrial fibrillation, premature ventricular contractions, and tachycardias.
The patient was medically converted with quinidine and she improved.
57. Rhonchus is a continuous dry rattling in the throat or bronchial tube due to a partial obstruction, heard on auscultation.
Occasional rhonchi are present in the chest
58. Sinus is a cavity or channel.
ECG was done and appears to be normal sinus rhythm.
59. Stenosis is the narrowing or contraction of a body passage.
A carotid sonogram documents an 80% to 99% stenosis in the left internal carotid artery.
60. Syncope is a temporary suspension of consciousness; fainting.
The patient denies dizziness, lightheadedness, or syncope.
61. Tachycardia is an abnormal rapid heart rate.
The physician ruled out supraventricular tachycardia.
62. Thrombosis is the formation of a blood clot within the vascular system.
The question of deep venous thrombosis has been raised.
63. Venous pertains to the veins.
Venous pulses are unremarkable.
64. Verapamil is a generic name for a coronary vasodilator.
He has been on verapamil therapy.
65. Capoten is the trade name for an antihypertensive.
The patient's medications included Capoten 12.5 mg t.i.d.
66. Cardiolite is the trade name for myocardial perfusion agent for cardiac SPECT imaging.
Persantine IV Cardiolite shows anteroapical and inferolateral ischemia.
67. Cardizem is the trade name for a calcium channel blocker for atrial fibrillation.
His medications include Cardizem 60 t.i.d. and aspirin.
68. Coumadin is the trade name for an anticoagulant.
She has a history of paroxysmal atrial fibrillation, chronic atrial fibrillation and is on Coumadin at home.
69. Cytotec is the trade name for an antisecretory, gastric protectant for the prevention of nonsteroidal anti-inflammatory drug induced gastric ulcers.
The patient's current medication is Cytotec 100 mg daily.
70. Ecotrin is the trade name for an analgesic, anti-inflammatory.
Her medications include Ecotrin 1 q.d.

71. Indocin is the trade name for nonsteroidal anti-inflammatory drug.
    The patient's current medications are Indocin 25 mg daily and Cytotec 100 mg daily.
72. Isordil is the trade name for an antianginal.
    His medications included Cardizem 60 mg t.i.d., Isordil 20 mg t.i.d., and aspirin.
73. K-Dur is the trade name for a potassium supplement.
    The patient's current medications are Capoten 12.5 mg t.i.d., K-Dur 20 mEq. b.i.d., and digoxin 0.125 mg daily.
74. Lanoxin is the trade name for a cardiac glycoside to increase cardiac output.
    The patient's medications included Coumadin per prothrombin times at home and, Lanoxin 0.25 mg o.d.
75. Lasix is the trade name for a diuretic.
    She will have her Lasix increased, and start on nitrates.
76. Lescol is the trade name for a reductase inhibitor for hypercholesterolemia.
    The patient's medications included Ecotrin, 1 mg q.d., Lescol, 20 mg q.d., and nortriptyline, 50 mg q.h.s.
77. Lotensin is the trade name for an antihypertensive.
    The patient was prescribed Lotensin, 1 tablet daily.
78. Mevacor is the trade name for a reductase inhibitor for hypercholesterolemia.
    The patient's current medications included Cardizem 60 mg t.i.d., Mevacor 20 mg, Isordil 20 mg t.i.d., and aspirin, which was stopped six days prior to surgery.
79. Persantine is the trade name for a coronary vasodilator.
    Persantine IV Cardiolite shows anteroapical and inferolateral ischemia.
80. Premarin is the trade name for estrogen replacement therapy.
    Her current medications include Premarin.
81. Provera is the trade name for progestin for secondary amenorrhea and abnormal uterine bleeding.
    Her current medications include Premarin and Provera.
82. Quinidex is the trade name for an antiarrhythmic.
    The patient's current medications include Capoten 12.5 mg t.i.d., K-Dur 20 mEq. b.i.d., Quinidex 300 mg b.i.d. and digoxin 0.125 mg daily.
83. Reglan is the trade name for a gastrointestinal stimulant; antiemetic.
    The patient had a history of intolerance to Reglan.
84. Senokot is the trade name for a laxative.
    Her medications included digoxin 0.125 mg daily and Senokot.
85. Synthroid is the trade name for a thyroid hormone.
    The patient's medications included Synthroid, 0.1 mg q.d., Ecotrin, 1 mg q.d., Lescol, 20 mg q.d., and nortriptyline, 50 mg q.h.s.
86. Tenormin is the trade name for a beta-blocker; antihypertensive agent.
    The patient's current medications are Tenormin 12.5 mg b.i.d., Indocin 25 mg daily, and Cytotec 100 mg daily.
87. Terramycin is the trade name for an antibiotic.
    The patient is allergic to Terramycin.
88. Theo-Dur is the trade name for a bronchodilator.
    The patient's medications included Coumadin per prothrombin times at home, Lanoxin 0.25 mg q.d., and Theo-Dur 300 mg b.i.d.
89. Trental is the trade name for an oral hemorrheologic drug.
    The patient's current medications are vitamin E, vitamin C, Trental, beta carotene, and Centrum Silver 1 tablet daily.
90. Vasotec is the trade name for an antihypertensive agent.
    She will be continued on her Vasotec, have her Lasix increased, and start on nitrates.
91. Xanax is the trade name for an antianxiety agent.
    Her current medications include Xanax, Premarin, and Provera.
92. Zyloprim is the trade name for an antigout agent.
    The patient's current medications are vitamin E, vitamin C, Trental, beta carotene, Centrum Silver 1 tablet daily, and Zyloprim.

CHAPTER 10 / PART I CHECK YOUR PROGRESS

1. a	24. a	47. a	70. a
2. c	25. b	48. b	71. a
3. b	26. a	49. b	72. d
4. d	27. c	50. d	73. b
5. d	28. b	51. b	74. a
6. a	29. a	52. a	75. c
7. b	30. a	53. d	76. a
8. a	31. a	54. a	77. c
9. d	32. d	55. d	78. a
10. d	33. b	56. a	79. a
11. c	34. b	57. a	80. d
12. a	35. c	58. c	81. a
13. a	36. a	59. d	82. a
14. a	37. d	60. b	83. b
15. a	38. b	61. c	84. d
16. c	39. d	62. b	85. c
17. b	40. d	63. c	86. c
18. a	41. d	64. a	87. b
19. b	42. d	65. a	88. b
20. c	43. c	66. c	89. d
21. a	44. a	67. d	90. a
22. b	45. b	68. b	91. b
23. d	46. b	69. c	92. c

CHAPTER 10 / PART II PRETEST (10T-2)

HISTORY AND PHYSICAL EXAMINATION

Patient Name: Horsh, Barbara

File Number: 78129

Date of Birth: May 1, 1942

Examination Date: *Current date*

Physician: Adam Valence, MD

HISTORY

CHIEF COMPLAINT: Precatheterization admission note.

HISTORY OF PRESENT ILLNESS: Mrs. Horsh underwent coronary artery bypass grafting on August 18, 1996 with right carotid endarterectomy at the same time. She has noted some intermittent visual symptoms in her left eye; however, I would not clearly call it amaurosis fugax. A carotid sonogram documents an 80% to 99% stenosis in the left internal carotid artery. Persantine IV Cardiolite shows anteroapical and inferolateral ischemia.

MEDICATIONS:
1. Synthroid, 0.1 q.d.
2. Ecotrin, 1 q.d.
3. Lescol, 20 q.d.
4. Nortriptyline, 50 q.h.s.

PHYSICAL EXAMINATION

NECK: Her examination shows a soft left carotid bruit. Neck veins are flat.

CHEST: Clear.

HEART: Regular, with grade I to II/VI systolic ejection murmur at the base with a soft aortic insufficiency murmur.

ABDOMEN: Soft.

EXTREMITIES: No edema.

---------------------- begin page 2 ----------------------

PLAN: The patient requires carotid angiography and coronary angiography. This will hopefully be done the same day.

_____

Adam Valence, MD/xx

FedDes Wellness Center
Cardiology Division, Suite 413
101 Wellness Way Drive
New York, NY 10036

Current date

Charles P. Davis, MD
FedDes Wellness Center
Family Practice Division, Suite 300
101 Wellness Way Drive
New York, NY 10036

Re: George Niehls
    Date of Birth: January 16, 19xx

Dear Dr. Davis

George Niehls is a 62-year-old man who was admitted for a cystectomy because of carcinoma of the bladder. He has a history of intermittent visual blurring. A routine physical examination revealed a right carotid bruit. A carotid sonogram was obtained which suggested high-grade stenosis of the right internal carotid. He is a longtime cigarette smoker and has moderate exertional dyspnea. There has been no definite angina pectoralis nor definite symptoms related to his right carotid lesion. There is a long history of hypertension, but drug therapy was discontinued in 1990.

Physical examination shows a blood pressure of 180/100 and a pulse of 80 and regular. Venous pulses are unremarkable. There is a long right carotid bruit. Occasional rhonchi are present in the chest, and there is a moderately slight prolonged expiratory phase. The heart is not enlarged. There are no significant murmurs or gallops. The abdomen contains no masses and no bruits. There is no peripheral edema.

Mr. Niehls would appear to have high-grade carotid artery stenosis. With contemplated major surgery, this should presumably be repaired preoperatively despite its essentially asymptomatic state. In addition, combined coronary arteriography with cerebral angiography would be appropriate. With his long history of hypertension, it would seem reasonable to also perform a renal arteriogram during the same procedure.

---------------------- begin page 2 ----------------------

We will arrange these studies and subsequent recommendations will be based on the results of the diagnostic findings. We appreciate the opportunity to participate in his care.

Sincerely

Lucas Site, MD

xx

HISTORY AND PHYSICAL EXAMINATION

Patient Name: Rolf, Nathan

File Number: 59025

Date of Birth: February 21, 19xx

Examination Date: *Current date*

Physician: Adam Valence, MD

HISTORY

CHIEF COMPLAINT: Shortness of breath.

HISTORY OF PRESENT ILLNESS: Nathan Rolf is a 35-year-old with documented idiopathic cardiomyopathy. He became symptomatic in 1995, and a subsequent cardiac catheterization was performed in 1997 at which time an ejection fraction of 25 was documented. His symptoms have progressed, and he was recently hospitalized several weeks ago for intravenous dobutamine therapy. He symptomatically improved, but in the past week he developed increasing dyspnea and orthopnea.

PHYSICAL EXAMINATION

VITAL SIGNS: Physical examination shows a blood pressure of 130/73 and a pulse of 112 and irregular.

NECK: Jugular venous pulse is slightly prominent.

CHEST: The chest is fairly clear.

HEART: The heart is moderately enlarged with an S3 gallop. No significant murmurs.

IMPRESSION: Mr. Rolf has severe cardiomyopathy. Parenteral inotropic agents will again be employed. Presumably his gastrointestinal symptoms are also indicative of congestive heart failure, but a complicating factor needs to be excluded as well.

PLAN: Admit to University Hospital due to his increasing dyspnea and orthopnea. He will again be assessed for a possible cardiac transplantation.

_____

Adam Valence, MD/xx

CHART NOTE

Patient Name: Jorshier, Fred

Date of Birth: October 27, 19xx

Examination Date: *Current date*

CHIEF COMPLAINT: Weakness. Chest and abdominal discomfort.

HISTORY OF PRESENT ILLNESS: Fred Jorshier presents today with weakness and some chest and abdominal discomfort. He has been on verapamil therapy. He has hyperkalemia with an elevated potassium at 7.7.

PAST HISTORY: Fred is a 51-year-old man with a long history of diabetes and renal failure as well as hypertension and pernicious anemia.

PHYSICAL EXAMINATION

VITAL SIGNS: BP 110/80, pulse 48 and regular.

NECK: Carotids are unremarkable. Jugular venous pulse is slightly distended.

LUNGS: There are rales at both bases.

HEART: The heart is moderately enlarged without significant murmur.

ABDOMEN: The abdomen is protuberant with some tenderness of the liver, which extends approximately 8 cm below the right costal margin.

EXTREMITIES: There is 3+ edema of the right leg and an amputation of the left leg.

DIAGNOSTIC TESTS: An electrocardiogram revealed bradycardia and a junctional rhythm was documented.

IMPRESSION: Mr. Jorshier's bradycardia is presumably related to his verapamil therapy as well as his hyperkalemia. His 12-lead ECG shows no evidence of transmural ischemia, but his chest discomfort could certainly be attributed to myocardial ischemia and infarction and this should be excluded.

------------------------ begin page 2 ------------------------

PLAN: If dobutamine and lowering his potassium does not correct his rhythm, a temporary pacemaker will be required.

A. B. Doner, MD/xx

HISTORY AND PHYSICAL EXAMINATION

Patient Name: Trilla, Patricia S.

File Number: 20145

Date of Birth: February 29, 19xx

Examination Date: *Current date*

Physician: Erica Purkinje, MD

HISTORY

CHIEF COMPLAINT: Chest pain.

HISTORY OF PRESENT ILLNESS: Patricia S. Trilla is a 49-year-old female who has been in good health. She is on estrogen replacement as well as occasional Xanax for rare panic attacks. During the past several days, she has noted intermittent aching and left chest discomfort that has not been precipitated by exertion. While eating lunch this afternoon, a persistent episode developed which was accompanied by nausea.

PAST MEDICAL HISTORY: Several years ago a diagnosis of mitral valve prolapse was made based on ECG tracing that showed an occasional premature ventricular beat.

MEDICATIONS: The patient has no known allergies. Her current medications include Xanax, Premarin, and Provera.

FAMILY HISTORY: The family history is noncontributory with the exception of a mitral valve prolapse.

SOCIAL HISTORY: The patient discontinued cigarette smoking five years ago. She does not drink to excess. The patient works as a legal secretary at B.W. Sharks, Ltd.

REVIEW OF SYSTEMS: Unremarkable.

PHYSICAL EXAMINATION

GENERAL: Physical examination shows a blood pressure of 139/70 and a pulse of 100 and regular.

NECK: Jugular venous pulse and carotids are unremarkable.

CHEST: Chest is clear. There is no chest wall tenderness.

------------------------ begin page 2 ------------------------

HEART: There is an apical systolic click.

ABDOMEN: The abdomen is unremarkable. Femoral pulses are palpable.

EXTREMITIES: There is no edema.

DIAGNOSTIC TESTS: Electrocardiogram is normal.

IMPRESSION: The patient's chest discomfort is atypical.

PLAN: Admit to University Hospital for cardiac assessment. Stress exercise testing will be performed later this afternoon if cardiac enzymes and electrocardiogram remain stable.

Erica Purkinje, MD/xx

See Pretest (10T-2).

CHAPTER 10 / PART III PRETEST (10T-5)

CHART NOTE

Patient Name: Forman, Beth

Date of Birth: May 3, 1953

Examination Date: *Current date*

CHIEF COMPLAINT: The patient presents with two episodes of her heart racing and some pain down her left breast for the last two nights.

HISTORY OF PRESENT ILLNESS: Beth felt that her heart was jumping around, somewhat irregularly, and she could not get back to sleep. This would last for about two hours. She denies any other symptoms. No dizziness or diaphoretic symptoms.

PAST HISTORY: Beth has a history of mitral valve prolapse. She really has not been symptomatic over the last few years. Her last real treatment for mitral valve prolapse was five years ago. Apparently she had an echocardiogram and Holter monitor exam at that time.

PHYSICAL EXAMINATION: BP 104/74, and pulse 76.
CARDIOVASCULAR: SI-SII with grade II-VI murmur. Ectopy is noted.
LUNGS: Clear to auscultation.

DIAGNOSTIC TESTS: ECG was done and appears to be normal sinus rhythm. I do not see any ectopy on the ECG.

ASSESSMENT:
1. Mitral valve prolapse.
2. Rule out supraventricular tachycardia.

PLAN:
1. I have ordered a Holter monitor and echocardiogram.
2. We briefly discussed the benefit of beta blockers and calcium channel blockers. I will determine their necessity based upon the results of the Holter monitor. She should probably have an echocardiogram every five years to monitor the valve and to ensure no deterioration of the valve.
3. She will follow up after the echocardiogram and Holter monitor exam is completed.

Erica Purkinje, MD/xx

CHAPTER 10 / PART III PRETEST (10T-6)

Current date

Charles P. Davis, MD
FedDes Wellness Center
Family Practice Division, Suite 300
101 Wellness Way Drive
New York, NY 10036

Re: Edward Chuk
    Date of Birth: June 19, 19xx

Dear Dr. Davis

Edward Chuk, an 84-year-old white male with a history of myocardial infarction in 1985, is scheduled for surgery next Thursday for diverticular disease of the colon. He has a history of an MI in the 1980s, chronic obstructive pulmonary disease, and diverticular disease. He has no known allergies and takes no medication. Mr. Chuk complains of dyspnea when taking out the garbage at home, but otherwise experiences no other chest pain.

On physical examination, his blood pressure is 129/79, pulse of 80, and a respiratory rate of 12/min. HEENT exam demonstrates brisk carotid upstrokes without bruits. He has normal heart sounds with normal S1 and S2, no S3, no S4, no rubs or murmurs. Lungs are clear. Abdomen is soft. I feel no abdominal aortic aneurysm. Right lower quadrant is tender. There are no abnormal bowel sounds. Extremities have no clubbing, cyanosis, or edema. Neurological exam is unremarkable. The electrocardiogram shows a left anterior hemiblock, normal sinus rhythm, and premature arterial contractions. Chest x-ray is negative. Laboratory data are unremarkable.

I think he should have a dobutamine echocardiogram prior to surgery due to his history of tobacco abuse and previous myocardial infarction. I have scheduled a dobutamine echocardiogram for next Monday morning. He should be ready for surgery if he is cleared by mid to late morning. Thank you very much for the opportunity to consult in Mr. Chuk's preoperative clearance.

Sincerely

Lucas Site, MD

xx

CONSULTATION REPORT

Patient Name: Isiaba, Naomi

File Number: 36902

Date of Birth: April 22, 19xx

Examination Date: *Current date*

Requesting Physician: Izzy Sertoli, MD

HISTORY OF PRESENT ILLNESS: Naomi Isiaba is a 19-year-old Asian female who is 32 weeks pregnant with twins. She has been in the hospital because of premature rupture of membranes. She was noted to have a swollen right leg with numbness and decreased sensation. The question of deep venous thrombosis has been raised. She has been in the hospital at bedrest for the past three days. She denies shortness of breath or pleuritic chest pain.

PHYSICAL EXAMINATION: Examination reveals a young, anxious, Asian female who looks her stated age. There is swelling of the right leg. There is minimal erythema. There is mild tenderness with decreased sensation. Pulses are excellent.

Mrs. Isiaba's swollen right leg may well be due to DVT. At this junction, she is refusing to consider intravenous heparin or any form of IV therapy or blood work. She will be encouraged to have a Doppler study of the leg to look for evidence of DVT. She is tender in the thigh and thus an ultrasound study should demonstrate a thrombus if present.

We will follow along with you. Thank you for the opportunity to participate in the care of this patient.

_____

Adam Valence, MD/xx

HISTORY AND PHYSICAL EXAMINATION

Patient Name: Whitehead, Samuel

File Number: 10945

Date of Birth: May 3, 19xx

Examination Date: *Current date*

Physician: Adam Valence, MD

HISTORY

CHIEF COMPLAINT: Chest pain.

HISTORY OF PRESENT ILLNESS: The patient is a 58-year-old man without cardiac history. He developed sudden chest pain two hours ago with diaphoresis and nausea. He presented to the University Hospital Emergency Room, and an acute inferior infarction was noted by the ECG.

PAST HISTORY: Cardiac risk factors include positive cigarette smoking two packs per day, negative vascular accident or transient ischemic attack specifically.

ALLERGIES: He denies allergies.

MEDICATIONS: None.

PHYSICAL EXAMINATION

GENERAL: Anxious man in no acute distress. BP 100/60, pulse 80.

NECK: Neck veins flat without bruits.

CHEST: Scattered rhonchi.

CARDIAC: Regular, without murmur, rub, or gallop.

ABDOMEN: Soft, nontender.

EXTREMITIES: Without clubbing, cyanosis or edema. PULSES: 2+ and equal.

LABORATORY DATA: ECG shows acute inferior infarction with peaked Ts laterally as well. There is reciprocal depression in leads I and II. Chest x-ray is negative. Mediastinum looks normal size. WBC 20.2, hemoglobin 15.2.

----------------------- begin page 2 -----------------------

IMPRESSION: Acute inferior infarction, possible lateral involvement as well.

PLAN: The patient has no contraindication to the GUSTO trial, and this is planned for him.

_____

Adam Valence, MD/xx

HISTORY AND PHYSICAL EXAMINATION

Patient Name: Gallette, Clifford

File Number: 00925

Date of Birth: April 1, 19xx

Examination Date: *Current date*

Physician: A. B. Doner, MD

HISTORY

CHIEF COMPLAINT: Chest discomfort.

HISTORY OF PRESENT ILLNESS: Mr. Gallette is a 64-year-old male with a history of hypertension, who yesterday noted a new onset of chest discomfort. The patient describes development of pressure across the upper chest with associated severe dyspnea. This occurred while he was walking his dog. The patient stopped and rested with resolution of the chest discomfort. He then attempted several times to continue walking and had recurrence of chest discomfort. Today the patient awoke and shortly afterwards developed chest discomfort at rest. Under insistence from his wife, he now presents in our office.

PAST HISTORY: Cardiac risk factors include hypertension, obesity, and a positive family history.

MEDICATIONS: Lotensin, 1 tablet daily.

ALLERGIES: The patient is allergic to Terramycin.

FAMILY HISTORY: Both parents had heart disease.

SOCIAL HISTORY: He is a retired fork lift operator, having previously worked for Caterpillar Industries. He is a nonsmoker and nondrinker.

REVIEW OF SYSTEMS: Noncontributory.

PHYSICAL EXAMINATION

GENERAL: Obese man who is slightly dyspneic. His blood pressure is 144/88 with a pulse of 80. Respiratory rate is 16/min.

NECK: Examination was without carotid bruits.

------------------------ begin page 2 ------------------------

HEART: Heart was regular, without murmurs, rubs or gallops.

CHEST: The chest was clear.

ABDOMEN: The abdomen is benign.

EXTREMITIES: Without edema.

DIAGNOSTIC DATA: Electrocardiogram shows normal sinus rhythm. There is 1 mm of ST segment depression in leads II, III, and aVF and approximately 1 mm of ST elevation in leads I, aVL.

IMPRESSION:
1. Unstable angina.
2. Hypertension.

PLAN: The patient will be admitted to exclude an acute myocardial infarction and to initiate therapy with beta blockers, aspirin, and heparin. He will also undergo cardiac catheterization.

_____

A. B. Doner, MD/xx

CHAPTER 10 / 10T-10

HISTORY AND PHYSICAL EXAMINATION

Patient Name: Sosa, Lorraine

File Number: 431098

Date of Birth: July 2, 19xx

Examination Date: *Current date*

Physician: Erica Purkinje, MD

HISTORY

HISTORY OF PRESENT ILLNESS: This is a 45-year-old white female being admitted to the ICU from my office. She relates a two-month history of shortness of breath with exertion, a dry cough, and chest discomfort that she describes as "an ache in her left upper chest." The symptoms have progressed causing her sleeping pattern to go from completely flat in bed to sleeping on two pillows, to sleeping in a lounge chair the last several nights. She appears somewhat cyanotic in the office and is quite dyspneic.

PAST MEDICAL HISTORY: She is a two-pack-a-day smoker. Denies alcohol use. She denies hypertension, although she is on Vasotec and diltiazem at the time of her arrival in my office. She has been diabetic for two years and is unaware of her cholesterol level. Past hospitalizations include: (1) a tonsillectomy as a child, (2) a hysterectomy secondary to endometriosis, and (3) a traumatic laceration of her left arm which occurred while at work several years ago.

FAMILY HISTORY: She has a family history of atherosclerotic disease. An aunt died of a stroke, her mother died of an MI, and a sister died of an MI. Both the mother and sister were diabetic.

REVIEW OF SYSTEMS: Review of symptoms is positive for rheumatic fever as a child. She is presently being treated with Pepcid for peptic ulcer disease, although she states she has never had frank bleeding. She has hypertension, diabetes, and probable COPD. She has been wheezing over the last month or so, but she denies any wheezing prior to that time.

PHYSICAL EXAMINATION

GENERAL: This is a 45-year-old white female who appears older than her stated age.

NECK: There is no visible neck vein distension at 45 degrees. Her carotid pulses have adequate upstroke.

------------------------ begin page 2 ------------------------

HEART: Auscultation of her heart reveal a regular rhythm with an S4 and decreased heart tones. The point of maximum impulse is not palpable.

LUNGS: Auscultation of her lungs reveals decreased breath sounds with crackles in the right base and scattered wheezes.

ABDOMEN: Her abdomen is rotund, soft, and nontender. She states that her abdominal girth has grown appreciably in the last six weeks.

EXTREMITIES: Her extremities show no evidence of cyanosis nor clubbing. She has 4+ pitting edema of her lower extremities bilaterally.

IMPRESSION: Mrs. Sosa has clear demonstration of right heart failure and possible left heart failure as well. She has a history of hypertension, diabetes, and a family history of coronary disease. Her admission diagnosis is biventricular failure, rule out coronary insufficiency.

PLAN: She will be admitted to the ICU at University Hospital for treatment of failure. A ventilation perfusion scan is being ordered to rule out chronic pulmonary emboli or other etiology of her right heart failure. She will be continued on her Vasotec, have her Lasix increased, and start on nitrates.

_____

Erica Purkinje, MD/xx

HISTORY AND PHYSICAL EXAMINATION

Patient Name: Fellows, Michael

File Number: 00348

Date of Birth: July 4, 1945

Examination Date: *Current date*

Physician: Lucas Site, MD

HISTORY

CHIEF COMPLAINT: Swollen left leg.

HISTORY OF PRESENT ILLNESS: Mr. Fellows is a very pleasant gentleman who approximately two days ago prior to presentation had undergone a long drive and consequently after the drive began developing progressive problems of the left lower extremity. An ultrasound exam demonstrated deep vein thrombosis on the left side. The patient has no previous embolic phenomenon. He denies any chest pain or shortness of breath.

PAST MEDICAL HISTORY: Significant for open reduction internal fixation of the right hip for what sounds like slipped capital femoral epiphysis disease. He also had pinings of both elbows from what appears to be a congenital problem. The patient also has a history of mild hyperlipidemia and gout. He quit smoking 20 years ago. He has a family history of coronary disease, but he himself does not.

MEDICATIONS: Vitamin E, vitamin C, Trental, beta carotene, Centrum Silver 1 tablet daily, and Zyloprim.

REVIEW OF SYSTEMS: Unremarkable.

PHYSICAL EXAMINATION

GENERAL: The patient is alert and in no distress. The skin is warm and dry. Blood pressure is 110/70. His respiration rate is 18/min. He is palpably afebrile. His heart rate is in the 70s and regular.

HEENT: The head is normocephalic, atraumatic. The eyes are PERRL. The carotids are quiet. There are no bruits. The thyroid gland is not palpable.

HEART: Regular rate and rhythm.

- begin page 2 -

LUNGS: Clear.

ABDOMEN: Soft.

EXTREMITIES: No cyanosis. The left lower extremity is swollen and tender to palpation of the calf.

NEUROLOGICAL: Nonfocal.

IMPRESSION: Deep venous thrombosis.

PLAN: Begin heparin and Coumadin therapy.

_____

Lucas Site, MD/xx

Current date

J. Thomas Geiger, MD
FedDes Wellness Center
Family Practice Division, Suite 300
101 Wellness Way Drive
New York, NY 10036

Re: Marie Monyet
   Date of Birth: July 5, 19xx

Dear Dr. Geiger

Mrs. Monyet is a 75-year-old with a long past medical history. She has carotid artery disease, with a recent MRI angiogram showing a 50% right internal carotid artery stenosis and no disease on the left. She has a history of peripheral vascular disease and is status post left iliac angioplasty with good results and no residual claudication. A cardiac catheterization in 1991 showed minimal nonocclusive disease. She chronically has an abnormal electrocardiogram with anterior T-wave abnormalities and a Q-wave in lead III. She had a normal dobutamine stress test in 1997 and again in February of 1999.

She has a history of peptic ulcer disease and a bleeding duodenal ulcer. The bleeding has stopped since she stopped drinking alcohol with nonsteroidal anti-inflammatories. She has pseudomembranous colitis, degenerative joint disease, functional bowel disorder and chronic sinusitis.

Current medications are Tenormin 12.5 b.i.d., vitamin E 400 daily, Indocin 25 daily, and Cytotec 100 mg daily.

She has been diagnosed this hospitalization with acute cholecystitis and is scheduled next Wednesday morning for a laparoscopic cholecystectomy and possible open cholecystectomy.

Her liver function tests are within normal limits. There is mild elevation of her calcium at 10.2. A current ECG demonstrates normal sinus rhythm with Q-wave in lead III, ST-T wave abnormalities anteriorly. I see no change from the previous tracings. White blood count is slightly elevated at 12.

- begin page 2 -

On physical examination, vital signs are normal. Her blood pressure is 130/68 with a pulse of 84. HEENT exam is unremarkable. She has clear lung fields and normal heart exam. Abdomen is soft. Extremities have no peripheral edema. There is a carotid bruit on the right and none of the left.

ASSESSMENT: I feel she is a reasonable candidate to proceed with laparoscopic and possible open cholecystectomy. She is stable from a cardiovascular standpoint. She has not had angina.

I will follow along with you. Thank you very much for the consultation.

Sincerely

Erica Purkinje, MD

xx

See Pretests (10T-5) and (10T-6).

CHAPTER 11 / PART I PRETEST

1. a	11. a	21. a	31. c
2. b	12. c	22. c	32. b
3. c	13. d	23. c	33. a
4. d	14. b	24. a	34. a
5. b	15. a	25. c	35. d
6. a	16. c	26. b	36. c
7. c	17. c	27. a	37. a
8. c	18. c	28. c	38. b
9. d	19. b	29. c	39. d
10. a	20. a	30. b	40. a

CHAPTER 11 / PART I ACTIVITY 3 (11T-1)

1. Acromioclavicular describes the articulation between the acromial process of the scapula and the clavicle.
   Mild degenerative changes are present at the acromioclavicular joint, characterized by mild inferior marginal spurring.
2. Amorphous is having no definite form, or shapeless.
   There is an amorphous calcific deposit in the right side of the pelvis measuring 2.3 × 0.8 cm, of which the exact etiology is not determined.
3. Anteverted is the abnormal forward tilting of an organ.
   Real-time ultrasound examination demonstrates a normal size anteverted uterus, 10.3 cm in length, 4.1 cm in AP dimension.
4. Ascites is the effusion and accumulation of serous fluid in the abdominal cavity.
   There is no sonographic evidence of intra-abdominal mass, lymphadenopathy, or ascites.
5. Asymmetry is without symmetry, lacking similar form or relationship of parts.
   Asymmetry is therefore probably due to the superior position of unopacified bowel over the adnexa.
6. Bilateral is affecting both sides.
   Bilateral low dose film screen mammography is compared to the study of October 12, 1999.
7. Calculus is a stone.
   I believe there is a 4 × 2 mm nonobstructing calculus in the proximal right ureter at the level of L3.
8. Carpometacarpal is the joint spaces between the carpal and metacarpal bones.
   Examination of the hands and wrists demonstrate degenerative changes at the first carpometacarpal joints bilaterally.
9. Centrum semiovale is the white matter of the cerebral hemispheres that has an almost oval shape.
   The lesions are contained to the deep white matter of the cerebrum and predominate in the centrum semiovale, bilaterally.
10. Contraindicate is a factor that makes it undesirable to treat a patient in the usual manner.
    A regular exercise program to include weightbearing exercise is also to be encouraged if not clinically contraindicated.
11. Contrast medium is the pharmaceutical given to the patient to allow radiographic visualization of a body structure.
    Computerized tomography was performed from the diaphragm to the symphysis pubis with the use of oral and intravenous contrast medium.
12. Cricopharyngeal is pertaining to the cricoid cartilage and the pharynx.
    Cricopharyngeal function is normal.
13. Demarcated is to set limits or boundaries.
    An 18 × 8 × 20 mm well-demarcated simple cyst is demonstrated within the central 12 o'clock position of the right breast corresponding to the well-demarcated density noted on mammography in this region.
14. Etiology is the science concerned with the causes or origin of a disease or disorder.
    There is an amorphous calcific deposit in the right side of the pelvis measuring 2.3 × 0.8 cm, of which the exact etiology is not determined.
15. Hiatus hernia is the herniation of an abdominal organ through the esophageal opening of the diaphragm.
    There is a tiny sliding hiatus hernia measuring 2 cm, which is not associated with reflux.
16. Hydronephrosis is the distention of the renal pelvis and calices with urine, often as a result of obstruction of the ureter.
    A survey of the kidneys reveals no left or right hydronephrosis.
17. Infarction is the death of a tissue due to lack of blood flow to the area.
    There is no evidence of hemorrhage or signs of infarction.
18. Intrahepatic is within the liver.
    The common bile duct and intrahepatic and extrahepatic biliary ducts are normal.
19. Ischemic is the lack of blood in a body part.
    Small vessel ischemic changes are seen in the convexity regions bilaterally, particularly on the right.
20. Jejunum is the second section of the small intestine.
    The stomach emptied in normal fashion with visualization of the jejunum.
21. Joint mouse is the loose bodies in synovial joints.
    A 2 mm oval osseous density is identified in the medial patellofemoral joint space consistent with a small joint mouse.
22. Lacuna is the small cavity within or between other body structures.
    An old lacunar infarct is present in the basal ganglia on the right side and the thalamus on the left side.
23. Lymphadenopathy is the disease of the lymph nodes.
    There is no retroperitoneal lymphadenopathy or pelvic lymphadenopathy.
24. Osteopenia is the decrease in bone mass below the normal.
    The degree of osteopenia is worse in the left hip with the reading at 2.19 standard deviations below the mean.
25. Parenchyma is the general anatomical term to describe the functional elements of an organ, as distinguished from its structure.
    The remainder of the testicular parenchyma has an inhomogeneous texture.
26. Paresthesia is the sensation of tingling and numbness.
    The patient reports a spastic bladder over the past three years with paresthesia involving the right leg over the past six years.
27. Passavant's cushion is a ridge appearing on the posterior wall of pharynx during swallowing due to contraction of palatopharyngeal spincter.
    During swallowing, there is sufficient inferior motion of the soft palate and anterior movement of Passavant's cushion to prevent reflux into the nasopharynx.
28. Periarticular is situated around a joint.
    There are no periarticular calcifications.
29. Pericholecystic fluid is a coined term, meaning fluid around the gallbladder.
    I see no visible gallstones or pericholecystic fluid.
30. Reflux is a backward flow.
    There is no evidence of reflux or esophagitis.
31. Retroperitoneal is behind the peritoneum.
    There is no retroperitoneal adenopathy or ascites.
32. Stricture is an abnormal narrowing of a duct or passage.
    The ureter in the region appears mildly narrowed and somewhat variable, suggesting mild stricture or spasm.
33. Subluxation is a partial dislocation.
    There is no evidence of fracture or subluxation.
34. Thrombosis is a formation of a blood clot.
    There is no sonographic evidence of deep venous thrombosis.

35. Transducer is a device that translates one form of energy to another.
    In sonography, a transducer transforms a sound wave into electronically displayed image.
36. Vertex is the top or crown of the head.
    Transverse and longitudinal sonograms of the maternal abdomen were performed, revealing a single intrauterine gestation in vertex presentation.
37. Isovue is the trade name for a drug used as a contrast medium.
    Isovue was administered via intrathecal injection.
38. Lescol is the trade name for a drug that decreases LDL cholesterol.
    She lists her current medications and supplements as Synthroid and Lescol.
39. Provera is the trade name for a drug used in restoring hormonal imbalance.
    She lists her current medications and supplements as Estrace and Provera.
40. Synthroid is the trade name for a drug used as a replacement in decreased or absent thyroid function.
    She lists her current medications as Synthroid and pain medication, which she takes only as needed.

CHAPTER 11 / PART I CHECK YOUR PROGRESS

1. a	11. c	21. c	31. d
2. a	12. a	22. d	32. c
3. a	13. c	23. c	33. a
4. c	14. a	24. b	34. b
5. d	15. a	25. a	35. a
6. c	16. b	26. c	36. c
7. d	17. b	27. a	37. d
8. c	18. c	28. c	38. d
9. c	19. b	29. b	39. b
10. a	20. a	30. c	40. a

CHAPTER 11 / PART II PRETEST (11T-2)

Current date

Samuel Brunner, MD
Internal Medicine, Ltd.
903 West Orange Street
New York, NY 10035

Re: Larry Methembaum
     Date of Birth: July 6, 1941
     Examination: LUMBAR SPINE

Dear Dr. Brunner

Frontal, lateral, and oblique views were obtained. There are five lumbar vertebrae. There is no evidence of disc space narrowing. No destructive lesion is seen. There is mild degenerative arthritis involving the L3-4 through L5-S1 facet joints bilaterally. No other finding of significance is seen.

IMPRESSION: There is evidence of degenerative arthritis involving the L3-4 and L5-S1 facet joints bilaterally. No other finding of significance is seen.

Thank you for referring this patient to us.

Yours truly

Potter T. Bucky, MD

xx

FedDes Wellness Center
Diagnostic Imaging Division, Suite 157
101 Wellness Way Drive
New York, NY 10036

Current date

P.H. Waters, MD
FedDes Wellness Center
Family Practice Division, Suite 300
101 Wellness Way Drive
New York, NY 10036

Re: Robin Hatherode
     Date of Birth: December 19, 1953
     Examination: LEFT WRIST ARTHROGRAM

Dear Dr. Waters

Scout films are unremarkable.

Following appropriate preparation of the skin, a #22 gauge needle was inserted into the radionavicular joint and 2 cc of iodinated contrast media was injected. Films were then obtained after minimal manipulation of the wrist. An additional group of films were obtained following further manipulation of the wrist. Contrast is present in the distal radioulnar joint, indicating a tear of triangular fibrocartilage.

There is no evidence of contrast in the midcarpal joints to suggest the presence of a ligamentous tear. No additional findings of significance are seen.

IMPRESSION: Findings consistent with a tear of the triangular fibrocartilage.

Thank you for referring this patient to us.

Yours truly

Hounsfield T. Scanner, MD

xx

FedDes Wellness Center
Diagnostic Imaging Division, Suite 157
101 Wellness Way Drive
New York, NY 10036

Current date

Ida Gundrum, MD
Railroad Station Health Center
321 Trainmaster Boulevard
Reading, PA 19604

Re: Tonya Guerrero
     Date of Birth: May 24, 1981
     Examination: CT ABDOMEN AND PELVIS

Dear Dr. Gundrum

Computerized tomography was performed from the diaphragm to the symphysis pubis with the use of oral and intravenous contrast medium.

The liver and spleen are normal. I see no visible gallstones or pericholecystic fluid. There is no pancreatic mass or calcifications. The kidneys are both functional and unobstructed. There is no retroperitoneal lymphadenopathy or pelvic lymphadenopathy. The uterus is midline. There is some slight fullness in the right adnexa. An ultrasound was performed on June 9, 20xx that showed no adnexal pathology. Asymmetry is, therefore, probably due to the superior position of unopacified bowel over the adnexa. No other pelvic abnormality is seen.

IMPRESSION: Negative exam.

Thank you for referring this patient to us.

Yours truly

Hounsfield T. Scanner, MD

xx

FedDes Wellness Center
Diagnostic Imaging Division, Suite 157
101 Wellness Way Drive
New York, NY 10036

Current date

Izzy Sertoli, MD
Family Practice Division, Suite 300
FedDes Wellness Center
101 Wellness Way Drive
New York, NY 10036

Re: Melinda Williams
    Date of Birth: July 16, 1951
    Examination: BOTH KNEES

Dear Dr. Sertoli

There is slight narrowing of mediofemoral, tibial, and patellar joint spaces and both patellofemoral joint spaces. A 2 mm oval osseous density is identified in the medial patellofemoral joint space consistent with a small joint mouse. There are no erosive or destructive changes. There are no abnormal soft tissue masses.

IMPRESSION: There is slight narrowing of the mediofemoral, tibial, and patellofemoral joint spaces as described above. There are no destructive changes. There is no significant osteophyte formation.

Thank you for referring this patient to us.

Yours truly

_____

Potter T. Bucky, MD

xx

FedDes Wellness Center
Diagnostic Imaging Division, Suite 157
101 Wellness Way Drive
New York, NY 10036

Current date

Charles P. Davis, MD
FedDes Wellness Center
Family Practice Division, Suite 300
101 Wellness Way Drive
New York, NY 10036

Re: Nevin Dull
    Date of Birth: May 1, 1963
    Examination: CHEST X-RAY, PA AND LATERAL

Dear Dr. Davis

The trachea and mediastinum are in the midline. The heart is not enlarged. There is no mediastinal adenopathy. The lung fields are clear. The costophrenic angles are clear. The visualized bony structures reveal no gross abnormalities.

IMPRESSION: Normal PA and lateral chest radiographs.

Thank you for referring this patient to us.

Yours truly

William C. Roentgen, MD

xx

CHAPTER 11 / PART II CHECK YOUR PROGRESS

See Pretest (11T-2).

Current date

Richard Yavell, MD
Family Health Center
16 Manor Avenue
New York, NY 10025

Re: Anthony Coates
    Date of Birth: March 22, 1987
    Examination: CT HEAD AND BRAIN WITHOUT CONTRAST

Dear Dr. Yavell

HISTORY: Multiple falls. The study is compared to the previous CT of the head that was performed approximately one month ago.

An old lacunar infarct is present in the basal ganglia on the right side and the thalamus on the left side. Small vessel ischemic changes are seen in the convexity regions bilaterally, particularly on the right. There is soft tissue swelling over the frontal region on the right side without evidence of underlying fracture. The sinuses are aerated appropriately. There is evidence of a previously performed craniotomy. A large defect over the convexity and some metallic densities, which are apparently related to that craniotomy, are seen particularly in the left frontal area.

IMPRESSION: No acute infarct, mass or hemorrhage is seen.

Thank you for referring this patient to us.

Yours truly

Hounsfield T. Scanner, MD

xx

Current date

Izzy Sertoli, MD
FedDes Wellness Center
Family Practice Division, Suite 300
New York, NY 10036

Re: Alice Pravio
    Date of Birth: February 23, 1945
    Examination: UPPER GI SERIES

Dear Dr. Sertoli

A scout film of the abdomen shows an unremarkable bowel gas pattern.

The patient swallowed the barium without difficulty. Primary esophageal peristalsis was noted. A mild degree of gastroesophageal reflux was observed during the course of the examination. There is a mild mucosal irregularity of the distal esophagus just proximal to the GE junction, consistent with mild esophagitis changes. The stomach has no mucosal abnormality and is normal in its size and shape. The duodenal bulb and sweep are normal in appearance, with the exception of an incidental diverticulum from the second portion of the duodenum that measures approximately 1 cm. The visualized proximal jejunum is unremarkable.

IMPRESSION: Mild gastroesophageal reflux. Minimal esophagitis changes of the distal esophagus are demonstrated. No active ulcer disease.

Thank you for referring this patient to us.

Yours truly

Scott E. Film, MD

xx

Current date

David Campella, MD
Bay Point Family Health Center
4530 Oyster Avenue
Bayside, NY 15609

Re: Stephanie D. Vaughn
     Date of Birth: March 14, 1939
     Examination: RIGHT BREAST SONOGRAM

Dear Dr. Campella

Comparison is made to the prior mammogram dated
February 26, 20xx.

An 18 × 8 × 20 mm well-demarcated simple cyst is demonstrated
within the central 12 o'clock position of the right breast
corresponding to the well-demarcated density noted on
mammography in this region. The cyst exhibits posterior wall
enhancement and sound through transmission.

A second cyst measuring 6.1 × 7.0 × 4.4 mm is present in the
approximate 10 o'clock position of the breast projecting 6-7 mm from
the nipple corresponding to the density noted on mammography in
this region. No additional lesions are identified.

IMPRESSION: The two densities noted in the right breast on the recent
mammogram correspond to simple cysts as described.

Thank you for referring this patient to us.

Yours truly

William C. Roentgen, MD

xx

Current date

J. Thomas Geiger, MD
Family Practice Division, Suite 300
FedDes Wellness Center
101 Wellness Way Drive
New York, NY 10036

Re: Helen MacBride
     Date of Birth: September 10, 1937
     Examination: IVP

Dear Dr. Geiger

There has been a change since the previous study dated
February 11, 1999. I believe there is a 4 × 2 mm nonobstructing
calculus in the proximal right ureter at the level of L3. The ureter in
the region appears mildly narrowed and somewhat variable,
suggesting mild stricture or spasm.

There is also a series of small calculi within the distal right ureter, the
most distal of which measures 5 × 3 mm. There is a mild partial
obstruction of the distal right ureter. On the postvoid film, the right
ureter does drain. On prevoid films, the right ureter is mildly dilated
along its length. I do not see any delay function. Both kidneys and
the bladder appear otherwise normal. No renal calculi are noted.
There are two gallstones in the right upper quadrant. They average
about 2 cm in diameter.

IMPRESSION: Several calculi are noted within the right ureter. A
nonobstructing calculus associated with slight ureteral narrowing is
noted at the L3 level in the proximal right ureter. There are a series of
calcifications within the distal right ureter, associated with a mild
partial obstruction.

Thank you for referring this patient to us.

Yours truly

William C. Roentgen, MD

xx

Current date

Matthew D. Sponch, MD
Family Practice Division, Suite 300
FedDes Wellness Center
101 Wellness Way Drive
New York, NY 10036

Re: Elizabeth Nicholas
     Date of Birth: April 29, 1936
     Examinations: VIDEO ESOPHAGRAM AND GI SERIES
                    FLAT PLATE OF THE ABDOMEN

Dear Dr. Sponch

At your request, an esophagram and GI series were performed on this elderly patient who complains of food "getting stuck in her throat" when she eats and "difficulty swallowing."

The patient was studied with the aid of videotape that has stop-frame capacity using air contrast and conventional barium. The patient was examined and imaged in both prone and erect positions. Analysis of swallowing functions reveals:

1. There is no leakage of barium from the mouth into the pharynx at rest.
2. During swallowing, there is sufficient inferior motion of the soft palate and anterior movement of Passavant's cushion to prevent reflux into the nasopharynx.
3. There is adequate inferior tilt of the epiglottis and sufficient anterosuperior motion of the larynx to prevent aspiration.
4. There is normal contraction of the posterior pharyngeal-prevertebral muscles.
5. Cricopharyngeal function is normal.
6. There are no anatomic esophageal abnormalities. We see no web, stricture, mass, diverticulum, ulceration or erosion.

There is a tiny sliding hiatus hernia measuring 2 cm, which is not associated with reflux. There is a slight narrowing at the level of the esophagogastric junction which measures 13 mm at its widest part. The patient was able to swallow a 12.5 mm barium tablet without obstruction or delay.

---------------------- begin page 2 ----------------------

The stomach is normal in tone, contour, peristalsis and mucosal fold pattern. There are no filling defects or ulcerations. There is no pyloric obstruction. The duodenal bulb and sweep are normal. The visualized portion of jejunum is normal.

IMPRESSION: There is a 2 cm sliding hiatus hernia associated with minimal narrowing at the esophagogastric junction. However, this narrowing does not cause obstructional delay to the passage of a 12.5 mm barium tablet. There is no evidence of reflux or esophagitis. The remainder of the esophagram and GI series is otherwise normal.

FLAT PLATE OF THE ABDOMEN

The psoas margins and renal shadows are normal. There are no abnormal opacifications. The bowel pattern is normal.

Thank you for referring this patient to us.

Yours truly

William C. Roentgen MD

xx

Current date

J. Thomas Geiger, MD
Family Practice Division, Suite 300
FedDes Wellness Center
101 Wellness Way Drive
New York, NY 10036

Re: Terresa Rosario
     Date of Birth: October 5, 1951
     Examination: BILATERAL HANDS AND WRIST

Dear Dr. Geiger

Examination of the hands and wrists demonstrate degenerative changes at the first carpometacarpal joints bilaterally. There is no joint space narrowing, subluxation, and periarticular sclerosis at these joints. No other specific abnormality could be identified. The appearance is unchanged from May 12, 20xx.

IMPRESSION: Bilateral degenerative joint disease of the first carpometacarpal joint.

Thank you for referring this patient to us.

Yours truly

Scott E. Film, MD

xx

c: Leslie Albert, MD—Orchard Hills Rheumatology Associates

Current date

Matthew D. Sponch, MD
Family Practice Division, Suite 300
FedDes Wellness Center
101 Wellness Way Drive
New York, NY 10036

Re: Cathy Evanson
     Date of Birth: January 26, 19xx
     Examination: BONE DENSITY SCAN

Dear Dr. Sponch

The patient is a 73-year-old postmenopausal white female who today measures 5 ft 2 in. She states that at her tallest she measured 5 ft 3 in. Her self-history indicates that she has back pain, has had an ankle fracture and has a maternal history of hip fracture. On the positive side, she regularly includes dairy products in her diet. She does not indicate that she exercises on a regular basis. She lists her current medications and supplements as Synthroid, Lescol, and pain medication, which she takes only as needed.

Bone density scanning was performed on the lumbar spine, left hip and left forearm.

Scanning of the lumbar spine reveals a total bone mineral density of 99% compared to young normals which is 0.13 standard deviations below the mean, a normal reading. It is noted that L1 and L2 were eliminated from analysis because of osteophytosis, and it is suspected that osteophytosis is falsely elevating the readings in L3 and L4 as well.

Scanning of the left hip reveals a total bone mineral density of 84% compared to young normals which is 1.32 standard deviations below the mean. According to World Health Organization standards, this is consistent with a diagnosis of osteopenia (1.0-2.5 standard deviations below the mean). The degree of osteopenia is worse in the left hip with the reading at 2.19 standard deviations below the mean.

Scanning of the left forearm reveals a total bone density of 104% compared with young normals which is 0.39 standard deviations above the mean, a normal reading.

----------------------- begin page 2 -----------------------

IMPRESSION: Scanning of the lumbar spine, left hip and left forearm reveals osteopenia involving the left hip.

Thank you for referring this patient to us.

Yours truly

Scott E. Film, MD

xx

Current date

Ms. Pamela S. Bartholin, MA, RN, CRNP
Family Practice Division, Suite 300
FedDes Wellness Center
101 Wellness Way Drive
New York, NY 10036

Re: Nancy Spangler
     Date of Birth: March 18, 1959
     Examination: PELVIC SONOGRAM

Dear Ms. Bartholin

The patient presents with right pelvic pain. Real-time ultrasound examination demonstrates a normal size anteverted uterus, 10.3 cm in length, 4.1 cm in AP dimension. The endometrial stripe is normal in appearance measuring 5 mm. No uterine lesions are identified. Both ovaries are normal in size and appearance, the right 2.2 × 1.9 cm, the left 3.0 × 1.9 cm. There is no free pelvic fluid. A survey of the kidneys reveals no left or right hydronephrosis. Imaging of the right lower quadrant of the abdomen with compression fails to demonstrate a mass or fluid collection to indicate appendicitis.

IMPRESSION: Normal uterus and adnexa. No right lower quadrant abdominal pathology or hydronephrosis evident.

Thank you for referring this patient to us.

Yours truly

Potter T. Bucky, MD

xx

Current date

Charles Davis, MD
Family Practice Division, Suite 300
FedDes Wellness Center
101 Wellness Way Drive
New York, NY 10036

Re: Eileen Bunny
     Date of Birth: December 4, 19xx
     Examination: BONE DENSITY SCAN

Dear Dr. Davis

The patient is a 67-year-old postmenopausal Caucasian female who today measures 5 ft 4 in. She states that at her tallest she measured 5 ft 6 in. Her self-history indicates that she regularly includes dairy products in her diet. She does not indicate that she exercises on a regular basis. She lists her current medications and supplements as Estrace and Provera.

A bone density scan was performed on the lumbar spine and left hip.

Scanning of the lumbar spine reveals a total bone density of 71% compared to young normals which is 2.79 standard deviations below the mean. According to World Health Organization standards, this is consistent with a diagnosis of osteoporosis.

Scanning of the left hip diagnosis of osteoporosis (greater than 2.5 standard deviations below the mean) reveals a total bone density of 62% compared to young normals which is 3.09 standard deviations below the mean, also consistent with osteoporosis.

IMPRESSION: Bone density scanning of the lumbar spine and left hip reveals readings consistent with a diagnosis of osteoporosis. As the patient is already taking hormone replacement therapy, consideration should be given to adding bisphosphonate therapy to her treatment. Consideration should also be given to placing the patient on 1000-1500 mg of calcium and 400-800 IU of vitamin D per day. A

----------------------- begin page 2 -----------------------

regular exercise program to include weightbearing exercise is also to be encouraged if not clinically contraindicated. If therapy is altered, a follow-up study is suggested in 12-18 months to evaluate for efficacy.

Thank you for referring this patient to us.

Yours truly

William C. Roentgen, MD

xx

Current date

Matthew D. Sponch, MD
Family Practice Division, Suite 300
FedDes Wellness Center
101 Wellness Way Drive
New York, NY 10036

Re: Donald Nathan Helix
     Date of Birth: February 15, 1948
     Examination: ABDOMINAL SONOGRAM (REAL-TIME IMAGING)

Dear Dr. Sponch

Real-time sonography of the upper abdomen was performed utilizing a 3 mHz transducer. Multiple longitudinal and transverse sonograms reveal the liver to be normal in size, position, configuration, and sonographic architecture. There are no solid or cystic masses. The gallbladder is normal. The common bile duct and intrahepatic and extrahepatic biliary ducts are normal.

The pancreas, spleen, and the abdominal vessels are normal. Examination of the right kidney reveals the presence of two clear, sharply defined, parapineal cysts measuring 1.1 and 1.3 cm. The left kidney also contains a single 1.3 cm cyst in the lower pole. The kidneys are otherwise normal. There is no sonographic evidence of intra-abdominal mass, lymphadenopathy or ascites.

IMPRESSION: Small bilateral renal cysts. There are no further abnormalities seen on abdominal sonography.

Thank you for referring this patient to us.

Yours truly

Potter T. Bucky, MD

xx

Current date

Charles P. Davis, MD
Family Practice Division, Suite 300
FedDes Wellness Center
101 Wellness Way Drive
New York, NY 10036

Re: Laura Dobbins
     Date of Birth: October 2, 1971
     Examination: MAMMOGRAPHY

Dear Dr. Davis

Low dose mammography fails to reveal any dominant mass, suspicious cluster of microcalcifications or area of architectural distortion. The skin and subcutaneous tissues are normal.

IMPRESSION: Radiographically normal mammogram.

NOTE: IT SHOULD BE NOTED THAT THERE IS A 10% FALSE-NEGATIVE RATE IN MAMMOGRAPHIC DETECTION OF BREAST CARCINOMA. MANAGEMENT OF A PALPABLE ABNORMALITY SHOULD BE BASED ON CLINICAL GROUNDS.

A NEGATIVE REPORT SHOULD NOT DELAY BIOPSY IF A CLINICALLY PALPABLE OR SUSPICIOUS MASS IS PRESENT.

Our mammography facilities are accredited by the American College of Radiology.

Thank you for referring this patient to us.

Yours truly

Potter T. Bucky, MD

xx

Current date

Kate Cobalamin, MD
Gastroenterology Division, Suite 279
FedDes Wellness Center
101 Wellness Way Drive
New York, NY 10036

Re: Allison Lapinski
     Date of Birth: May 14, 1952
     Examination: UPPER GI SERIES

Dear Dr. Cobalamin

A preliminary AP film of the abdomen is unremarkable. The swallowing function is intact. There is a 3 cm sliding hiatus hernia, which is not associated with reflux or esophagitis.

The stomach is normal in tone, contour, peristalsis, and mucosal fold pattern. No filling defects or ulcerations are seen. The duodenal bulb is slightly spastic and irritable. There is no persistent deformity or ulcer crater or outlet obstruction. The remainder of the duodenal sweep is normal. After an interval of approximately 20-25 minutes, the stomach emptied in normal fashion with visualization of the jejunum, which appears normal.

IMPRESSION: There is a 3 cm sliding hiatus hernia which is not associated with reflux or esophagitis. The duodenal bulb is slightly spastic and irritable. There is no persistent deformity or ulcer crater.

Thank you for referring this patient to us.

Yours truly

Hounsfield T. Scanner, MD

xx

Current date

Anna Bolism, MD
Gastroenterology Division, Suite 279
FedDes Wellness Center
101 Wellness Way Drive
New York, NY 10036

Re: Timothy Lavage
     Date of Birth: April 1, 1977
     Examinations: UPPER GI SERIES
                    FLAT PLATE OF THE ABDOMEN

Dear Dr. Bolism

The esophagus is normal. There is no hiatus hernia. The stomach is normal in tone, contour, peristalsis, and mucosal fold pattern. There is no pyloric obstruction. The duodenal bulb is spastic, irritable, and persistently deformed in association with the presence of a 7 mm ulcer niche projecting from the lesser curvature aspect of the base of the bulb. The ulcer is surrounded by a smooth ulcer collar. The second, third and fourth portions of the duodenum are normal as are the visualized portions of the small intestine.

IMPRESSION: Active duodenal ulcer as described above. There is no pyloric obstruction.

FLAT PLATE OF THE ABDOMEN

The intestinal gas pattern is not unusual. There is no evidence of a mass. There are no abnormal soft tissue calcific deposits. The visualized bony structures reveal no gross abnormalities.

IMPRESSION: Normal flat plate of the abdomen.

Thank you for referring this patient to us.

Yours truly

Scott E. Film, MD

xx

Current date

Gwenn Maltase, MD
Gastroenterology Division, Suite 279
FedDes Wellness Center
101 Wellness Way Drive
New York, NY 10036

Re: Barbara Whitefelter
     Date of Birth: July 3, 1960
     Examinations: BARIUM ENEMA, KUB

Dear Dr. Maltase

Per your request, a barium enema examination was performed on this patient. She presents complaining of right lower quadrant pain.

There is free flow of barium from the rectum to the cecum. The terminal ileum is visualized and is normal. There are no narrowed or dilated segments. No organic filling defects are seen. There is no evidence of an inflammatory process. There are no diverticula.

The postevacuation films and the air contrast studies revealed no further abnormalities. On the air contrast studies the colonic mucosa is featureless.

IMPRESSION: Normal barium enema.

KUB

There is an amorphous calcific deposit in the right side of the pelvis measuring 2.3 × 0.8 cm of which the exact etiology is not determined.

Thank you for referring this patient to us.

Yours truly

Scott E. Film, MD

xx

Current date

See Pretests (11T-5) and (11T-6).

Charles P. Davis, MD
Family Practice Division, Suite 300
FedDes Wellness Center
101 Wellness Way Drive
New York, NY 10036

Re: Sarah Fleb
      Date of Birth: August 19, 1943
      Examination: DOPPLER STUDY OF THE DEEP VEINS OF THE RIGHT
                   LEG

Dear Dr. Davis

The deep veins of the right leg were studied from the level of the
common femoral vein through and including the calf vessels utilizing
real-time imaging, duplex doppler and color-flow doppler imaging.
There is no sonographic evidence of deep venous thrombosis. The
veins are freely compressible with spontaneous flow throughout as
well as augmentation of flow on distal compression. There is no
evidence of soft tissue mass.

IMPRESSION: There is no evidence of deep venous thrombosis
involving the deep veins of the right leg from the level of the
common femoral vein through and including the calf vessels.

Thank you for referring this patient to us.

Yours truly

Scott E. Film, MD

xx

Glossary

Medical Terminology

Abduction (ab-<u>duk</u>-shun) is the movement of an extremity away from the midline.

Acromioclavicular (<u>ah</u>-kro-me-o-klah-<u>vik</u>-u-lar) describes the articulation between the acromial process of the scapula and the clavicle.

Acromion (ah-<u>kro</u>-me-on) is a spinous projection off the scapula.

Adduction (ad-<u>duk</u>-shun) is the movement of an extremity toward the midline.

Adenocarcinoma (ade-no-kar-si-<u>no</u>-mah) is a malignant tumor of the glands.

Adenoma (ad-ah-<u>no</u>-mah) is a benign tumor in which cells are derived from glandular epithelium.

Adenomatous (ad-e-<u>no</u>-ma-tus) relates to some types of glandular hyperplasia.

Adenopathy (ad-ah-<u>nop</u>-ah-the) is the enlargement of the glands, especially the lymph nodes.

Adnexa (ad-<u>nek</u>-sa) are the tissues or body parts that are near or next to one another.

Aeration (aer-<u>a</u>-shun) is the exchange of carbon dioxide for oxygen by the blood in the lungs.

Afebrile (a-<u>feb</u>-ril) is without fever.

Amaurosis (am-aw-<u>ro</u>-sis) is the loss of sight without the apparent lesion of the eye.

Amenorrhea (ah-men-o-<u>re</u>-ah) is the absence of the menses.

Amorphous (ah-<u>mor</u>-fus) is having no definite form, or shapeless.

Anastomosis (a-nas-to-<u>mo</u>-sis) is an opening created by surgery, disease, or trauma between two or more organs or structures.

Aneurysm (<u>an</u>-u-rizm) is a localized dilatation of the wall of a blood vessel.

Angiography (an-je-<u>og</u>-rah-fe) is the radiography of an artery after injecting a contrast agent.

Anteverted (<u>an</u>-te-<u>vert</u>-ed) is the abnormal forward tilting of an organ.

Apophysis (ah-<u>pofi</u>-sis) is any outgrowth or swelling; a process or projection of a bone.

Arrhythmia (ah-<u>rith</u>-me-ah) is the variation from the normal rhythm of the heartbeat.

Arteriogram (ar-<u>te</u>-re-o-gram) is the radiographic visualization of an artery after injection of a contrast medium.

Arteriography (ar-te-re-<u>og</u>-rah-fe) is the radiography of an artery after injection of a contrast medium in the bloodstream.

Arthroplasty (ar-<u>thro</u>-plas-te) is the reconstruction surgery to repair or reshape a diseased joint.

Arthroscopy (ar-<u>thros</u>-ko-pe) is the examination of the interior of a joint with an arthroscope.

Ascites (ah-<u>si</u>-teez) is the effusion and accumulation of serous fluid in the abdominal cavity.

Aspirate (as-<u>pi</u>-rat) is to draw in or out by suction.

Asymmetry (a-<u>sim</u>-e-tre) is without symmetry, lacking similar form or relationship of parts.

Asymptomatic (a-<u>simp</u>-to-mat-ik) is without symptoms.

Atelectasis (ate-<u>lek</u>-tah-sis) is the collapse of a portion of the lung.

Atherosclerotis (ath-er-o-skle-<u>ro</u>-sis) is the hardening of an artery due to deposits of plaque within the vessel.

Atrial (a-<u>tre</u>-al) pertains to the atrium.

Atrioventricular (a-tre-o-ven-<u>trik</u>-I-lar) pertains to an atrium and the ventricle of the heart.

Auscultation (aw-skul-<u>ta</u>-shun) is the act of listening for sounds produced within the body with an unaided ear or with a stethoscope.

Avulsion (ah-<u>vul</u>-shun) is a tearing away forcibly of a part or structure.

Bilateral (bi-<u>lat</u>-er-al) is affecting or relating to two sides.

Biliary (<u>bil</u>-e-ar-e) relates to bile or the biliary tract.

Bimanual (bi-<u>man</u>-u-al) is using both hands.

Bleb (bleb) is a bulla or blister.

Blepharospasm (<u>blef</u>-ah-ro-spazm) is a spasm of the orbicular muscle of the eyelid.

Bradycardia (bard-e-<u>kar</u>-de-ah) is the slowness of the heartbeat.

Bronchodilator (brong-ko-di-<u>la</u>-tor) is any drug that has the capacity of increasing the capacity of the pulmonary air passages and improve ventilation to the lungs.

Bruit (broo <u>e</u>) is a sound or murmur heard on auscultation.

Buccal (<u>buk</u>-al) pertains to the cheek.

Calcaneus (kal-kay-nee-us) is the heel bone or os calcis.

Calculus (<u>kal</u>-ku-lus) is an abnormal concretion; stone.

Callus (<u>kal</u>-us) is the new growth of bony tissue surrounding the bone ends in a fracture; part of the repair process of a fractured bone

Cardiomyopathy (kar-de-o-mi-<u>op</u>-ah-the) is the disease of the myocardium due to the primary disease of the heart muscle.

Cardioverter (<u>kar</u>-de-o-ver-ter) is a device used to administer electrical shocks to the heart.

Caries (<u>ka</u>-re-ez) is the condition of decay and destruction of a tooth.

Carotid (kah-<u>rot</u>-id) relates to the principal artery of the neck.

Carpometacarpal (<u>kar</u>-po-met-ah-<u>kar</u>-pal) is the joint spaces between the carpal and metacarpal bones.

Cecum (<u>se</u>-kum) is the cul-de-sac about 6 cm in depth lying below the terminal ileum, forming the first part of the large intestine.

Centrum semiovale (<u>sen</u>-trum <u>sem</u>-i-o-<u>val</u>) is the white matter of the cerebral hemispheres that has an almost oval shape.

Chlamydia (klah-<u>mid</u>-e-ah) is a widespread genus of gram-negative, nonmotile bacteria.

Cholecystectomy (ko-le-sus-<u>tek</u>-to-me) is the surgical removal of the gallbladder.

Cholecystitis (ko-le-sis-ti-tis) is inflammation of the gallbladder.

Claudication (klaw-di-ka-shun) is cramping pains of the calves caused by poor circulation to the leg muscles.

Coapt (ko-apt) is to bring together, as suturing a laceration.

Colitis (ko-li-tis) is the inflammation of the colon.

Collateral (ko-lat-er-al) is a secondary or accessory blood pathway.

Colonoscope (ko-lon-o-skop) is an elongated endoscope, usually fiberoptic.

Colonoscopy (ko-lon-os-ko-pe) is the visual examination of the inner surface of the colon by means of a colonoscope.

Colostomy (ko-los-to-me) is the establishment of an artificial opening into the colon.

Colporrhaphy (kol-por-ah-fe) is the suture of the vagina.

Concomitant (kon-kom-I-tant) refers to taking place at the same time.

Continent (kon-ti-ent) is the ability to control urination and defecation urges

Contraindicate (kon-trah-in-di-kate) is a factor that makes it undesirable to treat a patient in the usual manner.

Contrast medium (kon-trast med-e-um) is the pharmaceutical given to the patient to allow radiographic visualization of a body structure.

Contusion (kon-to-shun) is commonly called a *bruise*, where there is trauma to the body part but no break in the skin surface.

Cor pulmonale (kor pul-mona-le) is an abnormal heart condition characterized by the increased size of the right ventricle.

Coude' (koo-dae) is bent or elbowed.

Creatine kinase is an enzyme whose presence in the blood is strongly indicative of a recent myocardial infarction.

Creatinine (kre-at-I-nin) is a normal alkaline constituent of urine and blood.

Crepitus (krep-i-tus) is the grating sound of bone fragments rubbing together.

Cricopharyngeal (kri-ko-fah-rin-je-al) pertains to the cricoid cartilage and the pharynx.

Crohn's disease is inflammation of the terminal portion of the ileum.

Cyanosis (si-ah-no-sis) is the bluish-purple discoloration of the skin due to lack of oxygenated blood.

Cystitis (sis-ti-tis) is the inflammation of the urinary bladder.

Cystocele (sis-to-sel) is a hernia of the bladder, usually into the vagina and introitus.

Cystometrography (sis-to-me-trog-ra-fe) is the graphic record of the pressure in the bladder at varying stages of filling.

Cystoscope (sis-to-skop) is an endoscope especially designed for passing through the urethra into the bladder to permit visual inspection of its interior.

Cystourethroscope (sis-to-u-re-thro-skop) is an instrument for examining the posterior urethra and bladder.

Debridement (da-bred-maw) is the removal of dead or damaged tissue.

Decubitus (de-ku-bi-tus) is the state of lying down.

Demarcated (de-mar-ka-ted) refers to set limits or boundaries.

Dentition (den-tish-un) refers to the position and condition of the teeth.

Diaphoresis (di-a-fo-re-sis) is perspiration.

Digit (dij-it) is a finger or toe.

Distal (dis-tal) is the farthest from any point of reference; remote.

Diuresis (di-u-re-sis) is an increased excretion of urine.

Diuretic (di-u-ret-ik) is a substance that promotes the excretion of urine.

Diverticulitis is inflammation of the diverticula of the colon.

Diverticulum (di-ver-tik-u-lum) is a sac or pouch in the walls of a canal or organ.

Dobutamine MUGA scan is multiple gated acquisition (nuclear medicine imaging).

Dobutamine stress test is a generic name for a synthetic catecholamine administered parenterally for inotropic support in short-term treatment of adults with cardiac decompensation.

Doppler scanning is a technique used in sonography to image and analyze the behavior of a moving substance such as blood flow or a beating heart.

Doppler study is an ultrasound flowmeter used in assessing intermittent claudiation, thrombus obstruction of deep veins, and other abnormalities of blood flow in the major arteries and veins.

Dorsiflexion (dor-si-flek-shun) is to bend or flex backward.

Duodenal (du-o-de-nal) relates to the duodenum, the first division of the small intestine.

Dysmenorrhea (dis-men-o-re-ah) is painful menstruation.

Dysphagia (dis-fa-je-a) is difficulty in swallowing.

Dyspnea (disp-ne-ah) is labored or difficult breathing.

Dyspneic (disp-ne-ah) pertains to labored or difficult breathing.

Dysrhythmia (dis-rith-me-ah) is a disordered rhythm.

Dysuria (dis-u-re-ah) is painful or difficult urination.

Ecchymosis (ek-I-mo-sis) is a skin discoloration caused by a hemorrhage.

Echocardiogram (eko-kar-de-o-gram) is a diagnostic procedure using ultrasound to study heart structure and motion.

Edema (ede-mah) is the accumulation of excess fluid in the tissues of the body.

Effusion (e-fu-zhun) is the escape of fluid from blood vessels because of rupture or seepage, usually into a body cavity.

Electrolytes (e-lek-tro-lit) is any solution compound that conducts electricity.

Embolus (em-bo-lus) is a mass brought by the blood from another vessel that obstructs blood circulation.

Emesis (em-e-sis) is the act of vomiting.

Empiric (em-pir-i-kl) is treating a disease based on observation and experience rather than reasoning alone.

Endarterectomy (end-ar-ter-ek-to-me) is to excise the diseased endothelial and part or all of the media of an artery.

Endoscopy (en-dos-ko-pe) is the examination of the interior of a canal or hollow viscus by means of endoscope.

Epiphysis (e-pif-I-sis) is the center for ossification at the proximal and distal ends of a long bone.

Erythema (er-I-the-ma) is redness of the skin due to capillary dilatation.

Etiology (e-te-ol-oj-e) is the science concerned with the causes or origin of a disease or disorder.

Evert (e-vert) is to turn inside out.

Exacerbation (eg-zas-er-ba-shun) is an increase in the severity of a disease or symptoms.

Exostosis (ek-sos-to-sis) is an abnormal, benign growth on the surface of a bone, also called *hyperostosis.*

Expiratory ek-spi-ra-to-re) relates to exhalation.

Extravasation (eks-trav-ah-za-shun) is a discharge or escape of fluid from a vessel into the tissues.

Exudate (eks-u-date) is an accumulation of fluid in the tissues.

Fasciculations (fa-sik-u-la-shun) are the uncontrolled twitchings of a group of muscle fibers.

Fibrillation (fi-bri-la-shun) is the exceedingly rapid contractions of muscular fibrils.

Flank (flangk) is the side of the body between the ribs and ilium.

Flexion (flek-shun) is the movement by a joint that decreases the angle between the two adjoining bones; the bending of a joint.

Flora (flo-rah) are normally occurring microrganisms that live within the body and provide natural immunity against certain organisms.

Folate (fo-lat) is folic acid.

Formalin (for-ma-lin) is a 37% aqueous solution of formaldehyde.

Fossa (fos-ah) is a hollow or depressed area.

Fulguration (ful-gu-ra-shun) is the destruction of living tissue by electric sparks generated by a high-frequency current.

Fundus (fun-dus) is the bottom or base of an organ.

Fusiform (fu-zi-form) is a spindle-shaped structure tapered at both ends.

Gallop (gal-op)is a disorder in the rhythm of the heart.

Ganglion (gang-gle-on) is a knot or knotlike mass.

Gastritis (gas-tri-tis) is an inflammation of the stomach, especially the mucosal.

Gastroesophageal (gas-tro-e-sof-a-je-al) relates to both the stomach and the esophagus.

Gastrointestinal (gas-tro-in-tes-tin-al) relates to the stomach and the intestines.

Gastroparesis (gas-tro-pa-re-sis) is a slight degree of gastroparalysis.

Gastrostomy (gas-tros-to-me) is the establishment of a new opening into the stomach.

Gellhorn pessary is an inflexible device made of acrylic resin or plastic in the form of a large collar button. It has a canal through the stem that allows drainage of vaginal sections.

Genitourinary (jen-I-to-u-ri-ner-e) pertains to the genitalia and urinary organs.

Genu varum (je-nu va-rum) is bowleg

Gluteus medius ((gloo-te-us me-de-us) is one of three muscles that form the buttocks; it acts to abduct and rotate the thigh.

Gout (gowt) is a disorder associated with an inborn error of uric acid metabolism that increases production or interferes with the excretion of uric acid.

Granuloma (gran-u-lo-mah) is a small nodular tumor or growth.

Greater trochanter (tro-kan-ter) is the large projection at the proximal end of the femur.

Guarding (gahr-ding) is a body defense method to prevent movement of an injured part.

Hematemesis (he-ma-tem-e-sis) is to vomit blood indicating upper gastrointestinal bleeding.

Hematochezia (he-ma-to-ke-ze-a) is the passage of bloody stools.

Hematuria (hem-ah-tu-re-ah) is the discharge of blood in the urine.

Heme (hem) is the nonprotein, insoluble, iron constituent of hemoglobin.

Hemiblock (hem-e-blok) is the failure to conduct an impulse down one division of the left bundle branch.

Hemicolectomy (hem-e-ko-lek-to-me) is the removal of the left or right side of the colon.

Hemoptysis (he-mop-ti-sis) is the coughing or spitting up of blood from the respiratory tract.

Heparin (hep-a-rin) is a generic name for an anticoagulant.

Hepatosplenomegaly (hep-ah-to-sple-no-meg-ah-le) is the enlargement of the liver and spleen.

Hiatus hernia (hi-a-tus her-ne-ah) is the herniation of an abdominal organ through the esophageal opening of the diaphragm

Homans' sign (ho-manz sin) is a calf pain with dorsiflexion of foot.

Hydrate (hi-drat) is a compound containing water molecules.

Hydrocele (hi-dro-sel) is the accumulation of fluid in a sac-like cavity.

Hydronephrosis (hi-dro-ne-fro-sis) is the distention of the renal pelvis and calices with urine, often as a result of obstruction of the ureter.

Hypercholesterolemia (hi-per-ko-les-ter-ol-e-me-a) is the presence of an abnormally large amount of cholesterol in the cells and plasma of the blood.

Hyperkalemia (hi-per-kal-e-ma-a) is the greater than normal concentration of potassium ions in the blood.

Hyperlipidemia (hi-per-lip-i-de-me-ah) is the elevated concentrations of any or all lipids in the plasma.

Hypertrophy (hi-per-tro-fe) is an increase in the size of an organ or structure.

Hypotensive (hi-po-ten-siv) is characterized by low blood pressure or causing a reduction in blood pressure.

Icterus (ik-ter-us) is jaundice.

Idiopathic (id-e-o-path-ik) is a disease of unknown cause.

Iliac (il-e-ak) relates to the ilium.

Impingement is an abnormal contact or pressure between two structures.

Incontinence (in-kon-ti-nens) is the inability to control excretory functions.

Infarction (in-farkt-shun) is the death of a tissue due to lack of blood flow to the area.

Inferolateral (in-fer-o-lat-e-rak) pertains to a location situated below and to the side.

Infiltrate (in-fil-trat) is when fluid, cells, or other substances pass into tissue spaces.

Inotropic (in-o-trop-ik) influences the contractions of the muscular tissue.

Interarticular (in-ter-ar-tik-u-lar) is between two joints.

Interosseous (in-ter-os-e-us) is situated or occurring between bone.

Intimal (in-ti-mal) relates to the inner coat of a vessel.

Intrahepatic (in-trah-he-pat-ik) is within the liver.

Intrauterine (in-trah-u-ter-in) means within the uterus.

Ischemia (is-ke-me-ah) is a decreased supply of oxygenated blood to a body part.

Jejunum (je-joo-num) is the second section of the small intestine.

Joint mouse (joint mows) is loose bodies in synovial joints.

Ketone (ke-ton) is any compound containing carbon oxide.

Labyrinthitis (lab-i-rin-thi-tis) is the inflammation of the internal ear, or otitis interna.

Lactic dehydrogenase is an enzyme present in elevated concentrations when these tissues are injured.

Lacuna (lah-ku-nah) is the small cavity within or between other body structures.

Lamina (lam-i-nah) is a thin, flat layer.

Laminectomy (lam-I-nek-to-me) is the surgical excision of the lamina.

Laparoscope (lap-ah-ro-skop) is an endoscope for examining the peritoneal cavity.

Leukocytes (loo-ko-sit) are colorless blood corpuscles.

Lingula (ling-gu-lah) is a small tongue-shaped anatomic structure.

Lipoma (li-po-mah) is a benign tumor composed mostly of fat cells.

Lipomatous (li-po-mah-tus) is affected with or of the nature of lipoma.

Lithotomy (li-thot-o-me) is an incision of a duct or organ for the removal of calculi.

Liver function test is a series of laboratory procedures that measure some aspect of liver functions including serum protein electrophoresis and one-stage prothrombin time.

Lumen (lu-men) is the cavity or channel within a tube.

Lymphadenopathy (lim-fad-e-nop-ah-the) is a disease of the lymph nodes.

Lymphedema (lim-fi-de-ma) is edema due to obstruction of lymph vessels.

Malaise (mal-az) is a feeling of uneasiness.

Malleolus (mah-lee-o-lus) is either of the two rounded projections on either side of the ankle joint.

Marshall test is performed to determine stress-related urinary incontinence.

Meatus (me-a-tus) is an opening.

Meclizine (mek-li-zeen) is an antiemetic especially effective for control of nausea and vomiting with motion sickness.

Mediastinum (me-de-ah-sti-num) is the mass of tissues and organs separating the sternum in front and the vertebral column behind.

Melena (me-le-nah) is the darkening of the feces by blood pigments.

Meniscectomy (me-ni-sek-to-me) is the surgical removal of a meniscus.

Meniscus (me-nis-kus) is the crescent-shaped fibrocartilage in the knee joint.

Metastasis (me-tas-tah-sis) is the transfer of disease from one organ or part to another not directly connected with it.

Metatarsus (met-a-tar-sus) is any of the five long bones of the foot between the ankle and the toes.

Motility (mo-til-I-te) is the ability to move spontaneously.

Mucosa (mu-ko-sah) is the mucous membrane.

Myalgia (mi-al-je-ah) is muscular pain.

Myocardial (mi-o-kar-de-al) pertains to the muscular tissue of the heart.

Myringotomy (mir-in-got-o-me) is an incision of the tympanic membrane

Nebulization (neb-u-li-za-shun) is a treatment by a spray.

Nephrectomy (ne-frek-to-me) is the surgical removal of the kidney.

Nocturnal (nok-tur-nal) is something that occurs at night.

Normocephalic (nor-mo-se-fal-ik) is having a normal size head; mesocephalic.

Nystagmus (nis-tag-mus) is the involuntary, rapid, rhythmic movement of the eyeball.

Occlude (o-klood) is to close tight.

Occlusion (o-kloo-zhun) is the act of closure or state of being closed.

Occult (o-kult) is a specimen hidden from view.

Odynophagia (o-din-o-fa-je-ah) is the painful swallowing of food.

Oophorectomy (o-of-o-rek-to-me) is the excision of one or both ovaries.

Orthopnea (or-thop-ne-ah) is the ability to breathe easily only in an upright position.

Os (os) is an opening, mouth, or bone.

Osteopenia (os-te-o-pe-ne-ah) is the decrease in bone mass below the normal.

Osteophyte (os-te-o-fit) is an outgrowth of bone that is usually found around a joint.

Palpitation (pal-pi-ta-shun) is an unusually rapid, strong, or irregular heartbeat.

Panendoscope (pan-en-do-skop) is a cystoscope that gives a wide-angle view of the bladder.

Parenchyma (pah-reng-ki-mah) is the general anatomic term to describe the functional elements of an organ, as distinguished from its structure.

Paresthesia (par-es-the-ze-ah) is the sensation of tingling and numbness.

Parkinson's disease is a slowly progressive disease characterized by degeneration within the nuclear masses of the extrapyramidal system.

Paronychia (par-o-nik-e-ah) is the inflammation involving the folds of tissue surrounding the nail.

Paroxysm (par-ok-sim) is the sudden recurrence of symptoms.

Partial thromboplastin time is the period required for clot formation in recalcified blood plasma after contact activation and the additon of platelet substitutes. It is used to assess the pathways of coagulation.

Passavant's cushion (pas-a-vants koosh-un) is a ridge appearing on the posterior wall of pharynx during swallowing due to contraction of palatopharyngeal sphincter.

Pectoralis (pek-to-ra-lis) pertains to the chest or breast.

Pedal (ped-al) is a term relating to the foot.

Periarticular (per-e-ar-tici-u-lar) is situated around a joint.

Pericholecystic fluid (per-I-ko-le-sis-tic) is a coined term for fluid around the gallbladder.

Peripheral (pe-rif-er-al) is occurring away from the center.

Perirectal (per-i-rek-tal) is around the rectum.

Periumbilical (per-e-um-bil-I-kal) is around the umbilicus.

Pessary (pes-ah-re) is an instrument placed in the vagina to support the uterus or rectum.

Phalanx (fa-langks) is the general term for any bone of a finger or toe.

Phallus (fal-us) is the penis.

Pinna (pin-ah) is the projecting part of the ear lying outside the head.

Pisiform (pi-si-form) is pea shaped; smallest carpal bone.

Pitting (pit-ing) is the formation of a small depression.

Plantar (plan-tar) is relating to the sole of the foot.

Pleura (ploo-rah) is the serous membrane investing the lungs and lining the walls of the thoracic cavity.

Pneumonectomy (nu-mo-nek-to-me) is the surgical removal of all or a segment of the lung.

Pneumothorax (nu-mo-tho-raks) is the presence of air or gas in the pleural cavity.

Polycythemia (pol-e-si-the-me-ah) is an increase in the total red cell mass of the blood.

Polyp (pol-ip) is any growth or mass protruding from a mucous membrane.

Polypoid (pol-y-poid) resembles a polyp.

Postprandial (post-pran-de-al) is after a meal.

Postvoid film is a film of the bladder area taken after the patient has emptied his bladder.

Prevoid film is a film of the bladder area taken before the patient has emptied his bladder.

Proctitis (prok-ti-tis) is the inflammation of the rectum.

Prophylatic (pro-fi-lak-tik) is an agent that tends to ward off disease.

Prostate (pros-tat) is a male gland that surrounds the neck of the bladder and urethra.

Prothrombin time is a test to measure the activity of factors I, II, V, VII, and X, which participate in the extrinsic pathway of coagulation.

Pruritus ani (proo-ri-tus a-ni) is the intense chronic itching in the anal region.

Pulmonary toilet (pul-mo-ner-e toi-let) is the cleansing of the trachea and bronchial tree.

Purulent (pu-roo-lent) means containing pus.

Pyelogram (pi-e-lo-gram) is an x-ray study of the renal pelvis and uterus.

Pyelonephritis (pi-e-lo-ne-fri-tis) is the inflammation of the kidney and renal pelvis.

Pyuria (pi-u-re-ah) is pus in the urine.

Radiation (ra-de-a-shun) is the process by which energy travels through space or matter. In clinical medicine, it often refers to the divergence of pain from the site of injury to other areas of the body.

Radiculitis (rah-dik-u-li-tis) is the inflammation of a spinal nerve root.

Rale (rahl) is an abnormal crackle sound heard on chest auscultation.

Raphe (ra-fe) is a seam or ridge noting the line of junction of halves of a part.

Real-time ultrasound is a rapid imaging that produces a video display of organ motion.

Rebound (re-bownd) is a reversed response occurring upon withdrawal of a stimulus.

Rectocele (rek-to-sel) is a hernia protrusion of part of the rectum into the vagina.

Reflux (re-fluks) is a backward or return flow.

Resect (re-sekt) is to cut off or cut out a portion of a tissue or organ.

Retroflexion (ret-ro-flek-shun) is the bending of an organ so its top side is thrust backward.

Retroperitoneal (ret-ro-per-i-to-ne-al) is behind the peritoneum.

Rhinitis (ri-ni-tis) is the inflammation of the mucous membrane of the nose.

Rhonchus (rong-kus) is an abnormal sound heard on chest auscultation due to an obstructed airway.

Rub (rub) is a sound caused by two surfaces rubbing together.

Saphenous (sah-fe-nus) pertains to the two main superficial veins of the lower leg.

Sclera (skle-rah) is the tough white outer coat of the eyeball.

Sequela (se-kwel-lah) is any abnormal condition that follows and is the result of a disease, treatment, or injury.

Sigmoidoscope (sig-moi-do-skop) is an endoscope for use in sigmoidoscopy.

Sigmoidoscopy (sig-moi-dos-ko-pe) is the direct examination of the interior of the sigmoid colon.

Sinus (si-nus) is a cavity or channel.

Somnolence (som-no-lens) is drowsiness.

Spironolactone (sper-o-no-lak-ton) is the generic name for a diuretic.

Sputum (spu-tum) is the mucous secretion from the lungs, bronchi, and trachea that is ejected through the mouth.

Staghorn (stag-horn) is the calculus of the renal pelvis usually extending into multiple calices.

Stasis (sta-sis) is an abnormal slowing or stopping of fluid flowing through a vessel.

Stenosis (ste-no-sis) is the narrowing or contraction of a body passage.

Stent (stent) is a mold for keeping a skin graft in place.

Stricture (strik-chor) is an abnormal narrowing of a duct or passage.

Subluxation (sub-luk-sa-shun) is a partial dislocation.

Suprapubic (soo-prah-pu-bik) is above the pubis.

Supraventricular (soo-prah-ven-trik-u-lar) refers to situated or occurring above the ventricles.

Symptomatology (simp-to-mah-tol-o-je) is symptoms of a specific disease.

Syncope (sing-ko-pe) is a temporary suspension of consciousness; fainting.

Synovia (si-no-ve-ah) is the lubricating fluid of joints.

Tachycardia (take-kar-de-ah) is an abnormally fast heartbeat.

Tendinitis (ten-di-ni-tis) is the inflammation of a tendon, or tendonitis.

Thoracentesis (tho-rah-sen-te-sis) is the aspiration of fluid from the chest cavity.

Thrombosis (throm-bo-sis) is the formation of a blood clot within the vascular system.

Thyromegaly (thi-ro-meg-ah-le) is the enlargement of the thyroid gland.

Titrate (ti-trat) is to analyze a given solution component by adding a liquid reagent.

Trabeculation (trah-bek-u-lah) is a small beam or supporting structure.

Transducer (trans-doo-ser) is a device that translates one form of energy to another; in sonography, it transforms a sound wave into electronically displayed image.

Trapezius (trah-pee-zee-us) is the muscles of the back of the neck and shoulder.

Trigone (tri-gon) is a triangular area.

Turgor (tur-gor) is the normal resiliency of the skin.

Ulna (ul-nah) is the long, medial bone of the forearm.

Urethrocele (u-re-thro-sel) is the prolapse of the female urethra through the urinary meatus.

Urethrotrigonitis (u-re-thro-tri-go-ni-tis) is the inflammation of the urethra and trigone of the bladder.

Urogram (u-ro-gram) is a diagnostic x-ray study of kidneys, uterus, and bladder.

Urosepsis (u-ro-sep-sis) is the poisoning from retained and absorbed urinary substances.

Uvula (u-vu-lah) is a small soft structure hanging from the free edge of the soft palate.

Valsalva's maneuver (val-sal-vahz) is an attempt to forcibly exhale with the glottis, nose, and mouth closed.

Vas deferens (vas def-er-ens) is the excretory duct of the testis.

Vasculature (vas-ku-lah-tur) is the supply of vessels to a specific region.

Venous (ve-nus) pertains to the veins.

Vertex (ver-teks) is the top or crown of the head.

Verumontanum (ver-oo-mon-ta-num) is the elevation on the floor of the prostatic portion of the urethra where the seminal ducts enter.

Volar (vo-lar) pertains to the palm of the hand or sole of the foot

Vulva (vul-vah) is the external genital organ in women.

Drugs

Aldactone (al dak-ton) is the trade name for a diuretic.

Amoxicillin (ah-moks-i-sil-in) is the generic name for an aminopenicillin antibiotic.

Amoxil (ah-moks-il) is the trade name for a preparation of amoxicillin, an antimicrobial.

Ancef IV (an-sef) is the trade name for an cephalosporin antibiotic.

Ascriptin (ah-skrip-tin) is the trade name for a preparation of aspirin with Maalox, an analgesic and antiinflammatory.

Aspirin is a generic name for an analgesic, antipyretic, antiinflammatory; antirheumatic.

Ativan (at-I-van) is the trade name for an anxiolytic.

Atrovent (at-ro-vent) is the trade name for a nasal spray, bronchodilator.

Augmentin (awg-men-tin) is the trade name for a preparation of amoxicillin, an antimicrobial.

Axid (ak-sid) is the trade name for an antagonistic for the treatment of gastric and duodenal ulcers.

Azmacort (az-ma-kort) is the trade name for a corticosteroid for the prevention or treatment of bronchial asthma.

Bacitracin (bas-I-tra-sin) is a generic name for an antibacterial.

Bactrim (bak-trim) is the trade name for an antibiotic.

Bactrim DS is the trade name for an antibiotic.

Beta blocker is a generic name for a drug that blocks the action of epinephrine at beta-adrenergic receptors on cells of effector organs. It is used to treat angina pectoralis, hypertension, and cardia arrhythmias.

Beta carotene is an ultraviolet screen; vitamin A precursor.

Betadine (bat-ah-den) is the trade name for a topical antibacterial, antiseptic.

Biaxin (bi-ak-sin) is the trade name for an antibiotic.

Botox (bo-toks) is the trade name for a powder for extraocular muscle injection.

Bumex (bu-meks) is the trade name for a loop diuretic.

Calan (kal-an) is the trade name for an antianginal, antiarrhythmic, antihypertensive.

Capoten (kap-o-ten) is the trade name for an antihypertensive.

Captopril (kap-to-pril) is a generic name for an angiotensin-converting enzyme inhibitor.

Cardiolite (kar-de-o-lit) is the trade name for a myocardial perfusion agent for cardiac SPECT imaging.

Cardizem (kar-di-zem) is the trade name for a calcium channel blocker for atrial fibrillation.

Cardura (kar-du-rah) is the trade name for an antihypertensive, antiadrenergic.

Centrum Silver is a trade name for a geriatric vitamin/mineral supplement.

Cephalosporin (sef-ah-lo-spor-in) is a generic name for any of the large group of broad-spectrum antibiotics.

Chem-7 is the trade name for a profile of seven different chemical laboratory tests.

Cipro (si-pro) is the trade name for a fluoroquinolone antibiotic, antibacterial drug.

Claritin (klar-i-tin) is the trade name for a nonsedating antihistamine.

Codeine (ko-den) is a generic name for an opioid analgesic.

Colace (ko-las) is the trade name for a stool softener.

Compazine (kom-pah-zen) is the trade name for a tranquilizer and antiemetic.

Copolymer (ko-pol-i-mer) is the trade name for one of the immune modulating drugs.

Cortisone (cor-ti-son) is the generic name for a corticosteroid used to treat inflammations.

Coumadin (koo-mah-din) is the trade name for an anticoagulant.

Cytotec (si-to-tek) is the trade name for a drug used for the prevention of NSAID-induced gastric ulcers.

Darvocet (dar-vo-set) is the trade name for fixed combination preparations of propoxyphene napsylate and acetaminophen, an analgesic.

Darvon (dar-von) is the trade name for a narcotic analgesic.

Demerol (dem-er-ol) is the trade name for a synthetic narcotic analgesic.

Digoxin (di-jok-sin) is a generic name for a cardiotonic.

Dilantin (di-lan-tin) is the trade name for an anticonvulsant used in the treatment of epilepsy.

Diltiazem (dil-ti-a-zem) is the generic name for acoronary vasodilator.

Ditropan (di-tro-pan) is the trade name for an urinary antispasmodic.

Dobutamine (do-byu-ta-men) is a generic name for a cardiotonic agent.

Dolobid is the brand name for a drug classified as an NSAID, a nonsteroidal antiinflammatory drug.

Doxepin (dok-se-pin) is the generic name for an antidepressant.

Doxycycline (dok-se-si-klen) is a generic name for a broad-spectrum antibiotic active against a wide range of gram-positive and gram-negative organisms.

E.E.S. is the trade name for an antibiotic.

Ecotrin (ek-o-trin) is the trade name for an analgesic, antiinflammatory.

Elavil (el-ah-vil) is the trade name for an antidepressant.

Erythromycin (e-rith-ro-mi-sin) is a generic name for a broad-spectrum antibiotic.

Estrace is the trade name of an estrogen; classification as an antineoplastic

Evista (e-vis-ta) is the trade name for a selective estrogen receptor modulator (SERM) for the prevention of postmenopausal osteoporosis.

FiberCon (fi-ber-kon) is the trade name for a bulk-forming laxative.

Heparin (hep-ah-rin) is a generic name for an anticoagulant.

Humulin (hu-mu-lin) is the trade name for an antidiabetic.

Hydrochlorothiazide is a generic name for a diuretic, antihypertensive agent.

Hydrocortisone (hi-dro-kor-ti-son) is the generic name for a corticosteroid.

Hytrin (hi-trin) is the trade name for an antihypertensive used in the treatment of benign prostatic hyperplasia.

Imodium (I-mo-de-um) is the trade name for an antidiarrheal.

Indocin (in-do-sin) is the trade name for a nonsteroidal antiinflammatory drug, NSAID.

Isordil (I-sor-dil) is the trade name for an antianginal.

Isosorbide (i-so-sor-bid) is the generic name for a nitrate-based antianginal agent.

Isovue (is-o-vu) is the trade name for a drug used as a contrast medium.

K-Dur (Kay-dur) is the trade name for a potassium supplement.

Keflex (kef-leks) is the trade name for an antibiotic.

Klonopin (klon-o-pin) is the trade name for an anticonvulsant.

Lanoxin (lah-nok-sin) is the trade name for a cardiac glycoside to increase cardiac output.

Lasix (la-ziks) is the trade name for a diuretic.

Lesco is the trade name for a drug that decreases LDL cholesterol; classification as an antihyperlipoproteinemic.

Lescol (le̲-zkol) is the trade name for a reductase inhibitor for hypercholesterolemia.

Lidocaine (li̲-do-kan) is a generic name for a local anesthetic used as a cardiac antiarrhythmic.

Lipitor (li̲p-i-tor) is the trade name for an hypercholesterolemia; classification as an antihyperlipidemic.

Lo-Ovral (lo-o̲v-ral) is the trade name for an oral contraceptive.

Lopressor (lo-pre̲s-or) is the trade name for a beta-adrenergic blocker; antihypertensive.

Lorazepam (lor-a-ze̲p-am) is a generic antianxiety drug.

Lotensin (lo̲-ten-sin) is the trade name for an antihypertensive.

Macrobid (ma̲k-ro-bid) is the trade name for a urinary bacteriostatic.

Maxaquin (mak-sa̲-kwin) is the trade name for a fluoroquinolone antibiotic, antibacterial.

Maxzide (ma̲k-sid) is the trade name for a diuretic and antihypertensive.

Meclizine (me̲k-li-zen) is a generic name for an antiemetic, antihistamine, motion sickness relief.

Melatonex (mel-a-to̲-neks) is the trade name for a sleep aid.

Metamucil (met-ah-mu̲-sil) is the trade name for a bulk laxative.

Mevacor (mev-a ko̲r) is the trade name for a reductase inhibitor for hypercholesterolemia.

Naprosyn (na̲-pro-sin) is the trade name for a nonsteroidal antiinflammatory drug, NSAID.

Neosporin (ne-o-spo̲r-in) is the trade name for a topical antibiotic.

Neptazane (nep-ta̲-zan) is the trade name for a diuretic, antiglaucoma agent.

Nifedipine (ni-fe̲d-i-pen) is a generic calcium channel blocker drug.

Nitroglycerin (ni-tro-gli̲s-er-in) is a generic name for a vasodilator used to relieve certain types of pain.

Nitroglycerin paste is a generic name for a vasodilator used to relieve certain types of pain.

Nitroglycerin spray is a generic name for a coronary vasodilator, antianginal.

Nitroglycerin is a generic name for coronary vasodilator, antianginal.

Noroxin (no̲r-o-sin) is the trade name for an antibacterial, urinary tract antiinfective.

Nortriptyline (no̲r-trip-ti-lin) is a generic name for an antidepressant.

Norvasc (no̲r-vask) is the trade name for an antianginal, antihypertensive.

NPH (neutral protamine Hagedorn) insulin is the trade name for an insulin that decreases blood sugar.

Ophthetic (of-the̲-tik) is the trade name for proparacaine hydrochloride, eye drops.

Ortho-Tricyclen (o̲r-tho-tri-si̲-klen) is the trade name for a triphasic oral contraceptive used in the treatment of acne vulgaris in women.

Partial thromboplastin time is the period required or clot formation in recalcified blood plasma after contact and the activation and the addition of platelet substitutes. It is used to assess the pathways of coagulation.

Paxil (pa̲ks-il) is the trade name for a selective serotonin reuptake inhibitor (SSRI) for depression, obsessive-compulsive disorder, and panic disorder.

Pencillin is the generic name for any of the large group of natural or semisynthetic antibacterial antibiotics.

Pepcid (pe̲p-sid) is the trade name for an acid controller for heartburn and acid indigestion.

Percocet (per-ko̲-set) is the trade name for an opioid analgesic (Schedule II).

Persantine (per-sa̲n-ten) is the trade name for a coronary vasodilator; antiplatelet agent.

Phenergan (fe̲n-er-gan) is the trade name for an antihistaminic.

Prednisone (pre̲d-ni-son) is a generic name for an antiinflammatory and antiallergic agent.

Premarin (pre̲m-ah-rin) is the trade name for estrogen replacement therapy.

Prilosec (pri̲l-o-sek) is the trade name a proton pump inhibitor for gastric and duodenal ulcers and other gastroesophageal disorders.

Procardia (pro-ka̲r-de-ah) is the trade name for a coronary vasodilator.

Proctocream HC (pro̲k-to-kreem) is the trade name for topical corticosteroidal antiinflammatory used as anorectal cream.

Propine (pro̲-pine) is the trade name for an antiglaucoma agent, eyedrops.

Proventil inhaler is the trade name for a bronchodilator, metered dose inhaler

Proventil MDI (pro-ve̲n-til) is a trade name for a bronchodilator, metered dose inhaler

Provera (pro-ve̲r-ah) is the trade name for progestin for secondary amenorrhea and abnormal uterine bleeding.

Pyridoxine (pir-o-do̲k-sen) is one of the forms of vitamin B_6.

Quinidex (kwi̲n-I-des) is the trade name for an antiarrhythmic.

Quinidine (kwi̲n-I-den) is a generic name for an antiarrhythmic agent used in the treatment of atrial flutter, atrial fibrillation, premature ventricular contractions, and tachycardias.

Reglan (re̲g-lan) is the trade name for a gastrointestinal stimulant; antiemetic.

Restoril (re̲s-to-ril) is the trade name for a sedative-hypnotic.

Ritalin (ri̲t-ah-lin) is the trade name for a mild central nervous system stimulant and antidepressant.

Senokot (se-no̲-kot) is the trade name for laxative.

Serevent (ser-e-vent) is the trade name for an aerosol bronchodilator.

Skelaxin (skel-aks-in) is the trade name for a skeletal muscle relaxant.

Slo-bid (slo-bid) is the trade name for an extended-release bronchodilator.

Sulfacetamide (sul-fah-set-ah-mid) is a generic name for an antibacterial sulfonamide, antibiotic.

Synthroid (sin-troid) is the trade name for a drug used as a replacement in decreased or absent thyroid function.

Tenormin (ten-or-min) is the trade name for a beta-blocker.

Terpin (ter-pin) is used as an expectorant.

Terramycin (ter-ah-mi-sin) is the trade name for an antibiotic.

Tetracycline (te-trah-si-klen) is the generic name for an antibiotic.

Theo-Dur (the-o-dur) is the trade name for a bronchodilator.

Theophylline (the-o-fil-in) is a generic name for a bronchodilator.

Tigan (ti-gan) is the trade name for an antiemetic.

Timoptic (tim-op-tik) is the trade name for a topical antiglaucoma agent; antihypertensive; beta blocker.

Tolinase (tol-I-nas) is the trade name for an antidiabetic agent.

Toradol (tor-a-dol) is the trade name for a nonsteroidal anti-inflammatory drug; analgesic for acute, moderately severe pain.

Trental (tren-tal) is the trade name for an oral hemorheologic drug.

Triamcinolone (tri-am-sin-o-lon) is the trade name for a corticosteroid.

Trimpex (tri-mip-eks) is the trade name for an antibacterial, antibiotic.

Vancenase (van-kan-az) is the trade name for a corticosteroid for bronchial asthma; pocket inhaler.

Vanceril (van-ser-il) is the trade name for a corticosteroid.

Vasotec (vah-o-tek)is the trade name for an angiotensin-converting enzyme inhibitor.

Ventolin (ven-to-lin) is the trade name for a bronchodilator.

Verapamil (ver-ah-pam-il) is a generic name for a coronary vasodilator.

Versed (ver-sed) is the trade name for a short-acting benzodiapine general anesthetic adjunct for preoperative sedation.

Vicodin is the brand name for the drug classification opioid analgesic

Vicoprofen (vik-o-pro-fen) is the trade name for a narcotic analgesic.

Vitamin C is ascorbic acid, anticorbutic, urinary acidifier.

Vitamin E is vitamin E supplement; topical emollient

Xanax (zan-aks) is the trade name for an antianxiety agent.

Xylocaine (zi-lo-kan) is trade name for an antiarrhythmic; local anesthetic.

Zantac (zan-tak) is the trade name for an acid controller for heartburn and acid indigestion.

Zocor (zo-kor) is the trade name for a reductase inhibitor for hypercholesterolemia and coronary heart disease.

Zyloprim (zi-lo-prim) is the trade name for an antigout agent.

Index

Index

Formatting—cont'd
  of statistical data
    on consultation reports, 31
    on diagnostic imaging reports, 27
    on history and physical examination reports, 23
    on operative reports, 30
    on procedure reports, 29, *29-30*

G

Gastroenterology, definition of, 241
Gastroenterology practice, office medical transcription
      from, 240-275
  keyboarding medical terms and definitions in,
      251-253
  proofreading and error analysis in, 264-268
  spelling medical terms in, 253-254
  transcribing medical sentences in, 254
  transcription tips in, 272-275

H

Heart in H&P report, 24
HEENT in H&P report, 24
History
  family, in H&P report, 24
  past medical, in H&P report, 24
  of present illness in H&P report, 23
  sample, *5*
  social, in H&P report, 24
History and physical (H&P) examination reports, 22-25
  formatting statistical data on, 23
  topics included in "history" heading of, 23-24
  topics included in "physical examination" heading of,
      24-25
History and physical (H&P) format for chart notes, 20-22,
      21-22
Homonyms, *81-82*
Hyphen, guidelines for use of, 56

I

Impression
  in diagnostic imaging report, 28
  in H&P report, 25

J

Journal of the American Association of Medical Transcription
      (JAAMT), 80

L

Laboratory data in H&P report, 25
Left lateral projection, 26
Left posterior oblique projection, 27
Letter(s)
  business, 32-33, *34*
  consultation, 32-33
    sample, *7*
  diagnostic imaging, sample, *6, 28*
LPO projection, 27
Lungs in H&P report, 24

M

Magnetic resonance imaging, 26
Medical dictionary(ies), 78
  electronic, 79
Medical documents
  outpatient, 19-33
  understanding, 12-43
Medical reports, 18-34
  typical, *4-7*
Medical spellers, electronic, 79
Medical terms
  keyboarding
    in cardiology practice, 285-287
    in diagnostic imaging practice, 316-317
    in family practice transcription, 117-119
    in gastroenterology practice, 251-253
    in orthopaedic practice, 152-154
    in pulmonary medicine practice, 214-216
    in urology practice, 181-183
  sound-alike, *81-82*
  spelling
    in cardiology practice, 288
    in diagnostic imaging practice, 318
    in family practice transcription, 119-120
    in gastroenterology practice, 253-254
    in orthopaedic practice, 154
    in pulmonary medicine practice, 217
    in urology practice, 184
Medical Transcription Guide Do's and Dont's, 79
Medical transcriptionist
  career outlook for, 4
  job description for, model, *8-9*
  knowledge needed by, 7, 10
  personal attributes of, 7, 10
  profile of, 4, 7
  skills needed by, 7, 10
  using *Essentials of Medical Transcription* method to become,
      10
Medications in H&P report, 24
Merck Manual, 78

N

Neck in H&P report, 24
Neurologic examination in H&P report, 24
Nuclear medicine, 26
Number expression guidelines, 53-55
Nursing Drug Handbook, 78

O

Objective findings in SOAP format, 20
Online resources, 79, *80*
Operative report, 30-31
Orthopaedic practice
  overview of, 144
Orthopaedic practice, office medical transcription from,
      143-172
  keyboarding medical terms and definitions in, 152-154
  proofreading and error analysis in, 161-165
  spelling medical terms in, 154
  transcribing medical sentences in, 155
  transcription tips for, 168-171

P

Pelvis in H&P report, 24
Period, guidelines for use of, 56
Perspectives on the Medical Transcription Profession, 80
Pharmaceutical references, 78
Physical examination, sample, *5*
Physician's Desk Reference, The (PDR), 78
Physicians' GenRx, 78
Physiology textbooks, 79
Plan
   in SOAP format, 20
   treatment, in H&P report, 25
Procedure reports, 28-30
Production for Pay summary, *84, 85*
Progress notes, 19; *see also* Chart note(s)
Projections in medical imaging, 26-27
Proofreading, 44-71
   abbreviation guidelines for, 52
   basic English usage review for, 51-52
   capitalization guidelines for, 52-53
   in cardiology practice, 297-302
   in diagnostic imaging practice, 323-327
   error analysis chart in, 49-51
   error analysis in, 51
   in family practice transcription, 129-134
   in gastroenterology practice, 264-268
   guidelines for, 49
   marks used in, 51
   number expression guidelines for, 53-55
   in orthopaedic practice, 161-165
   process of, 49
   in pulmonary medicine practice, 227-232
   punctuation guidelines for, 56-58
   in urology practice, 193-197
Pulmonary medicine practice, office medical transcription
      from, 205-239
   keyboarding medical terms and definitions in, 214-216
   proofreading and error analysis in, 227-232
   spelling medical terms in, 217
   transcribing medical sentences in, 218
   transcription tips in, 235-238
Pulmonologist, 206
Punctuation guidelines, 56-58

Q

Quotation marks, guidelines for use of, 58

R

Radiology, diagnostic, definition of, 311
Rectal exam in H&P report, 24
Reference initials, 33
Reference line, 33
Reference materials, 78-80
   electronic, 79
References, pharmaceutical, 78
Reports, medical, 18-34
Review of systems in H&P report, 24

S

Salutation, 33
Semicolon, guidelines for use of, 57
Signature line(s)
   of business/consultation letter, 33
   formatting, 18-19
      on consultation reports, 32
      on diagnostic imaging reports, 28
      on history and physical examination reports, 23
      on operative reports, 31
SOAP format for chart notes, 20, *21*
Social history in H&P report, 24
Sonography, 25-26
Spacing guidelines, 58
Spellers, medical, electronic, 79
Statistical data, formatting
   on consultation reports, 31
   on diagnostic imaging reports, 27
   on history and physical examination reports, 23
   on operative reports, 30
   on procedure reports, 29, *29-30*
Stedman's Medical Dictionary, 78
Style guides, 79
Subjective findings in SOAP format, 20
Symbols, guidelines for use of, 58

T

Templates, 33-34
Transcriber, 83, *84*, 85
Transcription
   guidelines for, 85-88
   preparation for, 82-83, 85
   process of, 72-103
   sound of, 78

U

Ultrasound, 25-26
Urology, definition of, 174
Urology practice, office medical transcription from,
      173-204
   keyboarding medical terms and definitions in,
      181-183
   proofreading and error analysis in, 193-197
   spelling medical terms in, 184
   transcribing medical sentences in, 185
   transcription tips in, 200-203
Usage guidelines, 87-88

W

Word books, 78
Word search, 80

X

X-rays, diagnostic, 25